*The Massachusetts
General Hospital
1955–1980*

The Massachusetts General Hospital

1955–1980

EDITED BY

BENJAMIN CASTLEMAN, M.D.
Chief, Department of Pathology (1953–1974)
Shattuck Professor of Pathological Anatomy, Emeritus,
Harvard Medical School

DAVID C. CROCKETT
Deputy to the General Director
Vice Chairman, Committee on Research

S. B. SUTTON
Author/Editor

Foreword by
John E. Lawrence, Esq.

Little, Brown and Company
Boston/Toronto

It is a great privilege for the editors to have the opportunity to dedicate this volume, the sixth chronologic history of the Massachusetts General Hospital, to the five chairmen of the board of trustees who actively participated in the affairs of the hospital covered in the 25-year period of this book.

The Right Reverend Henry K. Sherrill
Chairman of the Board of Trustees   1935–1947
Honorary Chairman of the 150th Anniversary Program 1961

Francis C. Gray, Esq.
Chairman of the Board of Trustees   1947–1964

John E. Lawrence Esq.
Chairman of the Board of Trustees   1964–1978

F. Sargent Cheever, M.D.
Chairman of the Board of Trustees   1978–1982

Francis H. Burr, Esq.
Chairman of the Board of Trustees   1982–

Contents

Part I. Administration and Physical Development

Part II. Medical Services

Part III. Children's Service

Part IV. Surgical Services

Part V. Clinical Departments

Part VI. Other Departments and Services

Foreword

In these pages will be found the story of the Massachusetts General Hospital during the past 25 years of its extraordinary growth and accomplishment in the long history of a hospital that has set a standard for American medicine.

The authors included in this volume have wisely chosen to characterize the achievements of the MGH during that period through a series of biographic sketches. The lives of physicians, administrators, researchers, trustees, and others who have contributed their talents to the MGH are portrayed here. Special credit for bringing the raw material of numerous authors into balance is due to the late Dr. Benjamin Castleman, with David C. Crockett and S. B. Sutton.

Ever since its earliest days, the MGH has been distinguished for its highly personalized and closely integrated clinical, teaching, and research activities. The purpose of the institution has remained, as always, the alleviation of suffering through the prevention, treatment, and conquest of disease. And it is in this spirit that all parts of the hospital are bound together in the one common cause of improving the quality of life for "the whole family of man."

This communality of purpose together with the impact of the close personal interdepartmental relationships on the quality of patient care will be dealt with extensively in the ensuing pages. That this tradition of personal service coupled with deep feelings of loyalty to the institution as a whole continues so strongly today despite the ever-increasing size and complexity of its affairs is due to the superb band of men and women who constitute the professional and support staffs of this hospital.

No account of any period of the MGH history, however, can be written without paying special tribute to the members of the public it serves and upon whose generosity it is completely dependent for the support of the physical plant and programs essential to its operations. Space is not available, unfortunately, for acknowledging all gifts of which it has been the grateful recipient during the past 25 years, but perhaps through mentioning a few it will be understood that it is our intent to honor the many.

During the period under review, with scientific and technologic advances of unprecedented proportions, substantial gifts from families such as the Coxes, Websters, Stevenses, and Grays have enabled the hospital to respond through four major building and renovation programs. Certain foundations like Kresge, Joseph P. Kennedy, Jr., and Mallinckrodt have also been large contributors to the erection of laboratories, equipment, endowment of positions and programs, as well as improvement of clinical areas. To accomplish these ends, contributions of considerable magnitude are required, but it is also to the tremendous numbers of small donors that we would like to express our eternal gratitude. These gifts mean a great deal to us. They are often given at considerable personal sacrifice to the donor, and the hospital could ask for no greater vote of confidence than that expressed through the 125,000 individual gifts received for the Cox Cancer Center.

As you read through the history, you will come to understand the truth of the following comment made by Dr. Oliver Wendell Holmes in the middle of the nineteenth century: "The hospital has always inspired the fervid attachment of those holding any relation to it whatsoever." This is the result of the dedicated effort of many people through the years. As one walks through the corridors one feels the presence of physicians and surgeons who have walked there before as well as administrators, nurses, technicians, and secretaries who in their day have served their fellow human beings. And one also feels the concern of the members of the community who have contributed whatever they could toward making the Massachusetts General Hospital what it is today.

John E. Lawrence, Esq.
President

Preface

With this volume the Massachusetts General Hospital continues a tradition, started in the 1850s by Dr. Nathaniel I. Bowditch, of publishing at more or less regular intervals historic accounts of its development. The current installment takes up the history where Dr. Nathaniel W. Faxon's volume left off, in 1955, and carries it forward through the next quarter century to 1980. Human events, however, do not dispose themselves so neatly. Some items and individuals that eluded Faxon's narrative, perhaps because their significance did not yet show clearly, present themselves here for attention.

The evolution of the science and practice of medicine, as well as the enormous growth of the MGH during the 25 years under review, suggested a different approach to preparing a manuscript than had been taken in the past. First, we decided not to include the McLean Hospital, in part because the new corporate structure sets it apart from the General Hospital, in part because the activities there are well documented in other publications. Next, we regonized that no single person could be expected to account for developments in specialties ranging from transplant surgery to computer technology. This history, therefore, became the work of many authors, an unknown number of consultants, many prevailed upon by us and some, no doubt, approached by the authors before the chapters came to us, and three slightly tyrannical editors. We read the contributions with an eye on balance, literary quality, continuity, and length of the entire volume. We reluctantly, but ruthlessly, excised lists of names of residents and fellows, or of research projects; the institution has grown too large, and such lists too long, to make good reading. We sometimes asked a second writer to supply additional information or biographic reflections to flesh out a chapter. We eliminated such repetitions of material as were bound to occur when several people worked independently. However, we never aimed for uniformity. We respected the voices and points of view of our contributors. Some used the first person; others preferred the third person, even when describing their own careers. Like the MGH itself, the history represents the combined efforts of gifted, unique men and women.

This perception of the hospital as an institution animated by the energies of supremely talented individuals guided the shaping of the manuscript. We tried to sharpen the focus on people and singled out for particular notice those who died or retired during this quarter century but who live in MGH memory as great mentors, innovators, and makers of policy.

This has been a substantial editorial task, and we owe thanks to many people. Rose Mooradian merits a special thanks for her indispensable administrative assistance. We are further beholden to many individuals beyond those identified with each chapter. Unfortunately, since we fear that no list could ever be complete—and in keeping with out strict policy about lists—we offer merely warm and general gratitude to all who shared their thoughts, reviewed chapters, and answered questions.

Our co-editor, Benjamin Castleman, died in June 1982, some four months before the manuscript was ready for the publisher. He had been an energetic editor, especially during the last six months of his life, beating the bushes for truant contributors, checking for scientific accuracy, reading second and third drafts, always suggesting improvements. He had been relieved to see, in May, that the work might be finished during the summer, but errant chapters were among his final thoughts. It was our pleasure to be his partners in this project.

David C. Crockett
S. B. Sutton

Contributing Authors

Raymond D. Adams, M.D.
Bullard Professor of Neuropathology (Emeritus), Harvard Medical School;
Senior Neurologist, Honorary Neuropathologist, Massachusetts General
Hospital, Boston

W. Gerald Austen, M.D.
Edward D. Churchill Professor of Surgery, Harvard Medical School; Visiting
Surgeon and Chief of the General Surgical Services, Department of Surgery,
Massachusetts General Hospital, Boston

H. Thomas Ballantine, Jr., M.D.
Professor of Surgery (Emeritus), Harvard Medical School; Senior
Neurosurgeon, Massachusetts General Hospital, Boston

Martin S. Bander
Director, News and Public Affairs; Deputy to the General Director,
Massachusetts General Hospital, Boston

G. Octo Barnett, M.D.
Professor of Medicine, Harvard Medical School; Physician and Director,
Laboratory of Computer Science, Massachusetts General Hospital, Boston

Marshall K. Bartlett, M.D.
Clinical Professor of Surgery (Emeritus), Harvard Medical School; Senior
Surgeon, Massachusetts General Hospital, Boston

Jacqueline D. Bastille
Director, Health Sciences Libraries, Massachusetts General Hospital, Boston

William S. Beck, M.D.
Professor of Medicine, Harvard Medical School; Physician and Director,
Hematology Research Laboratory, Massachusetts General Hospital, Boston

Irvin H. Blank, Ph.D.
Assistant Professor of Dermatology (Retired), Harvard Medical School;
Associate Biochemist, Massachusetts General Hospital, Boston

Thornton Brown, M.D.
Clinical Professor of Orthopaedic Surgery; Harvard Medical School; Senior
Orthopaedic Surgeon, Massachusetts General Hospital, Boston

John F. Burke, M.D.
Helen Andrus Benedict Professor of Surgery, Harvard Medical School; Visiting Surgeon, Chief of Trauma Services, Massachusetts General Hospital, Boston

Francis H. Burr, Esq.
Chairman, Board of Trustees, Massachusetts General Hospital, Boston.

Bradford Cannon, M.D.
Clinical Professor of Surgery (Emeritus), Harvard Medical School; Senior Surgeon, Massachusetts General Hospital, Boston

Edwin H. Cassem, M.D.
Associate Professor of Psychiatry, Harvard Medical School; Psychiatrist and Chief, Psychiatric Consultation-Liaison Service, Massachusetts General Hospital, Boston

Earle M. Chapman, M.D.
Associate Clinical Professor of Medicine (Emeritus), Harvard Medical School; Honorary Physician, Massachusetts General Hospital, Boston

Perry J. Culver, M.D.
Assistant Clinical Professor of Medicine, Harvard Medical School; Senior Physician, Massachusetts General Hospital, Boston

R. Clement Darling, M.D.
Associate Clinical Professor of Surgery, Harvard Medical School; Senior Vascular Surgeon and Chief of the Vascular Clinic, Massachusetts General Hospital, Boston

Leon Eisenberg, M.D.
Professor and Chairman, Department of Social Medicine and Health Policy, Harvard Medical School; Honorary Psychiatrist, Massachusetts General Hospital, Boston

Daniel S. Ellis, M.D.
Associate Clinical Professor of Medicine, Harvard Medical School; Senior Physician, Massachusetts General Hospital, Boston

Richard W. Erbe, M.D.
Associate Professor of Pediatrics, Harvard Medical School; Pediatrician, Assistant Physician and Chief of Genetics Unit, Massachusetts General Hospital, Boston

Daniel D. Federman, M.D.
Professor of Medicine, Harvard Medical School; Physician, Massachusetts General Hospital, Boston

Thomas B. Fitzpatrick, M.D., Ph.D.

Edward Wigglesworth Professor of Dermatology and Chairman, Department of Dermatology, Harvard Medical School; Dermatologist and Chief, Dermatology Service, Massachusetts General Hospital, Boston

Hermes C. Grillo, M.D.

Professor of Surgery, Harvard Medical School; Visiting Surgeon and Chief, General Thoracic Surgery, Massachusetts General Hospital, Boston

John W. Grover, M.D.

Associate Clinical Professor of Obstetrics and Gynecology, University of Illinois College of Medicine, Chicago; Chairman, Division of Obstetrics and Gynecology, Lutheran General Hospital, Park Ridge, Illinois

Walter C. Guralnick, D.M.D.

Professor of Oral and Maxillofacial Surgery, Harvard School of Dental Medicine; Visiting Oral and Maxillofacial Surgeon, Massachusetts General Hospital, Boston

Edgar Haber, M.D.

Higgins Professor of Medicine, Harvard Medical School; Physician and Chief of Cardiology, Massachusetts General Hospital, Boston

John Hedley-Whyte, M.D.

David S. Sheridan Professor of Anaesthesia and Respiratory Therapy, Harvard University; Anaesthetist-in-Chief, Beth Israel Hospital, Boston

Charles E. Huggins, M.D.

Associate Professor of Surgery, Harvard Medical School; Associate Visiting Surgeon and Director, Blood Transfusion Service, Massachusetts General Hospital, Boston

Homayoun Kazemi, M.D.

Professor of Medicine, Harvard Medical School; Physician and Chief, Pulmonary Unit, Massachusetts General Hospital, Boston

Sylvester B. Kelley, M.D.

Assistant Clinical Professor of Surgery (Retired), Harvard Medical School; Honorary Urologist, Urological Service, Massachusetts General Hospital, Boston

Samuel H. Kim, M.D.

Associate Clinical Professor of Surgery, Harvard Medical School; Associate Visiting Surgeon, Massachusetts General Hospital, Boston

Raymond N. Kjellberg, M.D.
Associate Clinical Professor of Surgery, Harvard Medical School, Visiting Neurosurgeon, Massachusetts General Hospital, Boston

Stephen M. Krane, M.D.
Professor of Medicine, Harvard Medical School; Physician and Chief, Arthritis Unit, Massachusetts General Hospital, Boston

Lawrence J. Kunz, Ph.D.
Associate Professor of Microbiology and Molecular Genetics, Harvard Medical School; Bacteriologist and Director of Bacteriology Laboratories, Massachusetts General Hospital, Boston

John E. Lawrence, Esq.
President, Massachusetts General Hospital, Boston

Alexander Leaf, M.D.
Professor of Medicine and Ridley Watts Professor of Preventive Medicine, Harvard Medical School; Physician, Massachusetts General Hospital, Boston

John W. Littlefield, M.D.
Given Professor of Pediatrics and Chairman, Department of Pediatrics, The Johns Hopkins University School of Medicine, Baltimore; Pediatrician-in-Chief, The Johns Hopkins Hospital, Baltimore

Ronald A. Malt, M.D.
Professor of Surgery, Harvard Medical School; Visiting Surgeon, Chief, Gastroenterological Surgery, Massachusetts General Hospital, Boston

Henry J. Mankin, M.D.
Edith M. Ashley Professor of Orthopaedics, Harvard Medical School; Visiting Orthopaedic Surgeon and Chief of Orthopaedic Surgery, Massachusetts General Hospital, Boston

Bucknam McPeek, M.D.
Associate Professor of Anesthesia, Harvard Medical School; Anesthetist, Massachusetts General Hospital, Boston

George L. Nardi, M.D.
Professor of Surgery, Harvard Medical School; Visiting Surgeon, Massachusetts General Hospital, Boston

John C. Nemiah, M.D.
Professor of Psychiatry, Harvard Medical School; Psychiatrist-in-Chief, Beth Israel Hospital, Boston

Edward C. Parkhurst, M.D.
Associate Urologist, Massachusetts General Hospital, Boston

John T. Potts, Jr., M.D.
Jackson Professor of Clinical Medicine, Harvard Medical School; Physician and Chief of the General Medical Services, Massachusetts General Hospital, Boston

John P. Remensnyder, M.D.
Associate Professor of Surgery, Harvard Medical School; Visiting Surgeon, Division of Plastic Surgery, Massachusetts General Hospital; Chief of Staff, Shriners Burns Institute, Boston

Sidney V. Rieder, Ph.D.
Senior Associate in Medicine (Biochemistry), Harvard Medical School; Director Clinical Chemistry Laboratories, Massachusetts General Hospital, Boston

Paul S. Russell, M.D.
John Homans Professor of Surgery, Harvard Medical School; Visiting Surgeon and Chief of the Transplantation Unit, Massachusetts General Hospital, Boston

J. Gordon Scannell, M.D.
Clinical Professor of Surgery, Harvard Medical School; Senior Surgeon, Massachusetts General Hospital, Boston

Cecil G. Sheps, M.D., M.P.H.
Taylor Grandy Distinguished Professor of Social Medicine, University of North Carolina at Chapel Hill School of Medicine, Chapel Hill, North Carolina

Lloyd H. Smith, Jr., M.D.
Professor and Chairman, Department of Medicine, University of California, San Francisco, School of Medicine, Chief at the Medical Service, Moffitt–University of California Hospital, San Francisco

John B. Stanbury, M.D.
Professor of Experimental Medicine, Emeritus, Massachusetts Institute of Technology; Senior Physician, Massachusetts General Hospital, Boston

John D. Stoeckle, M.D.
Professor of Medicine, Harvard Medical School; Physician, Department of Medicine, Massachusetts General Hospital, Boston

Morton N. Swartz, M.D.
Professor of Medicine, Harvard Medical School; Physician and Chief, Infectious Disease Unit, Massachusetts General Hospital, Boston

William H. Sweet, M.D., D.Sc., D.H.C.
Professor of Surgery (Emeritus), Harvard Medical School; Senior Neurosurgeon, Neurosurgical Service, Massachusetts General Hospital, Boston

Nathan B. Talbot, M.D.
Charles Wilder Professor of Pediatrics (Emeritus), Harvard Medical School; Consulting Visiting Pediatrician, Massachusetts General Hospital, Boston

Samuel O. Thier, M.D.
Sterling Professor and Chairman, Department of Internal Medicine, Yale University School of Medicine; Chief, Department of Medicine, Yale–New Haven Hospital, New Haven

Howard Ulfelder, M.D.
Joe V. Meigs Professor of Gynecology (Emeritus), Harvard Medical School; Deputy to the General Director for Cancer Affairs and Consulting Visiting Gynecologist, Massachusetts General Hospital, Boston

Chiu-An Wang, M.D.
Clinical Professor of Surgery, Harvard Medical School; Senior Surgeon and Chief of Endocrine Surgery, Massachusetts General Hospital, Boston

Claude E. Welch, M.D.
Clinical Professor of Surgery (Emeritus), Harvard Medical School; Senior Surgeon, Massachusetts General Hospital, Boston

Earle W. Wilkins, Jr., M.D.
Clinical Professor of Surgery, Harvard Medical School; Visiting Surgeon, Chief of Emergency Services, Massachusetts General Hospital, Boston

William C. Wood, M.D.
Associate Professor of Surgery, Harvard Medical School; Associate Visiting Surgeon and Medical Director, MGH Cancer Center, Massachusetts General Hospital, Boston

Paul C. Zamecnik, M.D.
Collis P. Huntington Professor of Oncologic Medicine (Emeritus), Harvard Medical School; Senior Physician, Massachusetts General Hospital, Boston

Nicholas T. Zervas, M.D.
Professor of Surgery, Harvard Medical School; Visiting Neurosurgeon and Chief, Neurosurgical Service, Massachusetts General Hospital, Boston

Part I. Administration and Physical Development

1. Trustees

FRANCIS H. BURR, ESQ.

Nearly every chapter of this volume addresses some facet of institutional increase—in manpower, in committees and their membership, in building facilities, in budget, in intellectual and educational endeavor, in community and health care responsibility, in red tape. It may, then, cause some astonishment to discover that the number of trustees who govern the Massachusetts General Hospital has remained constant since 1811 when the Great and General Court of Massachusetts provided in the hospital's charter for a board of one dozen trustees. As in most institutions, the trustees are responsible for setting policy and making major policy decisions. Since it is a small board, and by longtime custom a "working" board, it functions much like a directors' executive committee of a business corporation. The general director, who is the chief executive officer, reports directly to and consults frequently with the board. Of the twelve trustees, eight are elected by the corporation, and the remaining four are designated by the governor. The Commonwealth acquired this privilege in exchange for its gifts to the hospital of a building site (which the original trustees judged inadequate and leased until 1947 when it was sold for a handsome sum) and of the Chelmsford granite, cut by prisoners from the state prison, used to construct the Bulfinch Building.

To run a teaching hospital the size of the MGH with a board of 12 is rather unusual in the present day. Immediately after World War II, in 1946–1947, when the hospital was trying to reorganize its committees and to reach out into the community with the idea of raising funds on a continuous basis in order to rebuild clinical and research areas, it became obvious that more than twelve individuals would be needed to accomplish all this. Instead of increasing their own number (which would have required a revision of the charter) the trustees recommended enlarging the corporation. Since the corporation was composed principally of former trustees, its membership of that time was weighted heavily with retired governors' appointees. (At that time, when a Republican governor took over from a Democratic administration—and vice versa—he sacked the previous appointees and designated another four, usually his personal physician and three others; the retired four then became life members of the corporation.) The reason for expanding the corporation in the postwar years was to lighten the burden of the trustees' fund-raising duties, often the primary function of trustees in other hospitals with larger boards. The 12 MGH trustees—and it is true to this day—were so occupied with other assignments that they could not devote adequate time to raising money. Some trustees were explicitly told at the time of their appointments that they would not be expected to do so, which may account in part for the hospital's success in enticing very busy people to labor long hours on its behalf even though not only is there no financial compensation but also trustees are urged to make the MGH a prime object of their charitable giving.

And so the number of MGH trustees has remained at 12. The format has succeeded in large part because generations of board members have honored the spirit of the word *trust* and given immoderately of their intelligence and time. As Leon Eisenberg observes in a later chapter, "The quality as well as the quantity of trustee input to hospital policy was remarkable. It was not merely that the hospital had a distinguished group of trustees (many do, on paper) but that they contributed long hours to hospital affairs."

Community, ethnic, religious, or political representation have no bearing on the election of board members. The corporation has traditionally taken as its criteria individual quality, willingness to devote an enormous amount of time to the assignment, and, in some instances, professional knowledge of issues important to the hospital. In 1947, for example, the need was felt to include on the board someone with training and background in public relations, so Francis W. Hatch, Sr., vice-president and director of Batten, Barten, Dursten & Osborne was selected. At the same time it seemed important to infuse the board with some youthful blood, so young John E. Lawrence was invited to become a member. Lawrence has served the MGH ever since, both as a member of the board and its chairman. Meanwhile, the trustees determined a need for some scientific expertise. Since the corporation had already filled its slots, the then governor, Governor Bradford, was introduced to the idea of naming a scientist as one of his four appointments. He chose Francis O. Schmitt of the Department of Biology at MIT, whom every succeeding governor through Dukakis had the wisdom to reappoint and who still sits with the board, now as an honorary member, and makes a very real contribution to any scientific issue that comes before it.

It became customary during the forties and fifties to include the retired chief of an important clinical service on the board; Arthur W. Allen, a general surgeon, and William Jason Mixter, a distinguished neurosurgeon, served as trustees during that period. The custom, however, eventually lapsed. In the sixties and seventies, when the hospital faced many real estate problems, particularly with the development of the West End by the Boston Redevelopment Authority and the Boston Housing Authority and with the introduction of complexities in dealing with one's neighbors, the corporation asked Philip H. Theopold of Minot, DeBlois & Maddison, a real estate investment firm, to serve on the board, and his presence during this phase proved invaluable.

Because of the relationship between the MGH and the Harvard Medical School, it was not unusual to find a member of the Harvard Corporation sitting simultaneously on the board of the MGH. Robert Homans occupied both positions during the thirties. (Some time after his death his widow, Abigail Adams Homans, served as a governor's appointee until she reached retirement age.) The strong Harvard connection was continued with the election in 1962 of Francis H. Burr, a member of the Harvard Corporation, and in 1963 of George Putnam, currently treasurer of Harvard.

The trustees have full responsibility for all policy decisions of the hospital and for the selection of the general director. They also review the annual appointments of all staff members and manage the finances of the hospital. The endowment and all expenditures from its income, the annual operating budget, and all building plans and financing must be approved by the board.

The full board meets ten months of the year on alternate Fridays, from 9:00 A.M. to 10:00 A.M. (They meet only once a month in July and August.) There is little time for exchange of pleasantries; it is a solid hour of serious business.

Until such outside agencies as the Joint Commission on Hospital Administration began to require records, the board seldom bothered with the formalities of voting. They acted entirely by consensus. If one trustee disagreed, that person's view was heard with respect and the matter discussed in full; if the dissenter could not be convinced to join the majority, the item was usually carried over until the next meeting, allowing two weeks for further study. The new rules about voting did not really change this pattern; the trustees still work toward a consensus, and decisions are almost always unanimous. During the span of time covered by this history, there has never been a dichotomy between the eight corporation-appointed trustees and the four designated by the governor; at least two of the governor's appointees usually have had long years of service uninterrupted by changing administrations. (There may have been such problems in the past but, if so, they are lost to history because the written records of the trustees were so carefully understated that any internecine scraps do not appear.)

Clearly, however, the affairs of the hospital cannot be settled in one hour every second Friday morning. In an institution the size of the MGH—in 1981 the operating budget was approximately $250 million and there were about 10,000 staff and employees on the payroll—it is obvious that 12 trustees must delegate and divide responsibilities. Accordingly, the trustees do most of their work in various committees. Until 1978, when the structure of governance underwent a revision which will be discussed later, there were two forms of committees. The first, called the Standing Committees of the Trustees, included the Finance Committee, consisting of four board members, outside financial consultants, and the treasurer of the hospital who acted as chairman; the Legal Affairs Committee, including the treasurer of the hospital and the senior lawyer on the board; the Rules Committee, with a membership of two trustees; the Memorials Committee, also with two trustees; and a Visiting Committee for the McLean Hospital.

The second category of committees was known as the Combined Committees of Trustees and Staff. Of these the most important was the General Hospital Committee consisting of four trustees (one of whom presided at meetings), the general director, and staff representatives including the chiefs of Medicine and General Surgery and the chairmen of the Committee on Research and of the General Executive Committee (GEC, the premier professional staff committee); its meetings were also attended by frequent guests invited to discuss specific questions. The General Hospital Committee reviewed the recommendations of the GEC on appointments to the medical staff and passed on its advice to the board. In addition, the General Hospital Committee reviewed the activities of the Committee on Research (COR) which has the distinction of being the only professional committee in the hospital that reports directly to the trustees rather than through the GEC. Two to four trustees—among them, Professor Schmitt—serve on the COR and bring its recommendations to the General Hospital Committee or the full board.

A second combined committee, on planning and building, usually reported directly to the full board, occasionally soliciting advice of staff members on the General Hospital Committee when the planning of a major patient care, research, or educational facility raised larger policy issues. Other combined committees were the Phillips House–Baker Committee and advisory committees to the Volunteer Department, to the libraries, to the School of Nursing and the Nursing Service, and to the Social Service Department. All these committees had two trustee members as well as staff appointments of greater or lesser number. Trustees also sat on medical staff committees (Teaching and Education, Utilization Review) but not on the GEC. Complicated though it sounds, the committee system was really quite simple in operation. But it did—and does—demand an enormous amount of trustee time.

The change in the bylaws in the late seventies altered the committee structure to some extent. The 1978–1979 annual report listed Committees of the Board of Trustees as follows: Compensation and Personnel Practices, Education Division, Finance and Audit, General Hospital, Investment, McLean Hospital, Patent, Patient Care, Pension, Planning and Building, Research, and Resources and Development. These replaced the former standing and combined committees. The General Hospital Committee now consists of four trustees, the general director, the associate general director, the chiefs of Medicine and Surgery, the director of the Department of Nursing, the chairmen of the COR and GEC plus one other member of the GEC, the general counsel of the corporation, and "such other persons as the Chairman may appoint." The committee alternates with the full board in meeting every other Friday and delves into issues in considerable depth. It is now customary for the chiefs of services to report at least once a year to the trustees through this committee; each chief presents a written report in advance and then attends the meeting at which the achievements and the problems—if any—of the service and the outlook for the coming year are discussed.

The revision of the bylaws occurred in tandem with the administrative reorganization of the hospital (see Chapter 5) and was designed to mesh with it. At the same time there was an additional effort to reorganize the corporate structure of the hospital without tampering with the charter. Thus the Massachusetts General Hospital was set up, within the terms of the charter, as a holding company with three subsidiary corporations: the General Hospital Corporation, the McLean Corporation, and the Institute for Health Sciences, with leeway provided for other subsidiaries—it is possible, for instance, that research endeavors might be set up as separate corporations. This elaborate reorganization created new officers and new positions—the chairman of the General Hospital Committee became the president of the General Hospital Corporation, and the chairman of the McLean Hospital Committee the president of the McLean Hospital Corporation. But, for all intents and purposes, the functioning of the board remains the same.

Few outsiders have been in a position to observe the trustees for so long and at such close range as David Crockett who, in 1946 and 1947, as administrative assistant to the board, was privy to many of their deliberations. "Prior to the Second World War," he noted, "there were no observers except the general director and the secretary, who weren't members of the board. I think I was the first person other than a board member allowed to attend the meetings of the trustees. After I had been an observer for about a year, I was asked not to attend any longer and they went back to the closed meeting procedure. It wasn't until about 1960 that I was invited to join the meetings of the General Hospital Committee, of which I became a formal member, and was allowed to be an observer at full board meetings.

"It is an extraordinary tribute to the integrity of the men and women who made up the board that this system could function effectively for 172 years without any visible disruption, disagreement, or conflict. The only time that the trustees ever decided against the recommendations of its various joint committees or the General Executive Committee was on the question of whether or not the hospital should undertake heart transplantation. (See Chapter 5 for further discussion of this item.)

"To sum this all up, the strength of the ultimate governing body is due to the long tradition of service of trustees of the MGH and the small size of the board. New members of the board, whatever their background and regardless of whether they are governors' appointees or elected members, quickly become imbued with this sense of work and service.

"I don't think any other modern hospital can claim such high mutual regard as exists between the staff of the MGH—medical, nursing, and ancillary staff right down to the kitchens and the utilities—and its trustees."

A complete list of trustees during this period appears at the back of the book.

2. Dean Alexander Clark, General Director, 1949–1961

CECIL G. SHEPS

Dean A. Clark, appointed as the MGH general director in 1949, represented a radical departure in terms of background and experience from his predecessors in that office. While Clark brought a good deal of administrative experience in the organization and delivery of medical care, it had not been focused on hospital care. His orientation was basically toward the medical needs of the community as a whole rather than toward the role of the hospital, particularly the teaching hospital per se. All this became evident during his tenure in office and resulted in the adoption—often slowly and hesitantly—by the MGH of new program elements while previously existing programs and objectives were being reinforced.

Clark's private and professional history explains the attitudes that he brought to the task of running the MGH. Born in St. Paul, Minnesota, in 1905, he quickly showed a brilliant and incisive mind joined with a basic social concern and deep commitment to the problems of meeting the needs of all people so that they might function at full capacity. He ascribed the awakening of his interest in social justice, government programs to meet human needs, and the problems of the underprivileged to the influence of the Presbyterian Church in St. Paul, which he attended with his parents. As a child he was active in the Sunday School there; attendance at a "Y" camp during his adolescent years strengthened his interest in societal problems. Clark was still a boy in St. Paul when he befriended Roy Wilkins, who later became director of the National Association for the Advancement of Colored People. They spent a lot of time together. On one occasion, during a Sunday School conference, they shared a double bed—an unusual, if not daring thing to do at that time. It was that night that Wilkins, in response to Clark's question about his plans for the future, said, "I want to find a way to do something for my people." The statement had a profound effect on young Dean Clark.

Clark did his undergraduate work at Princeton University, qualified for Phi Beta Kappa, and graduated in 1927 as valedictorian of his class. His interest in community activities grew through his experiences at Princeton, stimulated largely by members of the faculty. Toward the end of his college career, when he was trying to decide whether law or medicine would equip him better to advance his interests in societal needs, one of his teachers helped him decide on medicine.

Following graduation from Princeton, Clark took advantage of a Rhodes scholarship and spent the years from 1927 to 1930 at Oxford University where he completed the basic science medical requirements. His experience in another great university in a different culture and social climate, along with the opportunity to work closely with a few distinguished scientists who took an interest in him, sharpened his mind and shaped the direction of his future. He received his M.D. degree from Johns Hopkins medical school two years later, and from

1932 to 1937 he did postgraduate residency work in medicine and neurology at Johns Hopkins and then at New York Hospital, returning to Hopkins for training in psychiatry. Meanwhile his interest in the application of medicine from the community point of view was always present, and he eagerly sought out people who might guide him in that direction.

In 1934, during his residency at New York Hospital, Clark attended a lecture on public health by Thomas Parran, then commissioner of health for the state of New York and later one of the most distinguished and farsighted surgeon generals of the U.S. Public Health Service. Clark later described the talk as "stupendous—a knock-out." He introduced himself to Parran, and they became colleagues and friends. About the same time, Clark also met Alan Gregg, a charismatic physician who was one of the great leaders on the staff of the Rockefeller Foundation, interested in medical education, research, and the social function of medicine. It was natural, given their overlapping concerns, that the two men met frequently. In 1937, while Clark was studying psychiatry at Hopkins, Gregg offered him a position on the staff of the Rockefeller Foundation. However, just at that time Clark fell ill with tuberculosis and spent a year in a sanitarium at Saranac Lake, New York.

Upon discharge, Clark and his wife Kay, who shared his interests, flew directly to the National Health Conference in Washington. This important event brought together national leaders, lay and medical, to address the health problems of the nation and to develop a program for national consideration. Though participation was limited to those who had been formally invited, the Clarks decided to go anyway. They were able to attend virtually all the sessions and were greatly stimulated by what they heard and learned. One presentation that particularly impressed them was made by a representative of the United Mine Workers who described the very poor health of the coal miners and the great difficulties they had in obtaining, and paying for, medical care. So affected were the Clarks by the account that they sought and acquired a foundation grant that enabled them to do a survey of this problem. They spent more than six months in coal fields and mining camps, visiting with miners, their families, and the local doctors. The Clarks completed a report, "Medical Care in Selected Areas of the Appalachian Bituminous Coal Fields," in March 1939. Though the study did not get wide circulation at the time, it produced enough interest so that, a few years later, a large-scale survey was conducted by Admiral Boone; this corroborated the Clarks' findings and led to the institution of a comprehensive national health and welfare program for the UMW membership through agreement between the union and the mine operators.

During the 1930s increasing numbers of Jews and other German citizens were fleeing Hitler's mounting persecution and murder. Alan Gregg asked Dean and Kay Clark to investigate potential locations for practice for refugee physicians from Nazi Germany as part of the Rockefeller Foundation's effort to assist them and other refugees. The Clarks carried out their survey in several states, mostly in the South where the shortage of physicians was most acute. In each community they met with citizens and doctors and were able to prepare a base for many of the physician refugees.

In 1939 Clark made his full professional commitment to public health and medicine for the community by joining the U.S. Public Health Service as a commissioned officer. In the six years that followed he was charged with a series of exciting and important responsibilities which broadened his understanding of the medical needs of the United States and sharpened his skills in analyzing the issues and developing programs to deal with them. He was chief of the Hospital Section of the U.S. Office of Civilian Defense in 1942–1943, then chief medical officer of the Office of Vocational Rehabilitation, and then medical survey officer of the American National Red Cross.

Shortly after the end of World War II, Clark accepted a position as medical director of a new organization, the Health Insurance Plan of New York. Developed mainly by George Baehr (with whom Clark was acquainted) and vigorously supported by Mayor LaGuardia, this infant program was a significant demonstration of a new approach to the delivery of medical care in this country. The plan incorporated principles of organization and financing that were adopted on the West Coast at roughly the same time; it combined a new approach to the actual delivery of care with a unique form of prepayment. A comprehensive range of services was to be provided by physicians and associated personnel organized into group practices rather than by a series of solo practitioners. Each group practice would undertake to provide medical care to a population specifically enrolled with it. The medical group would be paid for its services through annual capitation payments based upon the size of the enrolled population. Support for the entire program came from insurance premiums paid by, or in behalf of, the enrollees. As top administrative officer of this novel medical care plan, Clark's major task was the organization of services for the subscribers. His crucial leadership role in the pioneering program is acknowledged today by students of health care.

It was from this background of knowledge, experience, and commitment that Clark was invited to join the MGH in 1949 as its fifteenth general director. His report for the same year outlined the major planning effort that had been initiated and set forth some challenges for the institution which clearly reflected the new outlook he brought to MGH. Trustees and staff formulated a proposal outlining joint activities with the Harvard Medical School for the next decade. The project was undertaken "not only to review those areas which are directly concerned with the Medical School but also to attempt to draw a blueprint for the general development of the hospital during the next ten years." The study included a reexamination of the hospital's long-term objectives in research, education, patient care, and community service along with budgetary projections for salaries and facilities to implement the plan. Clark's report presented some challenging opportunities for the MGH in areas of patient care and community service which not only represented substantial new and relevant contributions but also provided settings for teaching and research, the importance of which was yet to be generally recognized in the academic medical community.

Clark based his recommendations upon the notion that the MGH was "in a strategic position to make an even greater contribution to the health care of the people. To accomplish this purpose the hospital's services must be put to work for a broader range of the community's population than has heretofore been possible." Among the new resources he recommended so that the MGH could "extend its services more effectively to the whole community" was the development of plans to establish a group medical practice unit which all members of the medical staff would eventually be invited to join. He conceived the purpose of the unit as follows: "to make organized professional care available to ambulatory patients of all income groups and, at the same time, to assist members of the medical staff in centering all the professional activities at the hospital . . . [so as to] . . . provide continuity of care for the patient whether at home, as an ambulatory patient of the medical group, or in a hospital bed."

Clark's first report also recommended the development, in collaboration with relevant agencies, of a rehabilitation center at the hospital, "conducted, however, as a general community enterprise rather than strictly as an activity of the hospital." He further noted that an attempt was being made, in conjunction with the United Community Services of Boston, to organize a complete health care service for families in the area surrounding the hospital. "By organizing a health care service available to neighborhood families at home, as well as in the clinic and the hospital, preventive medicine may be integrated into curative medicine. . . . By means of such steps, and others of the same general character—notably regional coordination of medical and hospital services—the hospital can rise to its point of maximum effectiveness in health service of the entire community."

This account is being written 30 years later. In the light of the perceptions held by the public and the health professions today, these program objectives seem cogent, important, timely, sensible, and even feasible. This was, however, not the case in 1949; at that time they were generally considered to be visionary, perhaps even diversionary, although possibly desirable. Such objectives were not viewed as fundamental issues by the leading figures in medicine or by the community and political leaders on the whole. From today's vantage point, it is interesting to note that in his 1949 description of proposed family health service, Clark pointed out that among the potential benefits "the general health of the community can be improved, and its need for the most expensive medical commodity—hospitalization—reduced." It was not until the late seventies that such concepts became the conventional wisdom. Note the watch words: regional coordination, continuity of care, organization of professional care, the community as a whole, health care of the people, putting the hospital's services to work for a broader range of the community's population, the hospital as the most expensive commodity—these are today's widely recognized and most pressing challenges. They represent fundamental approaches which, though recommended 30 years ago by a few like Dean Clark, were not then considered relevant by most people in medicine or in hospital administration.

Though these issues and the plans prepared to tackle them were all directed toward the accessibility, quality, effectiveness, and cost of health services per se, Clark was convinced, as were a few others at that time, that such programs of care also held promise for new and needed developments in education and research. Now, a quarter century later, there is a slowly growing recognition that the tertiary care referral center hospital cannot provide the full range of learning experiences essential for the most effective practice of medicine. Also there is accumulating appreciation among medical researchers that many important challenges in biomedical research require access to people and patients over long periods in the normal courses of their lives. Thus the powerhouse represented by the tertiary care teaching hospital cannot alone provide all that is needed for medical education and research and, therefore, must enhance its role by becoming an integral part of a community/regional organized set of comprehensive services.

Clark identified all these needs clearly. He came to the MGH because he saw an opportunity to develop programs to meet these challenges in one of the world's most prestigious hospitals. The pattern of administration of the hospital permitted him to devote most of his energies to the objectives he had outlined. There was an expert staff under the direction of Ellsworth T. Neumann, charged with the day-to-day hospital operations. The general director, of course, had the ultimate responsibility for overall administrative performance, and Clark met with the top administrators each workday morning and at other times for planning purposes or to deal with emergency situations. In all his relationships Clark started with a deep innate respect for each human being combined with an assumption that the knowledge, skills, and experience of others were essential to success in a complex enterprise. His contacts with his staff were, accordingly, most agreeable.

In the 12 years of Clark's tenure as general director, the activities and the facilities of the MGH increased substantially. New facilities were built to house expanding clinical and research programs. There were three major additions to the physical plant: a research building, a nurses' dormitory, and the Warren Building. The latter included a significant feature, relatively new on the hospital scene: Five floors of the structure were designated as office accommodations for the practices of approximately 75 physicians. Clark considered this provision essential to bringing the hospital in closer proximity to the delivery of care before and after the episode of inpatient care for all classes of people.

Research, which had long been a feature of the MGH program, quadrupled in expenditures from $1.3 million in 1949 to $5.2 million in 1960. Teaching programs in medicine, both undergraduate and graduate, were expanded and strengthened. For example, the size of the resident staff increased from 100 to 115 in 1949; by 1961 it had been enlarged to 140.

Special attention was given to education in health professions other than medicine. This effort included a review of the hospital's involvement in nursing education. In this connection again Clark's views were in the forefront of developments yet to become more widely accepted. In the fifties, the MGH suffered—as did most hospitals in the country—from a nursing shortage, which resulted in some of its bed capacity, badly needed for patients awaiting admission, being closed down. In 1957 all patient care units were open, finally, for the first time in 14 years, an accomplishment of which Clark was justifiably proud. This success had been achieved—with the indispensable aid of Ruth Sleeper, the distinctive director of nursing at the MGH—by offering better wages and attracting more nurses. But Clark's experience with the situation led him to believe that better education for nurses and more effective leadership in nursing service administration were more desirable objectives than simple increases in numbers. (See Chapter 40 on the MGH Nursing Service for more on Clark's views.)

Soon after his arrival at MGH, Clark identified its ambulatory care activities as requiring improvement in scope, size, and effectiveness. The conditions for care in the outpatient department were characteristic of virtually all hospitals at the time: The physical setting was dismal and the framework for "doctoring" poorly organized. Clark determined to reshape this aspect of health care into a modern and effective form. It is an interesting commentary—and no exaggeration—that those objectives were almost revolutionary for hospitals at that time, i.e., to organize medical care services for ambulatory patients (then largely unable to pay full private fees) around the needs of the patients and to provide an atmosphere that took into account their convenience and personal sensibilities, thus putting scientific and clinical activities into a more appropriate balance with the social and human needs of the individuals being served. Two decades later, in the wake of the turbulent sixties, such priorities became fairly widely recognized.

Clark brought these ideas to the MGH as a member of a small vanguard of medical care leaders in the nation. He delineated the cogency of a comprehensive approach to the health needs of ambulatory patients of all income levels in his first report in 1949 and then began to develop and implement detailed plans to achieve these ends. John D. Stoeckle relates this complicated tale elsewhere in this volume; in brief, although environmental, programmatic, and organizational improvements in ambulatory care were implemented, Clark's dream of a new clinics building was frustrated. It wasn't until 1980 that such a facility was built. In the interval a number of new and modernized structures were put into place, a result, at least to some extent, of the priorities established by the institution as a whole. Moreover, in pressing for such developments, Clark was not only in the vanguard in the hospital field, but public sentiment for such changes was not yet available to add power to his argument.

In 1955 Clark found it necessary to take decisive action to improve the services of the hospital despite the vigorous opposition of key figures. The issue was the organization of the Emergency Ward. Starting in the mid-forties, the MGH, like similar urban hospitals, found the demands upon its Emergency Ward rising sharply in quantitative terms while changing significantly in scope. Increasingly people turned to the urban hospital for non-urgent medical as well as surgical or traumatic care. The numbers of patients presenting themselves at the MGH had increased about tenfold since 1940. The general public was coming to see the hospital as the single reliable, around-the-clock medical resource, and approximately 60 percent of the MGH patients did not present surgical problems at all. Geared as they were to expecting true emergencies, the medical staff in the emergency service demonstrated scant interest in dealing with non-urgent problems, despite the growing influx.

Given the original purpose of the Emergency Ward, it was appropriate that responsibility for its organization and operation should have belonged to the Surgical Services. Clark and a few others saw that, with the changes in usage, this no longer made sense and proposed a joint form of organization. He ran into tremendous difficulties. The logic of what was clearly indicated was not compelling enough to lead to a ready, rapid, or full solution for two reasons. First, it was the pattern of the day for each clinical department to have sole and autonomous responsibility for certain types of patients and medical service functions, and the departments believed deeply in the value of separate territorial rights. While the spectrum of needs presented by the patients simply could not be met by such an approach, there was little, if any, precedent for clinical departments to work in a fully and continuously coordinated fashion.

Second, the chief of surgery, E. D. Churchill, was of no mind to create one. He insisted that his department continue to have the full responsibility despite compelling evidence that the Emergency Ward was not addressing the problems of many patients expeditiously or well. This arbitrary posture temporarily caused Clark to limit the discussion of change to the involvement of only one additional department, Medicine. The chief of that service, Walter Bauer, was quite prepared to develop a coordinated approach, but Churchill remained adamantly opposed to giving up any authority. Clark, though characteristically patient, finally resorted to use of his full authority as general director—something he did rarely—and implemented a Solomon-like decision. The "final arrangement," as he referred to it in his annual report for 1955, placed the Emergency Ward under the alternate leadership of the surgical and medical services, with the responsibility shifting at 12-hour intervals. This solution opened a path that led over the course of time to greater participation of relevant sections of the medical staff in Emergency Ward services. Clark had taken an action he believed vital to improving the services of the MGH. Churchill's relationship with Clark suffered thereafter, so deeply did the former feel about his views having been overridden. Clark was sorry about the deterioration in their relations but did not take personal offense.

Years after he left the MGH, Clark continued to express deep regret about his failure (as he described it) to develop a prepaid group practice at the hospital along the lines of the Health Insurance Plan of Greater New York. Certain leading members of the medical staff such as James Howard Means and Allan Butler—chiefs of Medicine and Pediatrics, respectively—because of their expressed progressive views about the organization and delivery of medical care, could have been expected to support such developments. However, the anticipation of this achievement that Clark brought with him to Boston was never explicitly discussed in advance of his arrival. He had not explored the plan's feasibility or the degree of interest among the medical staff or the MGH trustees.

Clark discovered that a number of physicians on the staff, including Marshall K. Bartlett and Earle Chapman, had already expressed an interest in group practice. They and others had many informal discussions with Clark on the subject. Early in the fifties steps were being taken to enable doctors to practice in loose association with each other and at the hospital. However, unlike New York where Mayor LaGuardia and union leaders had supported HIP, Boston demonstrated little political or public interest in a prepayment system. Nevertheless, discussions regarding some form of associated practice for some MGH staff proceeded apace after Clark's arrival, and in 1954 the MGH Staff Associates was formally launched. Measured against Clark's aspirations, it represented only a very tentative step forward. (See pages 139–142 for further discussion of the MGH Staff Associates.)

Having always conceived of medicine, medical care, and hospitals in terms of public needs rather than as instruments of the medical profession, Clark viewed the teaching hospital broadly as a social artifact which must be fashioned to meet societal needs of patient care, teaching, and research. Along with a few others, he recognized these objectives as distinct, though related: Though one is affected by the others, they are not interchangeable, and there are problems of balance among them. The need to delineate the goals and costs of each function so that social and individual obligations could be appropriately allocated was clear to Clark long before the seventies, when such matters began to receive a great deal of anguished attention in teaching hospitals and medical schools.

Two examples, among many, will suffice. Clark's report for 1956 contains a pithy discussion of the special educational costs of voluntary teaching hospitals, a subject generally taboo in those days. "These are the costs incurred because they *are* teaching hospitals; in reality, they are the costs of education, not costs of hospital care at all. . . . If the community wants to have a sufficient quantity of top-notch physicians, nurses, and others in the future, it must find a way now to finance their education. . . . Whatever method of meeting these hospital educational costs is found, it should clearly not depend alone upon payments by the hospitalized individual or upon philanthropy. Properly, it seems to me, the whole community should be called upon." Later in this same report he develops a case for financial support from the federal government, among other sources. Two years later, Clark points to a set of developing forces in society which he predicts—again correctly—will render infeasible the time-honored reliance upon the indigent ward patient as the focal point of medical education. Those forces included the health insurance programs that were increasingly being provided as an employee benefit in industry and the expanded government programs for the poor which were in the offing. He then sets forth the kinds of changes needed in admissions procedures, in the handling of patients of all social classes, in the organization of the delivery of medical care, and in the arrangements for charging fees for services rendered. With regard to these issues, Clark was again ahead of the great majority of his colleagues by a decade or more.

Clark's interests in public health and the social function of medical care were continuously amplified, modified, and strengthened, not only by his work at the MGH but also by his involvement with other national figures in diverse consultation and development activities. Most notable, perhaps, was his participation in the preparation of a significant report, *Building America's Health,* as a member of a special group set up by President Truman, called the President's Commission on the Health Needs of the Nation. This group, which worked intensively during 1952, expressed the view that "access to the means for the attainment and preservation of health is a basic human right" and set forth principles for federal and state participation in the financing of medical care and the development of group practice—elements that formed the foundation of much of the social policy adopted in this country since that time.

This review of what Clark brought to the MGH and the hospital's reaction to his leadership reflects the usual response of successful institutions to suggestions for new and unusual approaches. The MGH, one of the world's leading teaching hospitals, was in the forefront of medicine in terms of its scientific approach to the biologic problems of sick patients and its teaching and research programs. To most of its leading figures, extending and expanding these activities appeared to be a more secure road to the future than moving out in an innovative direction.

While supporting effectively the ongoing activities that had brought the hospital to its high level of prestige, Clark concentrated upon developing its full potential in new areas: the organization of ambulatory care, creative attention to the role of the teaching hospital in relation to other services with an eye on containing costs, working closely with the community, concern with preventive as well as diagnostic and curative medicine.

Twenty years or more after Clark pressed these ideas, they seem valid and timely to the majority of the leadership in academic medicine. At MGH, as in many other centers in the nation, real progress along these lines is now underway. Clark advanced these arguments before the hospital was fully prepared to accept them. Though he received support from isolated individuals, recognition of the relevance to the MGH of the program developments he was urging was slow and halting. That he made unique and crucial contributions to the growth of the MGH and to the progressive development of medical care services in the nation generally is now very clear.

Though to some extent disappointed by the failure of the MGH to move as quickly as he would have liked, he accepted the role of administrator philosophically. About midway through his MGH career he was moved to observe that his job was like an enzyme. "For one thing," he said, "an enzyme is itself a part of a living organism—it is, in a manner of speaking, very close to the center of life itself. Its function is to *facilitate* chemical reactions of living things, to help them occur. At the same time, the reactions that occur are the *important* things. . . . It used to be thought that enzymes did this in a kind of passive way; did not themselves take part in the reaction, were not changed nor destroyed themselves. Now we know better: enzymes *do* take part in the reaction, actually *participate,* and enzymes are changed in the process, are destroyed little by little. Certainly this last is like the Administrator. Enzymes must be replenished."

Perhaps feeling that the moment for replenishing had arrived, Clark resigned as general director on September 29, 1961.

3. John Hilton Knowles, General Director, 1962–1972

In 1964 John Knowles stood before a room full of physicians and fellow administrators and told them: "Medical administration is difficult. It is designed not for the faint-hearted, the inarticulate, the immature, those seeking power or those who have failed in practice or research. It concerns itself with the activities of highly intelligent, usually highly motivated individuals, possessed of charisma, multiple masters and tenure. It calls for giant men to provide leadership for such people."

It was characteristic of Knowles that he could make such an audacious remark without sounding pompous or self-serving, that he could disarm an audience with wit and candor. In that speech he had, in a way, told a tale about himself. He was an excellent practitioner of medicine. After his elevation to the directorship of MGH he continued to assume the responsibilities of visiting physician on the Medical Service for one or two months every year. "Practice," he maintained, "keeps me honest and humble, and I don't get too fancy on paper from the front office because I still know what the problems are that surround sickness." ("*Humble?*" mused Henry Romney in his reflection on Knowles' life. " 'Modesty is, of course, my long suit,' Knowles would say mockingly, and in his brash and self-centered moments he could be exasperating. . . . But he was humble in that he abhorred sham and pomposity, indeed fought them tooth and nail when he encountered them.")

If maturity can be defined so as to embrace spontaneity and mischief and to allow for an occasional error, Knowles was a mature man, philosophically attuned to the times, decisive, willing to take risks and accept the consequences. He was extraordinarily articulate, elegant in thought, scrupulous and respectful of language. While other people tossed around the word *charisma* and debased it, Knowles bothered to trace its usage back to Max Weber and to note that it means "gift of grace." So highly did he prize clear and effective communication that he stated the problem of the hospital administrator as "articulating his institution with the wants and needs of society at large," with full consciousness of the dual meaning of the word *articulate*. But as for faint-hearted, no one who ever worked with John Knowles would accuse him of that!

The subject of power is more complicated. Being decisive, bold, and articulate, Knowles inevitably made enemies who believed him overly interested in power. It is true that during his tenure power gravitated towards the office of the general director. But power, like technology, is intrinsically neither good nor bad; all depends on the wisdom of its deployment. Knowles was an ambitious man who liked to control. The record of his ten-year leadership of the MGH demonstrates that he used power according to his concept of the best interests of the hospital, the medical profession, and society at large; that he guided the institution through a complicated phase of growth and change; that the MGH benefited from his guidance.

"Giant" is a bit of inflationary prose, another word devalued by overuse—and probably employed by Knowles on that occasion for the sake of humor. But Knowles was undeniably one of those rare creatures: a true leader of men.

John Knowles was born in Chicago in 1926. His family moved around, alighting in St. Louis and then Los Angeles before coming to rest in Belmont, Mass. Knowles graduated from Belmont Hill School and went to Harvard where he distinguished himself as an athlete: He pitched for the baseball team, tended goal for the hockey team, and played a wicked game of squash. He was also a jazz enthusiast who could often be found at the old Imperial Hotel in Scollay Square sharing a piano bench with Jack Lemmon, the two of them banging out some old tune. (Knowles' life teems with delicious anecdotes. As Romney wrote, "John Knowles was a very, very funny man. . . . Everyone has a favorite Knowles story." But most of them must be resisted here lest they obscure the present, serious purpose which is to describe his administration of the MGH.)

Scholarship took second place to extracurricular activities, and Knowles' academic record failed to impress the admissions office at the Harvard Medical School. Yet the range of his adult mind suggests that he had absorbed more during his undergraduate years than his grades revealed. He became a voracious reader, primarily of humanist philosophers and historians; he studded his writings with references to de Tocqueville, Commanger, Aristotle, Weber, Francis Bacon, Bertrand Russell, and other nonmedical thinkers; and he pleaded for greater exposure to the humanities and social sciences in medical education.

Spurned by Harvard, Knowles pursued his medical studies at Washington University in St. Louis and graduated at the top of his class. He arrived at the MGH as an intern on the Medical Service in July 1951, the same year that Walter Bauer succeeded James Howard Means as chief of that service. Knowles rose aggressively through the ranks—from assistant resident, to resident, to chief resident in 1958. Along the way he married Edith Morris LaCroix, a pretty lab technician whom he had met over a stomach pump in the Emergency Ward. He spent two years in the Navy as officer-in-charge of a cardiopulmonary laboratory at the U.S. Naval Hospital in Portsmouth, Va. and returned to the MGH as chief of the Pulmonary Unit in 1959, director for medical affairs in September 1961, and as general director on February 16, 1962. He was 35 years old!

Knowles assumed his new responsibilities at a time when the morale of the hospital staff was precariously low. Edward Churchill, chief of Surgery, was about to retire. The health of his counterpart in Medicine, Walter Bauer, was failing noticeably. (Bauer would shortly enter the hospital as a patient, there to spend the last 18 months of his life; he died in December 1963.) Dean Clark, citing reasons of health, had resigned the directorship prematurely. This trio, particularly Churchill, had effectively run the hospital and been its spiritual leaders. The loss of all three almost simultaneously put a tremendous strain on the institution, for, as has often been observed, institutions are constitutionally anxious about change.

Superficially the MGH continued to function so that patients did not notice anything amiss, thanks largely to the attentions of Ellsworth T. Neumann, who kept the administrative machinery in motion. But the staff worried about shifts in priorities, research programs that had received support from the old regime failing to find favor with the new, and the fate of clinical projects and jobs.

Uncertainty generated gossip, vague rumors, and general unease until even the maintenance crew felt demoralized.

The trustees' selection of Knowles was a deliberate response to this domestic crisis. They perceived a need for a home-grown product who knew the hospital intimately and was already known by the staff. Knowles had demonstrated administrative acumen—not to say eagerness—and was immensely popular. Whereas Clark had come from public health administration, Knowles was a hospital-based practicing physician. There was doubtless disapproval in some quarters of the notion of catapulting a young whippersnapper over the heads of his seniors. But it is perhaps germane that Knowles' appointment occurred while John F. Kennedy sat in the White House, making youthful leadership credible and attractive.

Knowles, then, took charge at a sensitive moment when a minor miscalculation could have precipitated a major disaster. But it was also a moment of unique opportunity owing to the combined departures of Churchill and Bauer. Knowles, after all, had achieved his medical maturity under Bauer's watchful eye and would have felt awkward as his superior. Instead of having to challenge the prestigious old guard, Knowles was able to participate in the nominations of new chiefs to form a congenial new team. Paul Russell became chief of Surgery in 1962, and Robert Ebert came from Western Reserve to take over the Medical Service in 1964. The latter's account of his arrival is a Knowles story worth repeating:

I had made arrangements for a laboratory to suit my needs, and, believing everything had been settled, I was startled and more than a little angered to receive a letter from John saying the arrangements we had made were too expensive. He suggested that I write him saying how my needs might be scaled down. Impulsively, I wrote back suggesting that instead of negotiating, I would stay in Cleveland, where I had a good job and an excellent lab. By return mail, I received a letter from John saying, "Spoken like a true MGH tiger," and, of course, I could have the lab we had originally planned. Naturally, I was won over by his response and thought how gracious to respond so quickly. Six months later, I learned that he had paid for the renovations for my new laboratory from a discretionary fund which was mine as head of the Department of Medicine. I learned then that John didn't like to lose and rarely did.

He was truly a remarkable administrator of a large and complex institution. . . . He was into everything and knew everyone from the janitors to the professors. But he was not simply a gadfly. He had a burning need to know everything he possibly could about the institution he had been called to lead, and, remember, he was the youngest general director ever chosen to head the MGH. John had succeeded a brilliant but erratic man as general director, and the hospital was in substantial disarray when he took over. Patiently he rebuilt not only the physical plant and the administration, but also the spirit of the place. He was a marvelously cohesive force.

Ebert's account of Knowles' impact on hospital morale finds numerous backers among MGH intimates. David Crockett and Ben Castleman remember the phenomenon well. "It was incredible," Crockett says. "Knowles turned this place around in a year!"

One cannot expect to find clues to this somewhat mysterious stuff in public documents. Leadership has less to do with policies or visible results than it does with human character, and that has never been expressed in a foolproof formula. Knowles' intelligence, energy, humor, curiosity, and compassion come to mind as attributes, yet any number of his MGH colleagues possessed these qualities without being leaders of his dimension. Nor does leadership depend on the friendship of janitors. But Knowles' own definition of administration as articulation invites further inspection. With this explanation he located the general director at the junction between the hospital and the outside world, acting as a conduit for information between the two. In this view, articulation consists of much more than the stringing together of words in proper syntactic order; it becomes an act of interpretation and representation, of creative dialogue. Knowles' statements in the press, at medical meetings, as an expert witness at congressional hearings, and in fund-raising efforts, defined an image of the MGH and its values. Meanwhile, his interpretations of the exterior world to the MGH community indicated which pieces of that world he thought were relevant to the institution and required a response.

That leadership depends substantially upon articulation becomes most apparent in a failure of leadership. Complaints begin to sound about conflicting signals, confused priorities, blurred images, a "credibility gap" which is more often a measure of distance between rhetoric and reality than a matter of deliberate falsification. For, in order to be effective, the leader's representations must be plausible, grounded in the perceptions of the institution as well as in the expectations of the noninstitutional public. The realities are forever changing, the dynamics shifting. As Knowles said, "I would hope that we would recognize that the truth is evanescent, plural and contingent and not absolute or singular."

As American presidents have often become students of past presidencies, so Knowles turned to hospital history to understand and articulate contemporary concerns. He wrote:

Better understanding of the hospital is necessary if the medical profession wishes to play the main role in shaping its future. The consuming public needs understanding also, or the hospital will begin to reflect something undesirable and distorted. For the present form of the hospital has been molded and shaped by the wants and needs of society as well as its beliefs, values, and attitudes. As such it mirrors society and reflects not only its culture, but its economy, and it has never pretended to be better or worse than the times and the environment in which it finds itself.

Historical perspective is necessary as we view the evolution of the hospital to its present central position in the provision of health services and its unique role as a social instrument.

Knowles wrote prolifically, was a willing and witty speaker, and made himself accessible to the press. Newsmen quickly discovered that Knowles made good copy. His brain was quick, his language pungent. Mary E. Macdonald, director of the Department of Nursing, told a typical Knowles story at the memorial service after his death:

His manner of expression has been accurately described as outspoken, hard-hitting, incisive, witty, humorous, colorful, and, on occasion, earthy. . . . His impatience with mediocrity and idleness, his versatility with the instant epigram, are traits which have been duly noted—such as his comment to the press on the occasion of his censorship by the Massachusetts Medical Society: "I am not going to diddle around with those jerks." He stopped by my office the next morning for coffee, as was his custom, and when I questioned him on the veracity of the headline, his response was, "Of course I didn't say that, Mary." And then, with a twinkle in his eye, he asked, "Do you really want to know what I did say?" I know I share with some present this afternoon the knowledge of his true retort—a most colorful epigram but hardly fit for chapel recitation.

Since Knowles delivered lively copy, the media returned the favor by giving him generous coverage. Of course the press gave more space to items like his battle with the American Medical Association or to his broad-ranging political pronouncements on such topics as Vietnam and civil rights than it did to his less sensational reflections on the nature of the voluntary hospital; the public therefore received a misshapen impression of him. As Ebert observed, "John was no radical and his battle with the AMA has frequently been misinterpreted. The American Medical Association objected to his appointment as assistant secretary of health not because of his liberal views but because he was unpredictable and always said exactly what he thought." However, as Neumann noted, the AMA and others "could have invariably predicted his actions and statements if they had simply recognized the fact that he did his research carefully and stated the truth as he saw it—whether or not it was politically advantageous for him to do so. If controversy developed, he enjoyed it because he had all the facts and could articulate them forcefully to the audiences of all news media."

Knowles never bothered to quibble about distortions of his political image but chose instead to use the press as best he could. After the highly publicized saga of his near appointment to HEW earned him mention on the popular television show "Laugh-In," he told an audience: "As long as I have achieved such a peculiar form of notoriety, I might as well try to influence the public." And so he did.

Communications within MGH mattered most of all to him. "Communications is the stuff that cements organizations together," he would say. He observed that the medical world tended to defend itself against communication rather than invite it. Doctors, he claimed—only half jokingly—are the enemy of bureaucracy because medical education has prepared them for individual action and attention to patients. Few of them are concerned with the hospital as a social instrument; they do not participate in administration, do not understand the hospital's problems, and are the first to criticize when something goes awry. Knowles set out to alter this state of affairs. He hired Martin Bander, a medical reporter from a Boston newspaper, to improve the house organ, the *MGH News;* he tended carefully to the bulletins to the staff that originated in his offices; and he made himself generally available. He recognized these as symbolic interventions, however, meaningless without changes in organizational structure: "Much of the communication occurs through the visible committee structure of the hospital, and this is perhaps the most effective mechanism that exists."

Knowles therefore undertook major alterations in committee design, notably a controversial enlargement of the General Executive Committee (GEC). The suggestion, like many others, actually came from Neumann, and Knowles alertly perceived its usefulness. The GEC, the hospital's most powerful policy-setting body, numbered ten in 1960, with Churchill as chairman—a position he occupied for eight years; the director, Clark, acted as its secretary and took notes on the proceedings.

Leon Eisenberg, former chief of psychiatry, applied his professional insight to some of the responses Knowles' changes evoked:

As a Service Chief, I was also privileged to sit on the MGH General Executive Committee during a period crucial to the development of the hospital. In the year before I arrived, John Knowles had drastically changed the system of governance. Membership on the Executive Committee had been restricted by tradition to a small and select group of Chiefs. John insisted that each clinical service, as well as the Departments of Nursing and Social

Service, should have direct representation. Those who read Machiavellian motives into everything John did interpreted his proposal as an effort to dilute the authority of the Chiefs of Medicine and Surgery in order to augment his own by making the Committee a less effective decision-making body. Whatever may have been intended, the actual result was a far more open and democratic structure. In the past, those who had been excluded felt paranoid about what was happening behind closed doors. Once they were able to participate, they had to face the competing demands on the hospital and the inevitable necessity for horse trading in order to attain a dynamic balance.

Knowles was not the least bit embarrassed to acknowledge that the office of the general director had gained in this redistribution of power. "It was established," he wrote, "that the General Director would draw up the agenda well in advance of each meeting and in consultation with the Chairman prepare the necessary background material for decision making. Finally, it was re-established that the General Executive Committee was a misnomer in that the committee was not truly executive but rather was primarily advisory to the Board of Trustees and its agent, the General Director." Numerous other committees (on utilization review, teaching and education, community extension programs, computers, abortion, patients' rights) were expanded or born during Knowles' tenure, and he was an irrepressible member of most of them. Overall, the proliferation did serve to draw many more staff into the business of hospital administration, to force them to see issues in their complexity, to communicate, and to take responsibility.

Knowles' ninth annual report is a remarkable document. The last few pages read more like social change theory than an account of the MGH during the fiscal year, and they reveal the quality of reflection he brought to questions of administration. Though they ought to be read in full, a brief quotation captures the essence of his argument:

We have passed from the age of individualism to that of the power of collectivism. Methods of administration and organizational structures must change with changing social conditions, changing intellectual activities, and changing technological capacities. . . .

I believe that 50 percent of the bureaucratic methods should be retained, i.e., that portion which simplifies and speeds communication and provides for the implementation of change. Policy and change will be determined not by the rigid requirements of defined roles in the pyramid but by *ad hoc* and constantly changing groups in and out of the institution who will provide the expertise and the intellect to solve shared problems rapidly, point the way for change, and make final decisions. The administrative head (and it is a sociological fact that any social group has a head!) becomes the coordinator—asking the right questions and knowing who to assemble to provide the best answers—using both the formal and informal power structure to communicate and implement change. . . . He must learn to occupy an ambiguous position and to obtain his pleasures vicariously—no small order for a "normal man". Democracy is upon us; free communication is a necessity and cements complex institutions, and influence will be exerted on the basis of knowledge and skill and not the prerogatives of bureaucratic power.

Restructuring the MGH organization was John Knowles' most distinctive act as director, the achievement for which he bears singular responsibility. Given ordinary institutional inertia, it was no trivial feat. Most other developments during his administration, however, belong to a more tangled evolutionary web. Grand old institutions like the MGH—or the Harvard Medical School, not to mention the venerable College—move at a stately pace. The comment that a man is ahead of his time is another way of saying that individual ideas are in advance of collective thought. Though frustrating to creative individuals, on the whole this is probably a healthy situation. Society requires continuity as well as invention and change. The best ideas generally do get assimilated into the collective wisdom, though by the time they become part of the institution everyone has usually forgotten their sources.

As Cecil Sheps emphasized in the previous chapter, Dean Clark was a man in the vanguard of medicine with respect to social programs. Though he could not implement many of the ideas he cherished, his preparation of the collective MGH mind during the fifties helped clear an institutional path for Knowles in the sixties. Inspiration for such innovations as the Logan Medical Station, the Bunker Hill Health Center, the Chelsea Health Center, the stations in Boston's North End, expansion of the in-town pediatrics and screening clinics—all developments of the Knowles era—can be traced to Clark's concern for public health. The absence of institutional hysteria before the fact of Medicare in 1966 also, in a sense, harkens back to Clark.

This, admittedly, is a gross simplification. The ideals that animated the innovations of the sixties were buried deep in hospital history, and Clark had never been a lone voice. James Howard Means, for example, exerted a powerful influence on the thinking of both Clark and Knowles. By Knowles' time, however, societal forces had gathered momentum, and monies were available for community-based health centers; the moment was ripe. And Knowles' role must not be minimized. As Lawrence Martin, associate director in both the Knowles and Sanders administrations, observed, "John truly was an innovator by accepting many of the suggestions made to him by his staff." He shared many of Clark's dreams, and by putting some of them into operation he made the MGH a leader in community care. Still, it is reasonable to speculate that the institution would have resisted this direction had it not been previously cultivated by Clark and others. Even Knowles failed to build a new ambulatory care facility, an item that had been on the agenda since the early fifties but was repeatedly shelved as other concerns were given priority. Charles Sanders, finally, would do that job.

The hospital's expansion into community medicine was a complicated political effort requiring the coordination of numerous interests and agencies as well as the hard work and imagination of several members of the MGH staff. (See pages 146–147 for more detail.) Knowles threw the full power of his office behind these projects, conscious that the commitment represented a significant change in the social function of the hospital. He defined this function as follows:

Medicine must concern itself with the larger field of social welfare and develop a holistic concept of a community's health if it is to prevent disease and maintain health and thereby enhance the quality of life, to say nothing of the national welfare. Such a concept will allow medicine to take its rightful place in the larger field of social welfare, and will considerably enhance the learning experience of *all* health personnel. . . .

It is the intention of the MGH to develop such a holistic plan in conjunction with all the organizations concerned with the health of a community—be they urban renewal, educational, welfare, religious, public health, visiting nurses, and so on. It is the overall aim of this program to develop a health service system which will represent all the skills, manpower, and resources required to cultivate high level physical, cognitive, and psychologic health and competence during the formative years of pregnancy, infancy, and childhood, and to prevent, detect, and treat disease as necessary to maintain optimal health throughout life.

Knowles' vision placed the teaching hospital some distance beyond its classic role as a "citadel of acute curative, scientific and technical medicine." He believed that the MGH must assume broad social responsibilities not only for the sake of the national welfare but equally for the vitality, possibly even the survival, of the hospital itself. "We can speak of 'institutional Darwinism,'" he wrote, "a survival of the fittest institutions through inheritance of tradition and through cultural adaptation to contemporary social needs."

Nevertheless, the great building project of Knowles' administration—the Gray Building with the Jackson and Bigelow towers—addressed classic, and urgent, hospital needs: modern operating rooms, postsurgical care units, research laboratories, medical wards, a diagnostic radiology center, and other facilities which brought the MGH physical plant up to date with the skills of its physicians and the technologic arsenal. It was a huge and daring undertaking, the biggest construction venture in the hospital's history, adding more than half a million square feet at a cost of $22 million.

Finally, one can ponder that "arid mass of barren figures" that Knowles included in his last report to review his ten years in office. "Unfortunately we live in an age of numeracy, not literacy, and I am a product of that age," he apologized. The statistics testify to exuberant growth, an acceleration of trends that started after World War II. The MGH was hardly unique in this respect; universities and medical centers all over the country flourished in a climate of optimism, government support, and foundation generosity. But at the MGH, as elsewhere, growth brought certain problems. Knowles presided over this expansion, but his responsibility for it and for the problems it created is limited because the large-scale events were beyond his control. Similar statistics from comparable hospitals tell the same story and support this view.

A synopsis of the statistics for the ten years of the Knowles administration is as follows:

The total budget increased from $23.8 to $88.0 million.
The number of employees increased from 3,633 to 6,266.
The research budget increased from $5.6 to $13.5 million (approximately two-thirds of the funds came from the NIH).
The patient care budget increased from $12.2 to $53.7 million.
Admissions increased from 26,099 to 28,675 annually.
The average total per day cost increased from $41.05 to $155.01.

It was Knowles' job to see that the MGH maintained its foothold on the advancing edge of medicine by sustaining an intellectual climate attractive to great teachers, clinicians, and researchers. The impressive growth of the research budget and the increase in research personnel during the decade suggest that he succeeded. "I believe the healthy balance of patient care, community extension, teaching, and research has been maintained," he concluded, "and today, they all exist in fruitful and, I say emphatically, *happy* symbiosis at the MGH."

The research budget was distinct from the irksome figures for patient care—research costs were, and are, not passed on to patients. The swollen patient care statistics reflect medical advances such as intensive care units (where the average cost per day was sometimes more than $300); sophisticated technology and personnel skilled in its use; complicated surgical procedures; more laboratory tests and x-ray examinations; increasing educational costs; and a number of external factors which added to the overhead. Hospital costs, which in one variation or another had troubled previous directors, became a national issue in the sixties. Knowles spent countless hours explaining where the figures came from. All those pie charts comparing hospital and hotel costs must have been very tiresome for him.

In addressing the issue, Knowles was quick to point out that "hospital workers were not paid the minimum wage in most hospitals until the late 1960s. . . . I am proud to say that the MGH has led the way in achieving wages, fringe benefits, and working conditions which are commensurate with the value a community must place on its health workers. . . . A large part of inflation in hospital costs has been due to our 'catching up' with the industrial (as contrasted with the service) sector—and the remainder has been due to increasing costs of supplies. When I was an intern in 1951, I was paid $18.75 a month and asked whether I wanted it in war bonds or cash! Today the intern starts at $808.33 per month." But articulate as he was, Knowles made little headway on this front. Patients remain astonished by hospital costs.

The cost problem was generic, not specific to the MGH. Knowles recognized it as such, noted that "the money pit is not bottomless," and supported the principle of regional planning for health services while remaining skeptical of the government commissions that were being created to oversee the process. There is a parenthetical but important point to be made about Knowles here: Contrary to what many people inferred from his statements on Vietnam and civil rights or from his arguments with the AMA, Knowles was very wary of government intervention in medicine. He was an ardent supporter of voluntarism because, in his view, it was the voluntary, individual assumption of responsibility that kept democracy democratic. "We hand over the sole resolution of social problems to government at our peril," he cautioned.

Knowles resigned from the MGH in 1972. During the period that he was being considered for many important positions including assistant secretary of HEW, Eisenberg observed that "it was apparent that John was gradually widening his horizons beyond MGH; he needed a new challenge. Few were surprised when he accepted the invitation to head the Rockefeller Foundation." The trustees recorded their regret at his departure and their great appreciation of his work at the MGH. But the surest sign of the mark of his presence was the deluge of staff which turned out to say farewell; he spent an entire day shaking hands.

When he became ill in early 1979, Knowles instinctively left New York and returned to the hospital he knew and trusted. Sadly, nothing could be done to cure his disease, pancreatic cancer. He died in March at the age of 52, cruelly cut in full flower. His death created a genuine sense of loss among his associates as well as thousands of people who had never met him. As Ebert said, John Knowles had been an "ornament to the profession."

With the assistance of *Edith Knowles Dabney, Lawrence Martin,* and *Ellsworth T. Neumann*

4. Benjamin Castleman: Acting General Director, January–August 1972

In 1971, shortly after John Knowles made known his intentions to move on to the Rockefeller Foundation, the trustees initiated a search for a new general director. There being no obvious candidate within the MGH family, the committee cast its net across the country. Meanwhile, Benjamin Castleman, chief of pathology and the hospital's ranking citizen, held the fort as acting director. Though this interim lasted only eight months, Castleman performed energetically and set a remarkable record of accomplishment. During his tenure the revised rules and regulations of the medical staff were ratified and put into effect; construction of the parking garages in front of the White Building was completed; the house officers were relocated in the Walcott Building, a development that made possible the demolition of the old Parkman Street houses; a group practice, the Internal Medicine Associates, was inaugurated; and, most significantly, a Certificate of Need was obtained for the Cox Building and construction was started. These items come from a longer list that proves that Castleman was not merely occupying a vacant director's chair for the sake of symbolism. Except for meeting the press, which, of course, had been spoiled by a decade of John Knowles—Castleman enjoyed the experience. (See Chapter 33 for a biographic sketch of Castleman and his activities as a pathologist.)

5. Charles Addison Sanders, General Director, 1972–1981

The trustees' quest for a permanent director came to an unexpected end early in 1972 when the name of Charles Addison Sanders was pressed to their attention. Sanders, a cardiologist by profession, was chief of the Catheterization Laboratory at the MGH. Born and raised in Texas, he had studied medicine at Southwestern Medical School and trained as an intern and resident at Boston City Hospital. After a one-year fellowship in cardiology at the MGH, he received an offer to return to Southwestern Medical but accepted instead the MGH's invitation to head its Cardiac Catheterization Lab. Later, Sanders also managed the huge Myocardial Infarction Research Unit with an annual budget of about $2 million as well as the MEDLAB evaluation project. (MEDLAB is a computer system for gathering and dispersing information about critically ill patients; it did not pass muster at the MGH.) Sanders was an associate professor at the Harvard Medical School and had served on the editorial board of the *New England Journal of Medicine*. These and other prominent features marked the geography of the man's career. In addition to impressive credentials, Sanders possessed the important quality of being politically acceptable to the various elements within the hospital, and so, in 1972, the trustees appointed him the seventeenth general director.

As these words are being written, in September 1981, it has only been a few weeks since Sanders departed from the MGH to assume his new responsibilities as executive vice-president of E. R. Squibb & Sons. The hospital sent him off with balloons, flowers, good food, laughter, and a giant toothbrush at a party on the Bulfinch lawn, and he was to be missed. The man with the marvelous smile and the long, lanky Texas cowboy frame had gradually won their affection with his sense of humor, his diplomacy, and his quiet integrity. The ever-watchful Leon Eisenberg recalled the trustees' appointment of Sanders, "a staff member with whom I had had only a nodding acquaintance":

Perhaps the best way to convey the difference in style between John [Knowles] and Charles is a vivid personal recollection of the first meeting of the General Executive Committee after his succession. I had arrived a few minutes late; all of the chairs around the table were occupied; I sat in the second row unable to see those in front of me. I did not know that Charles was due that day and I did not discover he was present until he made his first comment, some five minutes before the end of the two hour meeting. Where John had expressed himself on almost every issue and had made it impossible to ignore his presence, Charles was reserved and didn't speak until he felt it was imperative. The difference between the two men was so dramatic that I was inclined for the first few months to underestimate Charles' capacity to tame the tigers who sat about the table. It didn't take me long to recognize my error. He went about it in a different way but one that was fully effective."

Sanders believed firmly in the process of building a consensus. "I listen a lot," he remarked. "You can't learn unless you listen. . . . I really do feel that if every-

27

body can come together and talk, then you can, in fact, come to the logical conclusion through the process of discussion."

It was very often said of Sanders that he was the right man for the times. Implicit in that expression was the understanding that the times had changed, that the exuberant abundance of the sixties had given way to a different, if not easily definable, political and economic climate. Sanders moved carefully to identify the issues that would determine the boundaries of his administration. In his first annual report he wrote:

As Mr. Lawrence E. Martin, our Comptroller, recently pointed out, it has come time for society to decide just exactly how much it is willing to pay to save a life. Obviously this is a difficult decision, but one which cannot be made unilaterally by the medical community.

In the years ahead, I believe we will look back on 1972 as a year of change for the health industry in general and for the Massachusetts General Hospital in particular. Many forces have been at work to influence our methods of delivering medical care, defining new responsibilities for the hospital, and threatening our ability to continue research into those factors producing human disease. Thus at this time it seems appropriate for us to ask what kind of hospital we are, and more importantly, what kind of hospital we want to be. . . . The mood of the country . . . is one to encourage—no, in fact, *to demand*—an increasing accountability of the actions of doctors and hospitals in delivering health care in an effort to improve health care delivery and to minimize cost. In addition, we are posed with the problems of applying existing knowledge to improving the delivery of health care without adding to costs.

At the end of his second year in office Sanders, having further surveyed the MGH terrain and the external forces that affect its functioning, continued this tangent of thought:

It is of interest that the expansive calls for a totally comprehensive health system through a government financing program have been modulated. I believe this has occurred primarily because it is now appreciated that comprehensive health care is an extremely expensive program, and inconsistent with the goal of tightly controlling the cost of health care. Thus the idealists who insist on a liberal comprehensive health care program and the economists who insist on cost containment have been on a collision course. Of great concern is that the realities favor the economists, and it may well be that in the near future health care will be financed on the basis of a limited number of dollars, rather than dictated by the actual needs of society.

In these times, then, we are stringently limited in our ability to grow and are held accountable for whatever growth does take place. This is not an atmosphere to which we have been accustomed, but it is by no means an environment in which we cannot live and prosper. To do so we must articulate to those who would regulate us those positive features about our health care system and in particular the necessity for great teaching hospitals like the MGH. . . . Equally important, we as an institution must be more sensitive to the allocation of limited funds. As one of my colleagues recently said in a speech relating to growth in the health care industry, it is a time to measure our goals and our resources.

Sanders thereby laid down some ground rules for guiding the MGH through the seventies. By contrast with the almost visionary tone of Knowles' holistic plan—a tone suited to the temper of a bygone decade—Sanders set his program within the context of more austere realities. Some of those realities proved even less manageable than he initially imagined. At his first news conference he promised to try to lower hospital costs, a feat later rendered impossible by the inflationary spiral of the decade. In 1974, for example, MGH costs for heat, light, and telephone doubled; steam purchased from Boston Edison rose from approximately $1 million to $2 million in a single year. That Sanders' administration moderated the rise in hospital costs was in itself a major achievement.

Early in his directorship Sanders discovered that the administrative apparatus he had inherited needed serious overhauling. Whereas Knowles had attended to expanding committees and creating communications channels, he had left the day-to-day administrative operations to Ellsworth Neumann (as had Clark before him). "Every time a new responsibility would come up," Sanders remembered, "the administrator would look at so-and-so, an assistant director, and figure out how many responsibilities he had. The one that had the least would get the new responsibility. It might have no relationship whatsoever to whatever else he was doing. . . . The place had gotten so big that something had to be done. I'm not saying that John failed to do that; he would have done it if he'd stayed longer, but he didn't." That this improvised system functioned at all depended upon Neumann's extraordinary knowledge and instincts about the hospital and on Martin's command of fiscal matters. When Neumann, after 24 years of service to the MGH, followed Knowles to the Rockefeller Foundation, Sanders and Martin got the trustees' blessing to reorganize the administration along corporate lines.

With the help of a consulting firm, programs and functions were identified and management responsibilities assigned accordingly. Assistant directors were placed in charge of specific functions such as personnel, medical and surgical support services, management services, clinical laboratories, fiscal affairs, and so forth. Whereas the old organization had been keyed to departments, services, or buildings, the new arrangement made horizontal cuts through the hospital. Sanders called it "keeping the M&Ms together, and the raisins together, and the peanuts together, and they all get together at the top in something called an Operations Committee." The reorganization made for more coherence in budget development as well as more efficient cost savings efforts. By 1975 the new system was in place, and Sanders reported that "there is sufficient cross-representation among all administrative committees to ensure the degree of communication necessary to keep the committees informed of one another's activities. The whole purpose of this reorganization has been to streamline the administration without adding substantial numbers of personnel, thus creating a bureaucracy with an inertia of its own. Although only in its early stages, the new administrative structure is already proving to be sensitive and responsive to the needs of the institution in a manner which recognizes its large size and extreme complexity." In the five or six years since this reorganization, the MGH has acquired a reputation as one of the best run hospitals in the country, and Martin, now associate general director, is looked upon as the dean of hospital administrators.

Economic considerations naturally played a strong part in the formulation of policy, sometimes forcing Sanders to make difficult choices. The most controversial, perhaps, was his opposition in 1974, and again in 1980, to heart transplant surgery at the MGH. Since the operation involves refined technology, additional beds, and some complicated logistics, Sanders viewed it as a policy decision in terms of resource allocation. When the General Executive Committee discussed heart transplants in 1974, no genuine consensus emerged. Although it was fully appreciated that no institution in the world had people better qualified than those at the MGH to perform such surgery, it was reluctantly recommended that cardiac transplantation should not be undertaken but that continued research was desirable.

By 1980, however, the GEC had moved into a position of almost unanimous support. When Sanders and the trustees solicited the opinion of the Committee on Research, they received an ambivalent response. "The net result was that they couldn't be sure it would contribute substantially to our research knowledge, but at the same time they couldn't be sure that it wouldn't," Sanders explained. He maintained the stance that the operation would not be in the best interest of the hospital as a whole. "The reason was not that we couldn't do it, not that the people who would have been involved weren't innovative and imaginative. But in terms of the balance of the hospital, in order to do *this,* we had to give up *that,* and giving up *that* wasn't something we wanted to do." Sanders' position, which the trustees backed by a final decision, did not rule out heart transplant surgery indefinitely; Sanders felt that such a program should be undertaken when it could be implemented without upsetting the balance of activities and resources.

While restraining development in some quarters, Sanders promoted it in others—in both instances with reference to a large-scale view of the institution—and the trustees wholeheartedly supported this perspective. His was the administration that finally built the Ambulatory Care Center that Clark had wanted so badly two decades earlier. No less committed to the concept of community care than his predecessors, Sanders put a new ambulatory facility at the top of his agenda early in his directorship; he pursued the matter obstinately, cutting his way slowly through the red tape strewn in his path by the Massachusetts Determination of Need process (estimated to have cost the hospital some $300,000 in direct expenses for information gathering plus another $3.5 million as a consequence of the delay in construction). The nine-story brick and glass structure flanking the main entrance of the White Building stands as Sanders' mark on the MGH landscape.

Another artifact of the Sanders years, the MGH Institute of Health Professions, does not so readily meet the eye. The institute, which began operation in 1980, is a hospital-based educational entity offering degree programs in various health care specialties such as nursing, physical therapy, and so on. The notion of acquiring degree-granting capability for the hospital surfaced in the Knowles administration but never advanced beyond the stage of interesting conversation. Sanders might have allowed the discussions to flounder and fade away in the less bountiful seventies; instead, he encouraged the project, set the appropriate committee mechanisms in motion, pursued state certification, and watched the institute come to life. "We were sending a lot of people out of here with certificates that they had done this, that, or the other," he explained. "They'd go to California, and that piece of paper wasn't worth a hill of beans. So I felt we had an obligation to offer those people a fairly professional course. Also, I felt uneasy about the failure to standardize or meet certain criteria in the educational process. We have an obligation to the rest of the industry."

During the early planning for the institute, it was generally believed that legitimation as an educational organization in its own right (by contrast with its affiliation with the Harvard Medical School) would open up new funding possibilities for the MGH. The argument lost power as the seventies ran down.

"Tuitions are going up. There are going to be a lot of people falling by the wayside . . ." Sanders observed gloomily. "As far as raising money for that kind of activity, and supporting it, I can't think of a worse time, and I worry about our ability to make it a sustained thing. But that doesn't make me less committed to its success than when we began." (See Chapter 44 for additional information.)

Early in 1981 Sanders announced a $114-million fund drive, earmarking the greater portion of the receipts for replacing antiquated inpatient facilities, whose turn it was since the Ambulatory Care Center was a reality. In the spring he made the stunning announcement of a ten-year $50-million-plus research contract between the MGH and Hoechst AG, a German chemical company, which will give rise to a new department of molecular biology at the hospital. Clearly both events will influence the affairs of the MGH for years to come and provide grist for the mills of the next generation of historians.

Shortly thereafter, Sanders startled the MGH by resigning. By September he had already moved to Princeton, New Jersey. His abrupt departure provoked nationwide comment and at least one historic observation: Washburn served as director for 14 years (not including a spell as director emeritus), Faxon for 14, Clark for 12, Knowles for 10, and Sanders for nine. Meanwhile, the MGH grew enormously. Its character evolved, and its health care responsibilities expanded. Government made its presence felt, largely through increasingly cumbersome regulatory agencies. Accordingly, the position of director grew more demanding every year. So perhaps it is not surprising after all that the terms of office have been shrinking or that the last three directors resigned before retirement age. While there is no reason to suppose the job will get any easier, Sanders' successor inherits a well-managed institution with its reputation intact, the morale of the staff healthy, and the foundations for exciting developments already in place.

With the assistance of *Charles A. Sanders*

6. The Committee on Research

In 1912 when he was a house officer—what we would now call a resident—George Minot had an inkling that pernicious anemia might have something to do with diet. Three years later he began to examine the eating habits of anemic patients. He cross-questioned them so exhaustively that some of the medical students considered him rather odd. Meanwhile he studied blood samples under the microscope. One student later recalled the first case of pernicious anemia ever cured with liver at the MGH: "When I was a senior, in the summer of 1926, George Minot one Sunday at lunch whispered in my ear to try large amounts of liver on the next pernicious anemia case I had. . . . The 'pup' at the time . . . was very disgusted at my ordering him to get a meat grinder, grind up tons of liver every day, and to pump it into this man with a nasal tube. He did it, however, and for several days nothing happened. The patient seemed to be getting worse. . . . [Then] old Mr. __ came out of his coma rather suddenly and, swearing in a rather feeble voice, complained that this was 'a hell of a place where they don't give you enough to eat.' He progressively and rapidly got better." Dr. Minot shared the 1934 Nobel Prize in Physiology and Medicine.

For the sake of contrast, imagine the seedling of some analogous hypothesis taking root in the brain of an insightful young MGH resident in the 1970s. Pursuit of this idea inevitably would lead to collection of preliminary data, formation of a team of relevant experts, designing a research strategy, writing a grant proposal, and anxious anticipation of a decision. Funding is essential, for without it one can purchase neither the skills nor the time (human and mechanical) necessary to the task.

The elaborate rituals of contemporary medical research are the consequences of several factors. The increase in the sheer quantity of information has generated smaller and smaller units of specialization; thus the need for the collective intelligence of a team comprising the appropriate shards of expertise. Meanwhile, the technology that can be usefully brought to bear on a research problem has become sophisticated and expensive. Lastly, there has been a massive financial investment, largely of public funds, in medical research. It is not necessarily easy to tease out cause from effect among these developments because they have occurred in tandem. Clearly, however, the availability of money has been a powerful stimulant. And, mindful of the suspicion in which the concept of progress is currently held, one can claim progress for medical science without embarrassment. The several chapters of this volume support that claim with examples of laboratory discoveries and improvements in patient care too numerous to list here. Those advances occurred within the framework of a large research structure, and it is the development of that support system that occupies us in this chapter.

In soliciting voluntary contributions, it is customary for fund raisers to cite instances of research discoveries that have been translated into better patient care. MGH history offers stunning object lessons, from the use of ether in 1846 to limb replantation in 1962, and so on. Though there is nothing wrong with the principle, such presentations tend to shorten the distance in time between research and application. Limb replantation did not happen overnight; it deployed decades of study and invention. The more immediate link between the quality of clinical care and research usually escapes attention. It lies in the simple fact that research is exciting. Research attracts imaginative minds, passionate explorers, people dissatisfied with the status quo; patients benefit from the character of intelligence and observation concentrated upon their illnesses.

The MGH has always appreciated this subtle connection. As the example of Minot's liver regimen suggests, research has been going on at the hospital in one guise or another since the Bulfinch Building opened its doors. By the late 1930s the notion of research as a legitimate function of the hospital had become valid intellectual currency. There was sufficient research volume to inspire the formation of a Hospital Research Council in 1938 "to keep all investigators in the Hospital constantly informed of the activities of their colleagues, to act as a clearing house, and to censor all reports prior to publication."

Nevertheless, by today's standards, the conditions of research were humble. Harvard Medical School financed most MGH projects, and investigators begged small grants from various other sources, but many inquisitive staff members effectively subsidized their own curiosity. Research space was chronically scarce. Thus, while paying lip service to the necessity for research, the hospital extended only meager support. In 1936, in mid-Depression, Paul Dudley White lamented that the Cardiac Clinic's "research balance is but a few dollars."

Research, then, did not really begin to secure equal footing with patient care and education at MGH until after World War II. Paul C. Zamecnik, writing in Faxon's volume of history, recalled the postwar mood:

The staff . . . returned one by one, each looking at the old and new buildings with a fresh pair of eyes and turning over the question of how to apply the lessons of wartime medicine to better patient care for the Massachusetts General Hospital of the future. The memory of the atom bomb was fresh and a spirit of confidence in science buttressed hopes for the conquest of unsolved diseases.

Penicillin had been a wartime wonder, and a train of newer antibiotics had followed in its wake. . . . At the luncheon table in the Doctors' Dining Room there was agreement that the infectious diseases were coming under control, but that a hard core of degenerative problems would remain to challenge the efforts of the coming generations. At this moment the hospital budget was in a delicate balance, with the possibility of a large deficit looming for the next fiscal year. . . . There was a suspicion that research costs would have to be pared radically in some way if a larger deficit were to be avoided.

The spirit of scientific optimism prevailed over the atmosphere of financial gloom. Trustees and staff committed their energies to fund-raising activities for research and, when supplementary energy seemed in order, appointed David C. Crockett to orchestrate the efforts. The Committee on Research (COR) supplanted the old Research Council in 1947, and the Scientific Advisory Committee was formed the same year. Edward D. Churchill is said to have suggested both groups, with trustees and staff warmly endorsing his inspiration.

The trustees charged the COR with the responsibility "to promote, facilitate, and guide research affairs at the Massachusetts General Hospital, in the belief that the staff would serve its cause better as partners than as individuals." The committee's duties were further outlined in its charter:

1. Evaluate all current research projects.

2. Recommend to the Board of Trustees the establishment of medical research units.
3. Review all grants-in-aid in accordance with the procedures approved by the Board of Trustees.
4. Recommend to the Board of Trustees the disbursements of all available research funds.
5. Appoint all committees essential for maintaining a strong research program.

Since its formation the COR has presided over the development of the MGH as one of the leading medical research institutes in the world. During the last quarter century, research has enjoyed a phenomenal expansion, no doubt exceeding even the wildest dreams of the postwar visionaries. Money has been the key to all this growth. Any description of the evolution of the genus research, as opposed to specific research projects, during the past 25 years ultimately returns to the subject of money—its quantity, the sources, the patterns of dispersal, and its influence upon the character of medical research. In 1955 the MGH research budget had just gone over the $2 million mark; by 1980 that budget had swelled to $28 million. A comparison of the composition of that budget shows that in 1955 the federal government's contribution (as represented by the U.S. Public Health Service, the Atomic Energy Commission, and the Armed Forces) accounted for less than half of the money committed to research at the MGH; ten years later the federal share was in the neighborhood of 75 percent, a level that was maintained through 1980. Meanwhile the hospital, which financed over 10 percent of research in 1955 from general funds, reduced its contribution to zero and can say, in this era of exaggerated health care costs, that the expenses of research are not passed on to patients.

Practically all the money in the research budget has been, and is, "soft." Federal and foundation grants run for a specific number of years after which they may or may not be renewed. Theoretically, the MGH research budget could wither away in a period of a few years if, by some crazy misalignment of the stars, all MGH grant applications were denied at the same time or if, in a somewhat less preposterous scenario, the federal government were suddenly to stop supporting medical research. (The latter possibility would not have seemed farfetched to COR members in the fifties; they had all lived through the Depression.) The other salient characteristic of the research budget is the extent to which it came to depend on federal tax dollars. Government agencies decide what kinds of research will or will not be funded; and government agencies are political entities, ultimately sensitive to public perception.

Given this potentially fickle climate, the COR's grand accomplishment has been the creation of a stable, long-range research capability at the MGH, a labor that absorbed its energies through the sixties. Committee reports from the mid-fifties, when the terrain was still being staked out, carried an undercurrent of excitement. "The fruitfulness of an interdisciplinary attack on medical problems in a hospital environment is becoming increasingly obvious both in the hospital and in the scientific world at large," read the report for 1955. By then *interdisciplinary* had assumed a broad meaning as the number of specialties relevant to medical science kept multiplying to include such fields as nuclear physics, electrical engineering, computer science, and chemical engineering, not to mention emerging disciplines of genetics, biostatistics, and their ilk.

As this picture of multifaceted research came into focus—and the Scientific Advisory Committee played a crucial role in encouraging that increase in scope—it suggested an orientation toward basic research, exploration of the fundamentals of biologic activity. This view was consistent with that already held by several senior members of the hospital staff; Walter Bauer, on one of his recruiting visits to the MIT Biology Department in 1948, was heard to growl to F. O. Schmitt, then head of the department, "If I can't build a strong basic research unit at the MGH, I am going to quit and raise chickens!" During the same period Churchill made the farsighted move of providing a laboratory home at the hospital for Fritz Lipmann, at the time a relatively young biochemist who some years later, while at the MGH, won the Nobel Prize. Also at the time Joseph Aub was building up a strong fundamental research capability in the Huntington Memorial Laboratory, having recruited Paul Zamecnik and a group of able young scientists, both M.D. and Ph.D. Bauer, Churchill, Aub, Crockett, and others beat the bushes for the funds needed to raise the first research building at the hospital. These examples of matching words with actions were greatly encouraged by the COR and the Scientific Advisory Committee.

As the development of nuclear energy depended upon comprehension and control of the atom and its particles, so essential medical advances require investigation of the cell and its components. The COR's commitment to this course represented a new research philosophy for the MGH. Traditionally, the hospital was a site of clinical applied research. To be sure, clinical investigators drew upon the knowledge stock of the theoretical or basic scientists, but basic science was primarily undertaken in research institutes and universities. By building a basic research component into the hospital, the COR sought to narrow the gap, geographic and intellectual, between the two endeavors. The committee expressed its view of the relationship in a policy statement drafted by Alexander Leaf:

The practice of medicine is clearly the application of knowledge toward practical ends. There is no clear dividing line between applied and basic research; basic research is aimed at increasing understanding, and applied research at utilizing this understanding to solve specific practical problems. The latter cannot long proceed without advances in the former. We are dealing with a continuum of understanding. Emphasis only on basic research would be denial of the social value of knowledge. Emphasis only on applied research in medicine would quickly exhaust the present levels of understanding and yield only inadequate solutions to major health problems. . . . Basic research is an investment in tomorrow's practical successes. Our understanding of life processes is yet so meager that we can ill afford to slacken our efforts to increase understanding.

Without any formal or deliberate plan, the research establishment began to grow within the departmental structure rather than as a separate institute or research department. The only exception to this one uncodified rule was the Laboratory of Biochemistry which developed under the direction of Lipmann and was perpetuated by his successor, Herman Kalckar. In those early days, young scientists, both M.D. and Ph.D., were recruited by department chairmen or unit chiefs, the selections usually being made on the basis of appropriateness of interests, competence, and scientific promise of the recruit. Thus the strength of the scientific enterprise depended upon the qualities of department chairmen and their senior investigators. The responsibility for determining the direction of research and the selection of particular problems resided with the individual scientists themselves and was not determined by any preexisting plan on a hospital-wide basis. The COR made every effort to ensure the quality of science at the hospital through its subcommittees, the local peer review of all grant applications prior to submission being a major factor. The committee frequently discussed various broad, and occasionally specific, research projects in progress but never attempted to plan, supervise, or determine the directions of research. It was accepted as an article of faith that no committee could know enough to take the responsibility for overall planning of science. The success or failure of the venture should depend on the quality of the scientists and the wisdom of their superiors. Collaboration was established strictly on a voluntary basis with no superimposition by the COR of planned interdisciplinary projects.

As research activity gained momentum at the MGH, so did the volume of work that fell to the COR and, accordingly, the size of the committee. In 1955, 24 people, including three trustees, sat on the COR; in 1970 there were 50; in 1980 the total was 88. (The research budget had increased by a factor of ten over the same period, so it cannot be said that committee expansion kept pace with the dollar growth; nevertheless, it did a reasonable imitation of the budget.) Fifty or 88 people may be able to pull rocks together, but committees of that size cannot accomplish much. Therefore the COR long ago evolved a smaller, functional executive committee and further distributed responsibilities among a number of subcommittees which were established as the need arose. A review of their functions permits insight into the world of MGH research.

The *Subcommittee on Research Planning and Policy* came into being in the late sixties as a consequence of the appearance of very large program project grants and also of interinstitutional research grants. It was clearly necessary to evaluate not only the quality of the proposed science but also the potential impact these very large commitments of money and people might have on the welfare of the institution as a whole. The COR also felt the strong need to "make every effort to convey to the public at large (via the press and other mass media) that biomedical science and research are integral parts of medicine and critically involved in the improvement of patient care." Subcommittee members also argued the research cause before congressional committees. During the seventies, this subcommittee took on an internal planning function ("Planning" was tacked on to its title), handling such policy-loaded matters as future space requirements and the desirability of certain proposed large-scale research commitments. It has the broadest mandate of all COR subcommittees.

The *Subcommittee on Review of Research Proposals* is the COR's quality control agent. It reviews all grant applications originating in the MGH. It is an advisory body rather than the ultimate authority, but its recommendations command attention. The committee's review process contributes to success of MGH research proposals in the various granting agencies. Because of the return of the detailed "pink sheet" of critique and suggestions for improvement to both the principal investigator and the department chairman, the former is assisted in improving proposals and the latter receives an evaluation of his scientific staff from colleagues (anonymously) on this committee. This subcommittee consists of 20 members of the scientific staff rotating on a yearly or bi-yearly basis and never includes a department chairman. The experience is valued greatly by, and is invaluable to, the participating staff members as well as the applicants. It is undoubtedly the hardest-working of the COR's subcommittees. The number of proposals that come up for review has proliferated every year; at last count it hovered around the 700 mark. Meanwhile, many of these proposals represent a staggering order of complexity and size. In 1973 the committee found itself confronted with an interinstitutional proposal that weighed 14 pounds and involved more than 100 investigators.

The *Subcommittee on Human Studies* further reviews all grant applications involving human subjects to ensure conformance with COR guidelines that protect the rights and welfare of individuals.

The *Subcommittee on Animal Farms,* later called the *Animal Care Subcommittee,* oversees and regulates that service to the research community.

The *Subcommittee on Research Colloquia* represents the COR's effort to solve the knotty problem of communication among diverse members of the MGH research community. The committee creates circumstances that encourage a more fluid dialogue between basic and clinical researchers and between researchers and practitioners. It publishes an annual register of research activities in the hospital, arranges evening colloquia, and organizes regular presentations to the full COR.

The now defunct *Subcommittee on Computer Service to Research* used to be responsible for seeing that MGH researchers had access to cost-effective, versatile, and appropriate computational capability—a straightforward task on the surface, but sometimes complicated. In 1970, for instance, the hospital terminated its rental contract for the XDS Sigma 2 because levels of utilization did not justify its costs; shortly thereafter the Harvard Computing Center, the alternate locus of computer hardware, dropped *its* contract for the XDS Sigma 7. Frustrated MGH researchers suddenly found themselves without access to a reactive computer for some months, and the subcommittee heard a great deal of grumbling. This subcommittee passed out of existence in 1973 when the Hospital Computer Center, attended by COR representatives, took over its functions.

The *Subcommittee on Bioengineering and Developmental Research* was conceived as a service organization. It spawned a financially independent consulting service, the Medical Engineering Group, in 1970. Two years later the subcommittee was reconstituted with the charge of advising on optimal use of MGH and neighboring bioengineering resources for research and patient care.

The *Subcommittee on Research Safety,* established in 1969, concerns itself with facilities for chemical storage, hazardous waste disposal, suitable building systems, and the like—matters of more than casual interest at MGH where many of the structures are old and subject to intensive use. In 1976 the subcommittee designated a special task force for biohazard containment to develop guidelines and review mechanisms for guaranteeing the safety of researchers, hospital personnel, and patients.

The *Subcommittee on Research Training* was appointed in 1977 to design a training program for MGH staff. It developed a combination of lecture courses and small tutorial seminars. The first lecture series, "Advanced Topics in Immunology," attracted over 100 people.

The review of COR subcommittees suggests the scope and character of concerns that research at the MGH generated over the past quarter century. However, it does not account for two items that dominated the COR's existence. The first problem, a practical one, followed naturally upon the initial commitment to basic science. The importation of basic scientists into the clinical setting made for some colossal headaches, the most obstinate of which was what the COR referred to as "finding a place in the academic sun, so to speak, for the new species: the full-time non-clinical research man in the hospital." Fuller discussion of that difficulty is included in the remarks on the role of the Scientific Advisory Committee because the SAC has a long history of involvement with the question of tenure. It is sufficient to say here that the discussions still go on.

The second issue with which the COR has had to grapple lies very near the heart of the MGH research organization. In the mid-sixties, when the federal share of sponsored research had reached the 75 percent level, changes began to appear in the funding pattern. By 1970 the new configurations provoked some alarm at the MGH and similar research institutions. In 1971 the COR commented formally upon the situation in its annual report to the trustees:

The scientific community has for some time been aware of a tendency to level off or even reduce Federal support for the biomedical research effort. Coupled with this has come an increased emphasis on targeted research as exemplified by the growing fraction of the total which is allocated to contractual research and large disease-oriented institutional or regional grants. There has been an increased tendency towards earmarking of funds by the Congress, the Executive Branch, and the individual Institutes, by dividing the national research budget into allocations designated by particular diseases. Many of us, though recognizing that the overriding goal of biomedical research is the solution of pressing health problems, question the assumption that by ordering research in terms of foreseeable relevance we can somehow accelerate the process. Furthermore, if the assumption is wrong, not only will medical progress be slowed, but changes will have taken place in the institutions from which this progress is expected which may be difficult to reverse. If conspicuous relevance rather than scientific excellence is to be the major criterion in the allocation of research support, there is a danger that academic and teaching hospitals may be polarized in directions which are incompatible with their long-term social goals.

Ironically, even as those words were being set to paper, construction crews were building the Cox Cancer Center, a controversial project for precisely the reasons stated above. The Scientific Advisory Committee, staunch advocate of basic research, had counseled against it. After much debate, the COR accepted the proposal only when sufficient proximity between basic and cancer-specific research had been demonstrated.

The COR had no quarrel with the principle of targeted research, but it objected to a pattern of sponsorship that supported it at the expense of basic science. Having worked hard to establish the nonclinical sciences in the hospital, the committee was ill disposed to surrender them to what it believed to be an ill-formed conception of biomedical research. At the same time, certain accommodations to financial reality seemed in order. The COR assigned its subcommittees on policy and grants to develop safeguards against proposals written to please funding agencies but lacking reference to the MGH research context. The groups were requested to create policies "to assure compatibility between large targeted research grants and the long-term goals of the institution to achieve balance, representation of the scientific community, increased communication, flexibility, and a broad interpretation of relevance, including that which is inherent in very fundamental research."

At present one of the most intriguing and serious questions that the COR faces is the rapidly developing interface with industry, which is now providing exponentially accelerating funding for a number of MGH research laboratories. Perhaps the most dramatic example is the recent (1981) $50 million Hoechst contract for the support of the new Division of Molecular Genetics chaired by Howard Goodman as part of the new Department of Genetics at the Harvard Medical School. This free-standing division is the successor to the Department of Biochemistry at the MGH under the leadership of Lipmann and Kalckar. This recent and important development at the hospital has led to the establishment of an Office of Technology Administration as part of the Research Office of the COR. The new full-time group, which works in coordination with the Trustees' Patent Committee, has written guidelines for patents and consulting arrangements and reviews all patent proposals from the hospital staff. In addition, the new Trustees' Advisory Committee on Industrial Relations, including three trustees, six senior professional people, and several from the administration, has recently been created to design guidelines and broader principles to ensure that collaborations with industrial organizations, whose motivations are quite different from those of the hospital, function in an effective and harmonious manner which does not do damage to academic freedom, the free flow of information within the hospital, the scientific community at large, and the organization of the institution. The COR should have a major role in helping this important association to develop in a healthy manner.

The COR's anticipation and policy development enabled the MGH to sustain its commitment to basic research during the seventies. But the inclination toward targeted research seems likely to increase in the economic climate of the eighties. Even those individuals at MGH—some of them sitting on the COR—who believe that the state of the art is such that targeted research is about to pay off handsomely do not want to abandon the basic sciences. The COR's argument rings with intellectual integrity. The outstanding question is whether it will continue to be politically viable in an atmosphere of intense competition for economic resources.

With the assistance of *Jerome Gross*

Growth and Dependence on Outside Funding: A View from Medicine

ALEXANDER LEAF

The mid-fifties were the beginning of the expansionist era in American Medicine-Science Unlimited. The funding of medical research that commenced with the National Institutes of Health (NIH) legislation of 1948 was reaching the academic center. Earlier, Walter Bauer had staunchly opposed the development of the intramural program of the NIH: "Give the money to the universities; we know how to do research; don't start up non-university non-affiliated research to compete with us for our funding and young scientists!" Despite these concerns—shared by several leaders of American academic medicine—there proved to be sufficient federal support to nourish not only its own baby but all of academia as well.

This author remembers the first grant, submitted to NIH for support of Ward 4, our clinical investigative center, which had previously been supported through the generosity of Edward Mallinckrodt, Jr. and had already bred a generation of clinical investigators starting with Aub, Bauer, Ropes, Short, Albright, Burnett, Bartter, and Forbes, whose studies began the interest in calcium metabolism at the MGH. Dr. Bauer called me into his office and told me his friend, Ralph Knutti, director of extramural research of the National Institute of Arthritis and Metabolic Diseases, had invited an application for support of Ward 4 and the investigators using it. I was instructed to write up the grant application, and the budget we submitted makes my mouth water now in these stringent funding times. The "Professors' Fund" included $50,000 and salary support for six physician-scientists with $6,000 supplements for each individual. No justification for any budget item was required. This marked the start of dependence of the Medical Services on large federal support for its major activities. The grant continued until December 1, 1979, as a program project grant supporting Ward 4 and units on the Medical Services engaged in research relating to calcium metabolism. On that date support of Ward 4 shifted to a Clinical Research Center grant which required that other services besides Medicine utilize the facility. The original Ward 4 grant was followed shortly by another large grant for support of cardiopulmonary research which joined the chiefs of Medicine (Bauer) and Surgery (Churchill) as coprincipal investigators. Their eventual successors, myself and W. Gerald Austen, preserved joint supervision of this grant.

But the largesse of the NIH nurtured many more research activities beyond the support of Ward 4 and the cardiac studies. In 1979 the total support for all MGH research had grown to $27 million of which more than 90 percent was federal. This has allowed many worthwhile projects to flourish and the Medical Services to be a beehive of exciting intellectual activity which, in turn, has attracted a large and gifted staff. In 1980 the total number of M.D. and Ph.D. professionals in the department exceeded 500. The situation creates a substantial dependence on "soft monies."

During his last illness James Howard Means, former chief of Medicine but then a patient in the Phillips House, called me to his bedside. Not one to proffer unsolicited advice to me, he nevertheless admonished me not to accept any money for the MGH from the government; that would lead only to loss of independence and governmental regulation. "He who pays the piper calls the tune," he warned. But his advice was much too late for the Medical Services; the die had been cast years before I became chief, by Walter Bauer. Without government support of research we could never have established and sustained our present position of preeminence. Though increasingly the direction of our research may have been affected by the categorical sources of funds and the intent of the funding agencies, our investigators nevertheless have managed to preserve their own options through avoidance of research contracts and dependence on investigator-initiated research proposals and peer review which ranks scientific quality above bureaucratic goals.

It should be added that not only the government but even more so foundations are attempting to set research priorities. Notices of funding are circulated by foundations to solicit applications for the support of the causes championed by the organization. The support will generally cover a three- to five-year period of development, with foundation support decreasing or terminating once the program has become established. Institutional funds are then expected to sustain the worthy project, and the foundation's funds are free to nurture some other meritorious cause. To assist in the choice of programs and their implementation, many foundations seek advice from prominent scholars who are themselves part of the academic culture, and this has helped keep funds flowing in to worthy and possible projects. But this is not invariably the case.

The Scientific Advisory Committee

By contrast with the Committee on Research, which is an internal organ, the Scientific Advisory Committee (SAC) consists of eminent scientists drawn from institutions beyond the MGH and has always included one representative each from Harvard University (though not necessarily from the Medical School) and MIT.

Since 1947 Nobel Laureates galore (Pauling, Gasser, Cori, Ochoa, Huggins, Luria, Medawar, Krebs, Tatum, Lipmann, Florey, Kornberg, and Gilbert), university presidents (Lowell J. Reed from Johns Hopkins; Karl Compton, Howard Johnson, and Jerome Wiesner from MIT), and other luminaries have assembled once each year for two days to advise the trustees on the "qualities, balance and direction of the research activities at the hospital." The committee originally numbered six individuals who served three-year staggered terms; the membership expanded to seven in 1977, eight in 1978, and there it has remained, still small enough to constitute a comfortable working group. In 1979 Elizabeth D. Hay, chairman of the Department of Anatomy at the Harvard Medical School, became the first woman to sit on the committee and presumably not the last.

The SAC occupies a position vis à vis the MGH research program akin to that of a university visiting committee, one whose observations have been taken very seriously. By virtue of its varied and distinguished membership, the committee can provide readings of the ever-shifting terrain of medical research, citings of the MGH position in that topography, and directional signals. In 1965, for example, it urged development of a strong program in human genetics. The SAC also acts as a disinterested and expert critic. While normally complimentary of the hospital's research efforts, it has on occasion issued gentle warnings. After one meeting, referring to presentations it had heard concerning the sociologic aspects of illness, the SAC remarked that the "methodologies brought to bear on the problems seemed to be feeble and the conclusions attempted were not novel," an evaluation that admonished against casual injections of the social sciences into biomedical research at an historic moment when "relevance" had become an issue.

Overall, the process of intellectual mapping helps the trustees and staff determine research priorities. In addition to its policy functions, David Crockett— the hospital's professional pragmatist—has seen the SAC as an ally in his fund-raising efforts. As he put it, "I always thought it a splendid idea that someone outside the hospital would be tooting the Mass General horn. It's not enough for *us* to go around saying how great we are!"

SAC meetings have customarily occurred in December when Boston's climate is often inhospitable. Though the committee has always confined its activities to two days, the agenda has become denser and more structured over the years, no doubt a reflection of the vastly expanded volume of research. The flavor of SAC meetings has varied, of course, with the personalities of its members, as has the quality of exchanges with trustees and staff.

Yet for all the human diversity, there has been a certain monotony to SAC deliberations. Two topics have monopolized the committee's attention for some 30-plus years: the role of basic science in medicine and the related question of tenure. The SAC responded to the MGH's need for advice about how to intro- duce and deploy basic science in the clinical environment in its very first report, in 1947, with the following recommendation:

The unique feature of a hospital is constant contact with patients and the stimulation afforded by their problems. Therefore, clinical investigation should always have the highest priority in the research work of a hospital. Yet there will often be research problems of a more fundamental character which are either stimulated by clinical investigation or are directed toward eventual clinical application. Such researches are not only important in themselves but will strengthen clinical investigation and medicine as a whole. Beyond this there are researches of a character so fundamental that they will be generally stimulating and illuminating to the entire staff even though not directly related to any specific disease at the present moment. Within limits the support of such research is highly desirable for the occasional man of truly outstanding ability and enthusiasm, even though it may be necessary to provide for him special laboratories of the type usually found in medical school departments of so-called "basic science."

This theme, subject to occasional variations in vocabulary, repeated itself again and again throughout the committee's history like a Wagnerian motif. And it gave rise to a natural, secondary set of considerations revolving around the ques- tion of tenure. For how, indeed, could the MGH hope to lure a person "of truly outstanding ability" away from some tenured or tenure-track position in aca- demia without extending the promise of equal job security? The hospital did not have tenured chairs; that privilege belonged to the Medical School which was ill-disposed to support a scientist down on Fruit Street rather than out on Long- wood Avenue. (And, as for untenured medical staff, private practice offered other avenues to financial security. Basic scientists had no such opportunities.)

The underlying issue, naturally, has been money. Government, foundations, and industry have proved willing to invest in medical research, and the hospital has been successful in attracting funds. Most of the money came in the form of short-term grants, while fund drives supported building projects to create re- search space. Meanwhile, endowed chairs being high-priced items, the tenure problem has never been resolved to the satisfaction of the SAC, which has con- sidered various schemes for bringing more basic scientists into the hospital fold.

The departure in 1956 of Fritz Lipmann (head of the Biomedical Research Laboratory, professor of biological chemistry at the Medical School and, most significantly, a 1953 Nobel prize winner) and the desire to replace him with a figure of commensurate ability dramatized the tenure quandry. Said the SAC: Tenure "is essential if capable young investigators are to be attracted and retained because the best of them can then look forward to receiving appropriate rec- ognition and security."

In 1959 Francis O. Schmitt, Institute Professor at MIT and a trustee of the MGH charged with advising on scientific matters, made the bold suggestion that the hospital form a pool of about 20 life-tenured positions, devise a ranking system for scientific personnel, and add several more units for basic biomedical research. He put a price tag of $5 million on the plan and suggested a novel approach to financing it: "What we used to call 'soft' money, i.e., government and foundation grants, is really 'hard' money today—it will continue in the foreseeable future—and what we used to call 'hard' money, i.e., endowment, is really 'soft' money now because of what seems to be permanent inflation." (That was written in 1959!) The SAC responded to Schmitt's plan more or less favorably—they were particularly captivated by his characterization of funds—while urging caution in the selection and composition of a scientific staff.

In 1974 there were eight tenured positions in research at the MGH, and the SAC advocated the creation of an additional five to ten tenure slots over a period of as many years. Moreover, the committee addressed the precarious status of the 146 researchers in temporary positions who, gazing into the future, could see little promise of achieving professional security at the hospital.

The SAC has considered a host of other items: Should the MGH be involved with classified research? No, said the committee; and the hospital was not. Should the MGH devote a special building to cancer? Probably not, opined the SAC; but the hospital raised the Cox Center. The committee discussed federal financing trends, the relationships between research and industry, and commented—usually favorably—upon various research initiatives at the hospital. Through it all, regardless of its membership, the SAC has persisted in pressing for a closer alignment between basic and clinical scientists, for a more lively dialogue between the two, and for a benign climate in which their joint efforts could flourish. The committee's reach has sometimes exceeded the hospital's grasp. Yet research now enjoys equal status with patient care and education at the MGH, the corps of basic scientists continues to increase, and there is a developing comprehension of the articulation between basic and clinical research.

The Committee on Research and the Individual

By the mid-1960s the advancing edge of medical research had moved into clinical areas of a particular delicacy. At the MGH new operating techniques were developing in neurosurgery, transplantation was an exciting enterprise, and there was interest in exploring the clinical applications of mind-altering drugs. (Remember, only a few years earlier, Harvard Professor Timothy Leary and his students had been experimenting with LSD over on Divinity Avenue in Cambridge!) The growing number of researchers involved with human subjects suggested the wisdom of articulating an ethical framework for such work at the hospital.

In his annual report for 1966 John Knowles observed that research engaging human subjects had traditionally been guided by a common set of assumptions. "Heretofore," he wrote, "the main safeguard for the rights of the patients or the subjects of human experimentation and research at the MGH has been the strongly felt and nurtured principle that the subject's personal interests come first, and that all our activities are always geared to his best interests. This basic principle has been as strong a guarantee of his rights and interests as any written set of rules could ever be."

Nevertheless, events exterior to the MGH—notably the civil rights movement—drew attention to the necessity for vigilance and, accordingly, for explicitness in matters bearing upon human rights. Furthermore, it had not escaped notice that Americans were becoming an increasingly litigious people, bringing all manner of complaints before the courts in the name of human rights. Together, the temper of the times and events along the frontiers of research prompted the trustees to create the Committee on Research and the Individual to advise on questions of human studies.

There have been multitudes of committees at the MGH during the past 25 years, and were one to account for all of them this volume would outweigh the average medical text. But this unique committee deserves notice because during its brief lifespan it performed the difficult task of designing an ethical superstructure for the conduct of human studies and its work became a model for similar groups throughout the country.

The trustees followed David Crockett's advice and appointed a committee which ensured that discussions would be well removed from hospital politics. Bishop Henry Knox Sherrill, a former chairman of the board and, therefore, a man familiar with the MGH as well as a figure of moral authority, agreed to act as chairman. Other committee members included Gordon Allport, professor of social ethics at Harvard; Mary Bunting, president of Radcliffe College; Paul Freund, and William Curran. Francis Schmitt of MIT, who counseled the trustees on scientific matters, represented the board; Ralph Meader, deputy director for research administration, and Henry Beecher, chief of Anesthesia, spoke on behalf of the hospital's research interests. Beecher, incidentally, was the only medical doctor in the group. He had long reflected upon the moral dilemmas that arise in medicine. As chairman of the COR's Subcommittee on Human Studies, he served this committee in an ex officio capacity. This particular mix of respected individuals gave the committee credibility with the public and, more importantly, influence within the hospital.

The committee based its deliberations on a draft written by Beecher; a final document entitled "Some Guiding Principles for Human Studies" was submitted to the trustees in January 1967 and accepted by them in March. Save for minor alterations of language which do not affect the substance, the document stands as the constitution for research involving human subjects. Recognizing the futility of anticipating all contingencies, the committee refrained from specifying research modes; rather, it addressed itself to the ethical responsibilities of investigators to their subjects: the obligations to inform subjects in understandable terms and to obtain consent, the right of subjects to overrule investigators as to what factors are or are not relevant to consent, the submission of difficult ethical questions to peers for advice, and the need to guard against coercion. The committee further recommended procedures for internal review of all proposals involving human subjects.

Ultimately, all guidelines rest on a single philosophical base expressed in simple, unambiguous language: "A study is ethical or not at its inception; it does not become ethical because it succeeds in producing valuable data. Ends do not justify means."

7. Physical Development

The architectural aspect of a hospital does not necessarily reflect the quality of medicine practiced therein. People do not choose to work or be treated in hospitals on aesthetic grounds. It has also been observed that hospitalized patients apply different criteria to their surroundings than do healthy people.

Bearing these caveats in mind, the time has come to face an essential truth: Massachusetts General Hospital is never going to win any architectural beauty contest. Its most handsome building, Bulfinch, is presently overwhelmed by neighboring structures, like some rare specimen plant in an overgrown garden. Buildings of different vintages representing various architectural intentions join for reasons of circulation and function but ignore one another's form, scale, and building materials. Nevertheless, the dense compound of mismatched buildings holds a peculiar fascination for the architecturally-minded historian—or the historically-minded architect. Salient developments in the life of the hospital can be read in its existing structures: Bulfinch, the original hospital, built in 1821; the old outpatient department (1903); Phillips House (1917); Baker Memorial (1930); the White Building (1939); Vincent-Burnham (1947); the Edwards Building (1950); and so on into the present era. Each of these buildings represents, in one fashion or another, the most advanced concepts of medical care and hospital architecture of its time.

A careful study of MGH construction history would reveal the forces that have shaped its physical form. Urgent demands for patient care and research facilities, budgetary and property constraints, government regulations, building codes, and functional necessities have all carried formal implications. On the architectural front building technologies have evolved while theories of hospital planning and design have been subject to transformations.

Before itemizing the building developments since 1955, a brief review of the overall strategy for physical growth of the hospital is instructive. Over the years long-range planning efforts were treated with varying degrees of interest. Finally, in 1948, planning became a formal piece of the MGH with the organization of the MGH Planning Office. Ten years later the planning division was separated from maintenance and became a Planning and Construction Office with Carleton N. Goff as resident architect and department head. His office was prepared to provide full architectural services for as much of the construction program as was possible with limited space, operating budget, and personnel, and was available to make feasibility and preliminary studies of the use of space, establish program budgets, assist in the selection of outside architects and, in all situations, act as a service department. Today the Planning Office, under the leadership of Burgess P. Standley, is deeply involved with the external authorities of certificate-of-need legislation, community planners, changing zoning regulations, and social legislation and pressures, as forecast by John Knowles in his 1969 report on "Progress and Planning at MGH." Planning is now appropriately recognized as a necessary part of any long-term decision making.

There has been more construction activity at the hospital over the past quarter century than during any comparable period in its history. The building facilities on the main campus have grown from 1,210,969 gross square feet to 2,519,898—more than double in area. Within the same time frame, however, the increase in property holdings has been relatively trivial. The demands upon the land, therefore, have been tremendous. The growth of the hospital has of necessity been skyward and at the expense of two landscaped quadrangles, one of them the formerly gracious Bulfinch courtyard. When the West End redevelopment project was being planned, the hospital briefly entertained hopes of acquiring land in that area to relieve some of the pressure. The hope never materialized, though it was of some consolation that physicians were permitted to rent office space on the ground floors of the apartment towers.

Along with the more obvious needs for space presented by greater numbers of patients and staff, modern medical technology (much of which cannot be plugged at random into old building systems), expanded research programs—in short, all those things that keep the MGH in the forefront of health care—hospital planners have had to contend with that ornery creature, the automobile. Parking became a major nuisance during the fifties and sixties; two garages on either side of North Grove Street were built in 1972 in an effort to alleviate the situation. Even so, there are only 1,300 parking spaces at MGH to serve more than 8,000 employees along with thousands of patients and visitors each day.

All new construction has taken place within the perimeters of Charles, Cambridge, and Blossom streets. The logistics have been complicated because, as comparison of the 1956 and 1980 plot plans demonstrates, old structures have constantly been demolished to make way for new. The old Domestic and Pathology buildings fell before the Gray-Jackson-Bigelow complex, Thayer and the Morgue before the Cox Center, Moseley and Walcott in the path of the Ambulatory Care Center. In every instance space had to be found for dislocated services pending completion of new quarters. Hence the appearance in 1965, when Gray-Jackson-Bigelow was getting started, of "temporary" buildings 1 and 2, which sprouted suddenly in the landscape like mushrooms after a spring rain and have been stubbornly persistent.

Faxon's history accounted for the Warren Building which went into construction in 1954 and was dedicated in 1956. Significant new buildings erected since then are listed below; more detailed references to these projects may be found in other chapters.

Pierce Cardiopulmonary Laboratories (1964). Occupying 9,078 square feet between Bulfinch and the Research Building, this structure includes a cyclotron. A large access panel in the roof was made to permit delivery and installation of the cyclotron, which took place about eight months after completion of construction. The panel is four feet thick, of solid concrete, and can be removed by crane; it must remain accessible to permit removal of the cyclotron from its vault.

Gray Building, Jackson and Bigelow Towers (1968). The biggest building project ever undertaken by the MGH, this $22 million complex added more than half a million square feet to the hospital. It provided desperately needed research and clinical laboratory space, a diagnostic radiology center, 21 modern operating rooms, and postsurgical critical care units. The construction program spanned several years and ended, finally, with the relocation of the medical wards, which had occupied the Bulfinch since 1821, to floors 6 through 11 of the Bigelow Tower.

The aforementioned *garages* (1972).

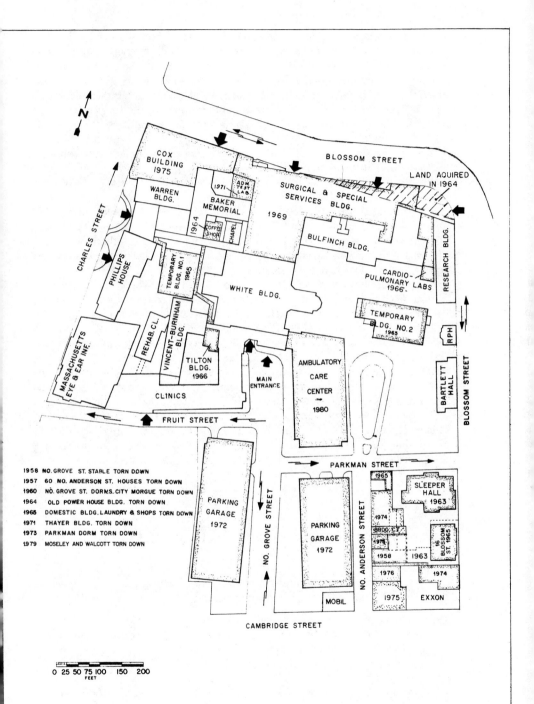

Plot plan for Massachusetts General Hospital, 1980.

The *Cox Cancer Management Center* (1974). The trustees authorized planning for a structure to house radiation therapy in 1964, and the plans matured into an ambulatory care center for cancer patients as well as clinical and research facilities. A generous capital gift to the building fund from Mrs. William C. Cox in 1970 added impetus to the project. The $22 million Cox Center was dedicated in 1975. The 111,000 square foot building houses medical and surgical oncology units, radiation medicine, and clinical and research laboratories; there are no beds in the building.

Ambulatory Care Center (1981). A nine-level brick and glass structure comprising 283,000 square feet and providing space for private doctors' offices, this long-needed facility sits on land formerly occupied by the Moseley and Walcott buildings.

In addition to raising new buildings, the MGH in 1965 acquired and recycled the old Winchell School for use by the School of Nursing (Sleeper Hall); and 16 Blossom Street, the West End House, wherein, among other things, the Planning Office is now located. There has also been uninterrupted remodeling activity within older hospital buildings.

Viewing the physical development of the MGH as a whole during the past 25 years, one cannot fail to note that research has enjoyed the greatest expansion, territorial growth consonant with its increasing share of the budget and the availability of outside funding. The second order of building activity occurred to accommodate modern technology—new operating rooms, clinical laboratories, radiation medicine, medical wards, and so forth. After much delay, outpatients were finally provided with new facilities. Conspicuously absent from this list are new accommodations for inpatients. Of the approximately 200 beds added to the hospital's capacity since 1955, 112 are in the Bigelow Tower and 24 in the Gray Building. Remodeling of the 12th floor of Baker-Warren and of Phillips House accounts for the remainder. Since Baker and White, which hold 635 of the total of 1,091 beds, date back to the 1930s, it is no wonder that new inpatient facilities have now floated to the top of the list of priorities.

> With the assistance of *Carleton N. Goff,*
> Resident Architect

Year-by-year Development of Hospital Facilities

1955   Operating Room No. 1 in White Building rebuilt to provide a
     complete shield against electromagnetic interference.
    White Building kitchen and cafeterias altered.

1956   New Cobalt machine installed on White 2.
    Second floor link between White, Baker, and Phillips House built over
     existing 1st floor corridor.
    New classroom for School of Nursing added in basement of Walcott
     House.
    Properties at numbers 20, 22, 24, 26, 28, and 30 North Anderson
     Street purchased and demolished. Doctors' parking lot off Parkman
     Street enlarged.
    Dedication of Warren Building.

1957 Open porches on south end of Baker enclosed on floors 4–10 for addition of 32 beds.
New laboratory facilities completed on 4th floor of Bulfinch for research in gastroenterology, endocrinology, and diabetes.

1958 Emergency power generators installed in Baker, Bulfinch, White, and Phillips House.

1959 Floors 3, 3A, and 4 added on northwest wing of White Building, together with 3rd floor connecting corridor between White elevator lobby and 3rd floor addition.
Open porches on south end of Phillips House removed and new rooms constructed on floors 2–8 to add 28 beds.
Northern Mortuary on North Grove Street purchased from city.

1960 Northern Mortuary and Nurses' Dormitory on North Grove Street torn down.
New Psychiatry Research Laboratory opened on Warren 6.

1961 Respiratory Intensive Care Unit completed on 2nd floor of Phillips House.
New Thyroid Laboratory completed in basement of Bulfinch.
Completion of 8th and 9th floors of Vincent-Burnham, dedicated as memorial to Joseph P. Kennedy, Jr.

1962 Ward B-3 in Bulfinch altered to provide a prototype Medical Intensive Care Unit.

1963 Emergency x-ray suite completed on White 1st floor.
Coffee shop completed on 1st floor near Chapel.
Completion of x-ray suites on 1st and 2nd floors of Baker.
Old Winchell School purchased from city.
Alterations started on all floors of Edwards Building. Construction completed in 1969. Laboratories for cardiovascular research, anesthesia, dermatology, pediatrics, psychiatry, neurology, physics, and animal physiology involved.

1964 Construction of Cardiopulmonary Laboratory: Pierce Building.
New Pediatrics Clinic completed on 3rd floor of Connecting Building.
Additional land acquired from city at northeast corner of site.

1965 Baker-Warren 12 completed with addition of 41 beds for postsurgical patient care.
Construction of Temporary Buildings.
Demolition of Domestic Building and Pathology Building.
Renovation of Winchell School to provide facilities for School of Nursing. (Renamed Sleeper Hall.)
Alteration of Rehabilitation Building for Occupational and Physical Therapy.
White 12 altered to provide improved dialysis facilities and new kidney transplant unit.
West End House (16 Blossom Street) purchased.
Completion of Neurosurgical Intensive Care Unit on White 11.

1966   Coronary Intensive Care Unit completed on 2nd floor of Phillips House.
      Tilton Building constructed.
      Construction started on Surgical and Special Services Building. (Gray Building, Jackson and Bigelow Towers.)

1967   New laboratory for myocardial infarction completed on Phillips House 1st and 2nd floors.
      Construction of tunnel under Blossom Street to Shriners Burns Institute.

1968   Occupancy begun on lower floors of Gray Building late in year.

1969   New General Store completed on 1st floor of Gray Building.
      Research Laboratories in Jackson Tower completed.
      Installation of new air conditioning for main kitchen and cafeterias in White Building started; completed 1971.

1970   Radiology service expanded into 2nd floor of Gray Building.
      New food stores and dietary administrative offices completed in basement of Gray Building.
      New Blood Gas Laboratory completed on 3A floor of Gray Building.
      New x-ray film storage in Gray sub-basement.
      New 14 bed recovery room, Gray 3A.
      New accounting and admitting areas, Gray 1st floor.
      Prototype Infant Intensive Care Unit, Burnham 6.

1971   New Admitting Test Laboratory, Gray 1st floor.
      Construction of two garages off North Grove Street started; completed 1972.
      Construction of new conference room for Radiology Department above Coffee Shop.
      Thayer Building and Morgue torn down to make way for Cox Building.

1972   Parkman Street dormitories torn down.
      Extensive remodeling and enlargement of Emergency Ward.

1973   Computer Science Laboratory completed on 13th floor of Gray.
      East wing of 3rd floor of White altered to provide two cystoscopy rooms.

1974   Purchase of additional lots in Blossom-North Anderson Street block; turned over to Cambridge Street Community Development Corporation for developmental planning.
      Construction begun to complete Gray floors 6–11, and White 8 and 10 for relocation of medical wards. Budget of $20,241,000 approved by trustees.

1975   Cox Building dedicated.
      Completed acquisition of land bordered by Cambridge, North Anderson, Parkman, and Blossom streets with the exception of #31 North Anderson and the Exxon station at the corner of Blossom and Cambridge Streets. Sites turned over to Cambridge Street Community Development Corporation for developmental planning.

1976   Bigelow 6 through 11 completed in May and occupied by patients from White 8 and 10 to permit full renovation of those floors.

1977   Completed Bigelow floors 6 through 11 occupied by the Medical,
            Urology, and Neurology services during summer months.
1978   Orthopedic Clinic completely renovated.
            New operating rooms in Gray 3, east wing, opened in spring.
1979   Alterations of Warren basement, 1st, 2nd, and 3rd floors completed for
            Pathology Department.
            Demolition of Walcott and Moseley buildings completed in December.
1980   Groundbreaking ceremony for Ambulatory Care Center, January 4,
            1980. Building closed in by end of year.
            Excavation for new tunnel in front of Bulfinch started in June.
            Installation of new CAT scanner in Cox basement completed in
            October.
            Renovations in Orthopedic Shop, Gray 1, completed in June.

8. David C. Crockett

BENJAMIN CASTLEMAN AND S. B. SUTTON

The story of the expansion of research and of the hospital's physical development since World War II cannot be told adequately without accounting for the activities of David Charless Crockett, a man whose skills and resourcefulness played a critical role in that growth. The MGH literature to date, however, offers but scant evidence of his presence. For instance, there were only six items listed under his name in Faxon's history; three of those entries referred to the same event: "Mr. David C. Crockett was appointed (beginning May 1, 1946) as Administrative Assistant to the Trustees, his duties to be the raising of funds for research and other activities of the Hospital. His success in this field, as evidenced by the Edwards Building, the Warren Building, the phenomenal support of research, and the growth of endowment funds, has amply demonstrated the wisdom of this move." Faxon also listed Crockett's appointment in 1951 as associate director for resources and development, his membership on the Committee on Research, and his participation in the planning of the fiftieth anniversary celebration of the Social Services Department.

Similarly, Crockett's name seldom turned up in MGH annual reports. Major gifts and grants were acknowledged, but Crockett's role in acquiring many of them for the hospital was not disclosed. Because he carried out his mission of promoting MGH interests behind the scenes, Crockett viewed this lack of personal recognition as entirely appropriate. Throughout his career he maintained the position that the institution's ability to attract financial support rested upon its excellence. "Backing me was an illustrious hospital with a devoted staff," he has said. "Someone simply had to mobilize them." In fact, so accustomed is Crockett to stepping outside the limelight that the other two editors of the current volume had to argue vigorously in favor of a chapter about him; it seems to them that a man who had helped raise approximately $300 million for the MGH was surely an integral part of its history.

Crockett's association with the hospital began in the winter of 1946. He was then just out of the armed services, recently married, and living on the family homestead in Ipswich. He was out of work and, as he remembered, "I was really hard put and had to hustle quickly to find a job. I was still in uniform. Actually, I couldn't afford to buy a new suit of clothes. My old suits looked a little tired and battered from attrition—moths had enjoyed them during my absence in the war." He was walking down Hereford Street in the Back Bay when he ran into Ralph Lowell rushing in the opposite direction. "I've been looking for you everywhere," Lowell said. "I have a job for you. Please get in touch with me right away. I'm now president of the Boston Safe Deposit and Trust Company. Come and see me in my office tomorrow morning." Without further elaboration, Lowell hurried off.

Crockett, of course, appeared on the designated premises as ordered. "Well, I have a job for you, Crockett," Lowell announced. "It's only good for about six months, but it will get you started. The Massachusetts General Hospital, of which I am now a Trustee, is planning, in October 1946, to celebrate the 100th anniversary of the first use of ether, and we need somebody to coordinate a national event that would focus on the MGH. I thought of you as somebody who might do this, but I didn't know where to find you and wasn't sure whether you were back from the war." Lowell had good reason to believe Crockett the right man for the task, for Crockett had already demonstrated considerable talents for both organization and fund raising.

Born in Ipswich in 1909, Crockett was raised there and in the Back Bay. He attended Milton Academy and graduated from Harvard College in 1932. His father, Eugene A. Crockett, a physician and one-time chief of staff at the Massachusetts Eye and Ear Infirmary, died that same year, leaving the family "without two nickels to rub together" during the Depression. Young Crockett found a lackluster job as a clerk with First National Stores and so quickly demonstrated his flair for organizing services and pleasing a select clientele that he was soon rising through the store ranks. Meanwhile he got his first taste of fund raising by collecting for the Emergency Relief Fund, parent organization of the United Way. He went from door to door on Beacon Street, soliciting the lady of the house in the upstairs parlor over a cup of tea—or a drink if he was lucky (Prohibition was in force)—and then went downstairs to ask for contributions from the cook and the maids.

Crockett enjoyed this work enormously. Years later, in an interview with *Boston Magazine,* he observed that "asking for money can be very good fun if you like people. If you listen to them say their piece. They don't want to listen to you. They have the money, you're trying to get it, and they like to have a little fun. They don't want to just sign a card or answer a mail appeal. There's nothing duller than that." It was that innate liking for, and understanding of, his fellow man—what William Sweet characterizes elsewhere in this book as "the combination peculiar to Crockett of tact, common sense, industry, and the necessary knowledge of people"—that underlay Crockett's staggering successes as a fund raiser.

The years between canvassing the Back Bay for the Emergency Relief Fund and the fortuitous encounter with Lowell found Crockett involved with the Red Feather appeal and raising money for symphony concerts on the Esplanade and "similar ventures of minor nature in the community." He was president of the Boston Society of Early Instruments and raised funds for their concerts. In 1939 he left First National Stores to work as the New England advertising representative of *Good Housekeeping Magazine,* a position which put him in touch with the business community; later he became Executive Secretary for a "world university" shortwave radio station, WRUL, which was to become the Voice of America. During the early 1940s Crockett led the bold campaign that launched the Friends of the Boston Symphony Orchestra and raised enough money for the Symphony to meet a serious deficit that had threatened suspension of the concert season. In short, he had a record of accomplishment that had not escaped the attention of people like Ralph Lowell. Crockett also had an adventuresome career with the OSS during the War and was experienced in accomplishing important secret missions without publicity.

The Ether Centenary, as Faxon wrote, was a grand success. When it was over, however, the terms of Crockett's initial agreement had expired and his status with MGH was unclear. He therefore asked for a meeting of the trustees' committee—consisting of Lowell, Phillips Ketchum, and Henry Guild—which had employed him. "We met in Mr. Lowell's office at the Boston Safe Deposit and Trust Company. Mr. Ketchum got rather excited and inquired what the problem was: What was the trouble? Was I unhappy? Didn't I like my job? Did I want a contract? I said I just wanted some assurance that I was employed by the hospital. After a great deal of shuffling about, Mr. Ketchum professed to be frightfully busy and rather annoyed that he had been called to this meeting. I was informed that if I was content, they were happy, and I could go along as I wanted to, but it wasn't a very specific arrangement."

The vagueness arose largely because the MGH had never before employed a full-time fund raiser or development officer—nor, for that matter, had any other Boston hospital, or even Harvard. That institutional position, which is by now a necessary feature of any sizeable teaching hospital or university, simply did not exist. Thus the MGH trustees demonstrated unusual foresight in keeping Crockett on the payroll even if they could not spell out his responsibilities. On his side, Crockett, now without the specific assignment of the Ether Centenary, applied his common sense and imagination to making himself useful to the MGH. He identified the potential and needs involved in developing basic research activities within the hospital and put his services at the disposal of those staff members, such as Walter Bauer, who were looking for ways to finance research efforts. Crockett pleaded the MGH case in Washington and before executives of pharmaceutical companies and encouraged voluntary health agencies such as the American Cancer Society and the Arthritis Foundation (of which he and Bauer were founders) to raise their own funds for research from which the MGH could draw on a competitive basis with other institutions.

Simultaneously, Crockett initiated aggressive direct mail and advertising campaigns to offset the hospital's deficit. "Mr. Lowell didn't think we would raise any money through direct mail," Crockett recalled with amusement. "One of our first returns was a check for $50,000 in a simple return envelope with no comment, from the Nathaniel and Elizabeth T. Stevens Foundation, the beginning of a long succession of gifts from that foundation. I remember Mr. Lowell's amazement when I showed him this check, without comment, from this fund which nobody had ever heard of." As one after another of Crockett's labors bore fruit, as the world of research sponsorship became more intricate, and as more capital was required to support building and other programs, the resources and development officer became a key figure in the functioning of the hospital.

Crockett summarized his first decade with the MGH as follows:

Since the war I have been holding down a fascinating but initially rather ill-defined job at the Massachusetts General Hospital. Now it is clear that my principal responsibility is to locate the wherewithal to supplement the income of the hospital from its endowment so that new ventures in research and teaching can be undertaken. The financial magnitude of these new projects has grown over the years so that the search for resources has kept me scurrying over the country exploring new charitable foundations and stimulating the activity of the voluntary health agencies and prodding various federal agencies to make more money available for research. In 1946 there was available for research projects underway at the hospital just over half a million dollars. In 1957 there [was] in the hospital's treasury two and a half million for specific research projects and broad research program support. Two new research buildings have been built as well as two other hospital buildings at a cost of over eight million dollars, in the last ten years. For these, new capital has been raised by the Trustees, and in this I have been quite active, too.

All this, however, has been possible because of the institution itself, that is: the Trustees, doctors, nurses and administrative personnel, past and present. Their collective enterprise and effort for nearly one hundred and fifty years have made the name, Massachusetts General Hospital, synonymous with good medical care.

Early in 1951 Dean Clark gave a speech entitled "MGH Pins Its Faith on 1961" in which he listed the hospital's needs over the next decade: an ambulatory care center, a radiation therapy building, a new facility with operating room suites, new quarters for diagnostic radiology, and facilities for the McLean Hospital. Crockett picked up this theme and used it extensively in preparation for the next major event, celebration of the 150th anniversary of the incorporation of the hospital. Though the MGH had opened its doors in 1821 and the centennial had been celebrated in 1921, both Crockett and Francis C. Gray, then chairman of the trustees, considered it important to capitalize on the earlier date, 1811, because, as Crockett explained, "there were rumblings at the Harvard Medical School that they were planning a major capital drive for all the hospitals in the Longwood Avenue area, and ours might have to be postponed if we didn't initiate activity in time."

The process of defining priorities within the context of the anniversary campaign was a coordinated program that extended throughout the MGH, stirred the staff, and involved them in active planning. Among the projects completed as a result of the drive were new research laboratories and clinical offices for the Orthopedic Service, the Joseph P. Kennedy, Jr. Laboratories for Pediatric Neurology and for the Study of Mental Retardation, the Bulfinch 3 Intensive Care Unit, the School of Nursing residence at 20 Charles Street, the Surgical Recovery Room, the James Howard Means Metabolic Research Laboratories, and adaptation of the Harvard cyclotron for neurosurgical procedures. Crockett orchestrated the development initiative and prepared much of the necessary groundwork by identifying sources of funding and matching departmental needs with appropriate sponsors.

Meanwhile, Crockett oversaw the preparations for the actual anniversary celebrations which were held during the last week of January 1961. The festivities began with panache because President Kennedy, who had just been inaugurated—and was a former member of the MGH Corporation—opened the ceremonies with an address from the White House, which was broadcast on the "Today Show." The scientific symposia got off to a poor start because a public transportation strike delayed the arrival of many people, but that proved to be the single snag in the entire event. "We pulled every trick in the book, I suppose," Crockett mused. "We gave honorary medals and certificates and had an alumni meeting; we had scientific sessions going all day, all over the hospital. We attracted people from all over the world. We also stirred up a large new component of interest in the community. People who had never been particularly active in either the fund raising or volunteer activities of the hospital were brought into the fold. The event drew attention to the MGH all over the country. Several scientific papers presented during the progam were reprinted in the *Lancet* and the *British Medical Journal* as well as in the *New England Journal of Medicine*."

The appointment of John Knowles as general director in 1962 brought a change in emphasis to the MGH. Whereas Clark had concentrated his fundraising effort on a new ambulatory care facility, Knowles was interested in a building to house new surgical areas, operating rooms, research laboratories, diagnostic radiology—in short, the facility that would be the Jackson-Bigelow-Gray complex. Accordingly, Crockett turned his attention to this project. He started by hiring American Mail Advertising to extend the drive by direct mail and build upon the good will that had been generated during the anniversary program. Crockett admits to "every known advertising gimmick and publicity trick we could pull, including putting Dr. Knowles on a number of radio and television programs—which he enjoyed enormously. We then started a very active massive campaign by direct mail to communities; the whole system was being handled by computers at the American Mail Advertising offices in Waltham. The courage and foresight of Mr. Gray, Mr. Bigelow, and Dr. Knowles, and the encouragement that they gave me in this plan benefitted the hospital enormously. This campaign developed a succession of annual gifts which continues to this day. But more than that, it paved the way for an active bequest program which I developed at the end of the period."

The magnitude of the effort is suggested first by the ultimate cost of the complex ($22 million) and even more so by the fact that it was constructed with funds provided by individual donations both small and large, family trusts, bequests, private foundations, and the National Institutes of Health. It was the single largest building project during Crockett's MGH career. Yet the facility had not been completed when the trustees authorized plans for a new radiation medicine accommodation under the direction of Howard Ulfelder, whose contributions, Crockett insists, "should never be underestimated in developing a plan and helping to raise the money." This was to be the Cox Cancer Center, and once again Crockett was busy behind the scenes. He also played an important role in the negotiations that brought the Shriners Burns Institute to the MGH, although he believes that Oliver Cope tends to give him too much credit for that accomplishment—credit that he emphasizes rests more properly with Cope himself.

Altogether, there were very few major research, building, or renovation projects at the MGH—not to mention the endowment—during this period in which David Crockett did not have a hand. Sometimes he acted as a guide, drawing on his vast experience of granting agencies to direct a proposal to a likely financial source; sometimes he was a social organizer, pairing potential donors with staff and trustees in an appropriate setting; sometimes he solicited in the offices of foundations or the National Institutes of Health or in a private house. Whatever the role, he played it with elegance and humor.

Crockett officially retired in 1973 so quietly that hardly anyone noticed. Aside from the likelihood that fanfare would have embarrassed him, the MGH really had no intention of losing him. He continues his appointment as deputy to the general director and works informally on behalf of the MGH and those it serves much to the gratification and benefit of all.

9. News and Public Affairs Office

MARTIN S. BANDER

To a degree hospital public relations both influences and reflects the growing maturity of medical writing. As late as the 1950s newspaper medical writing consisted of a city editor assigning a reporter "to find out about the cure for cancer" developed at a local hospital. That reporter might have just finished writing about a bullet-riddled body found in the Charles River. Ignorant of hospitals and medical terminology, he would typically alienate the doctor two questions into the interview, and the resulting news article would confirm the researcher's worst fears.

Even in those days there were exceptions. Pioneers like the Boston *Globe's* Frances Burns helped turn medical writing into an honorable specialty. By the late fifties many of the major dailies were employing full-time medical writers. Hospitals were starting to hire public relations practitioners who understood the problems of hospitals, doctors, and the news media. The better practitioners were able to walk the tightrope between facilitating the reporters' task and getting the hospital story to the public without compromising the patient or the physicians. Physicians who felt an obligation to help educate the public eased the public relations work. No one contributed more than the MGH's Paul Dudley White. In 1955, when President Eisenhower suffered his first heart attack, White bridged the information gap, turning every detail of the president's convalescence into an event of medical significance.

By the time (May 1962) an MGH chief surgical resident named Ronald A. Malt led a team in replanting a 12-year-old's arm, medicine was no stranger to the front page. That particular story exploded over the world news media. One of the participants in the news conference announcing the accomplishment was John Knowles, the new general director, who was to use the news media effectively throughout his career. As noted in Chapter 3, communication was an essential element in Knowles' theory of administration. Accordingly, in 1968 he convinced this author to foresake medical writing at the Boston *Herald-Traveler* to become the writer-in-residence at the MGH. Gradually I was to encumber all the hospital's public relations functions.

The News Office opened on March 25, 1968. It started as a two-person office, including Doris Schreckengaust, formerly of the *Herald-Traveler's* Science Bureau, and was charged with responsibilities to supervise the archives and to reformulate the external newspaper, the *MGH News*. Though the *News* had appeared episodically in the past, Knowles wanted it to be a regular publication. In 1980 it had approximately 25,000 readers including legislators, donors, libraries, staff (it is sent to homes so families can read it as well as professionals), and newspapers for which it serves as a press release. The *MGH News* is designed so that the lead story is usually a news item which, though it may have appeared in medical journals, has not yet been picked up by the press.

In December 1969 the News Office also began to publish the employee news-paper, the *Hot Line,* as the successor to the *World of the MGH* which Personnel had ceased publishing. The *Hot Line* serves 8,000 employees, inpatients, and other members of the MGH community. In July 1971 we assumed publication of the annual report and brochures. Three years later Dr. Sanders asked us to carry out all press contacts involving the Emergency Ward, a task which Mrs. Marjorie Reardon had performed ably for many years; Mrs. Schreckengaust assumed those duties. The News Office grew slowly until it had five full-time employees, still the smallest number in a major Boston teaching hospital.

Just as the fifties saw the emergence of medical writing as an important force, the seventies became the era of journalistic activism. The movement embraced medical writing with as much fervor as it did the State House and Capitol press rooms. Advances in research and triumphs in patient care took second place to high cost, medical fraud, and sundry medicosocial issues. Medical writers often injected opinion into their articles or fashioned them to favor their own view-points. Doctors and administrators bristled under intense scrutiny and what often seemed to be unfair articles. Thus the News Office had to intensify its efforts to see that the public received a balanced, accurate view of events within the MGH.

From its beginnings the News Office maintained a policy of actively seeking subjects to publicize. Increasingly, television became a vehicle to carry news about the hospital. But the office simultaneously promoted additional news and feature articles in newspapers and magazines and on radio stations. The overall result has been a substantive increase in the hospital's local and national exposure. A concerted effort has been directed toward presenting the MGH as a caring institution, an aspect often hidden behind the monumental facade of technology. In carrying out those missions of publicity, the support of the entire hospital community has been enlisted. As a result, large elements of the hospital not only provide leads but also involve this office when the news media telephone. The positive attitude that often follows such contacts helps combat the negativism that permeates the public view of health care. Even investigatory reporting or anti-MGH demonstrations are often blunted or sometimes turned into positive events by immediately confronting the complainers with facts.

All these thrusts have been advanced with one eye fixed on good taste, sensibilities, and patient confidentiality; the constant sensitivity to these needs has limited unintentional lapses both in degree and number. Frequently the News Office protects patients from news media interviews that would result in significant positive publicity for the institution.

One fallout from the consumer movement has been the increased emphasis on both public and patient education. The News Office tried to anticipate this trend first through the *MGH News,* then through brochures used by individual departments and through the news media. All these endeavors have involved the News Office in a variety of ways with other administrative, professional, and nonprofessional divisions of the hospital. Thus the office has become woven into the fabric of the institution.

While activism was a force outside, the News Office was evolving in different ways intramurally. Initially it served as a conveyor belt to carry news from the office to the general public. Knowles began the practice of placing the news office director on key committees; Sanders continued and accelerated this practice and began to hold regular meetings with me. These encounters provided a forum to discuss likely public reactions to envisioned actions and to explore hospital problems. Instead of having to convey negative news to an inquiring press, the News Office could on occasion prevent the event from occurring in the first place. This "activism" on the part of the News Office coincided with a national trend for public relations participation in the operation of a hospital.

In a sense, a well-coordinated public relations office has always performed rudimentary marketing functions, if only by making the public aware of the existence of a therapy or a clinic that had eluded its attention. Recently, two new MGH clinics went from a pre-publicity dearth of patients to heavy patient loads on the heels of an *MGH News* article or press release. Now the trend is clear to place such seat-of-the-pants marketing on a more scientific basis. In the eighties competition will drive hospitals to develop formal marketing programs that incorporate modern statistical methods to provide a data base for considered, step-by-step planning. Whether these programs remain within a given public relations office or not, it is clear that marketing and public relations functions will have to integrate closely.

Part II. Medical Services

During the years under review here, direction of the Medical Services fell to two chiefs, Walter Bauer, from 1951 to 1963, and Alexander Leaf, from 1965 to 1981. Between them, Robert Ebert occupied the position briefly before vacating it to become dean of the Harvard Medical School, and Alfred Kranes twice held the fort as acting chief. Essentially Bauer and Leaf presided, but the spirit of Bauer's predecessor, James Howard Means, extended well beyond his tenure.

10. James Howard Means

JOHN B. STANBURY AND EARLE M. CHAPMAN

James Howard Means succeeded David Edsall as the Jackson Professor of Medicine in 1923. His retirement in 1951 technically excludes him from this volume of the ongoing history of the hospital, but his contributions were of such magnitude as to require an appraisal in these pages. He was born in Dorchester in 1885, reared in the Back Bay, lived his mature years on Beacon Hill, and enjoyed his chosen exercise of walking to and from the scene of his life's work at the Massachusetts General Hospital and the Harvard Medical School. He was a true Bostonian: true in his heritage, his strength of purpose, his perceptive sense of social justice, his love of travel, and his appreciation of the need for freedom in education.

He was raised in an atmosphere of inquiry. He recalled that "my first great intellectual stimulus came not from school but from my father." He attended Noble and Greenough School, and at the age of 17, stimulated toward a career in science by his father, spent a year under the great biologist William T. Sedgwick at the Massachusetts Institute of Technology. He then attended Harvard College where he balanced the sciences with elective courses in philosophy and graduated cum laude in 1907. Four years later he received his medical degree at Harvard and was elected to Alpha Omega Alpha, the medical honor society. It was this background that gave him the firm belief that the education of physicians should include both the humanities and sciences integrated into secondary schooling, college, and medical school. Of the teachers who inspired him in his preclinical years, Means put at the top L. J. Henderson, whom he had already encountered in college; Walter B. Cannon, professor of physiology; and Otto Folin, professor of biochemistry, whom he perceived as the prophet of metabolism. He wrote of his personal philosophy in "Experiences and Opinions of a Full Time Medical Teacher," published in *Perspectives* (winter 1959).

Graduate education for Howard, as he was known to many people, began as a house pupil at the MGH (1911–1913), a 16-month straight medical internship. Halfway through this appointment, David Linn Edsall arrived to become a salaried professor of medicine at Harvard and chief of one of the two medical services at the MGH (there were East and West medical services at the hospital until 1921). Edsall began to build his full-time clinical staff by choosing some interns for exposure to research and sending them elsewhere upon graduation. Howard Means was one of those selected; he was given the Henry P. Walcott Fellowship. He first worked on calorimetry at the Carnegie Laboratory in Boston, and then studied blood flow with Krogh in Copenhagen and visited Barcroft in Cambridge, England.

Returning to Boston in 1913, Means resumed clinical investigation and the following spring attended a meeting of the "Young Turks" (American Society of Clinical Investigation) in Atlantic City. There he heard Eugene F. DuBois read a paper on basal metabolism. It was a pivotal event for him: He wrote in 1959, "This was right up my alley." Back in Boston he began metabolic studies in a small room under the present outpatient amphitheater using a Benedict respiration machine.

In 1916 Means spent three weeks with DuBois at Bellevue Hospital in New York, learning the technique of the respiration calorimeter and the method of determining the basal metabolic rate (BMR) based on the surface area of the body. It emerged that the BMR reflected the degree of thyroid hormone activity, a development that directed Means toward study of the thyroid and its disorders. All this came at a time when accurate or objective assays had scarcely found a place in medical diagnosis. As Means wrote, "For this development of mechanical perfection in an apparatus the profession owes in the first place a great debt to Professor E. F. DuBois; it also owes something to the competition among manufacturers which has found them to be continually inventing improvement." The statement reflected his recognition of both individual competence and the strength of our economic system.

Means' career was interrupted during World War I by overseas service in Base Hospital No. 6 in Bordeaux, France. He was Adjutant to Col. Frederic A. Washburn who had been resident physician at the MGH and who became its director from 1922 to 1934. The chaplain of Base Hospital No. 6 was Henry Knox Sherrill, who confirmed Means in France and was to become a lifelong friend. Sherrill was also to play an active role as a trustee of the MGH. These two men with Phillips Ketchum, a boyhood friend, were to be of great support during Means' 28 years as chief of Medicine. During this span he served as chairman of the Executive Committee of the hospital for 11 years.

After the war Harvard awarded Means an instructorship in medicine with a modest salary. Thus began for him the happy combination in medicine of practice, teaching, and pursuit of the thyroid that led to the creation of the Thyroid Clinic in 1920.

Means' great contribution to the profession of medicine came soon after his appointment in 1923 as Jackson Professor of Clinical Medicine at the MGH: This was the development of a hospital-based clinical research ward. Shortly before David Edsall left to become dean at the Harvard Medical School, he had secured funds for reconstruction of the east wing of the Bulfinch Building. Means inherited the task of the design and completion of the new unit which was to include a ward for clinical research. He received great inspiration from DuBois and from the special ward of four beds in Bellevue devoted to the study of energy metabolism. Planning and construction continued through 1924, and the unit, unique in concept, opened in the autumn of 1925. It contained ten beds and an adjoining chemical laboratory for the study of patients "both to their own benefit and that of others." It was called Ward 4. The ward continues as a focal point of the intellectual life of the hospital and is a lasting tribute to the tenacity of purpose and the creative energy of Howard Means. In 1949 the ward was renamed after Edward Mallinckrodt, Jr., of St. Louis in recognition of his repeated benefactions. This unit was the prototype for the huge clinical research center in Bethesda and for the 80-odd clinical research centers in the United States that are now supported by the extramural program of the National Institutes of Health.

Means' history of Ward 4 was published by the Harvard University Press in 1958. It is a remarkable volume full of anecdotes and insight, in which he not only describes the nuts and bolts of the operation but also synthesizes the main streams of research activity which took place over the years. The casual reader may fail to appreciate the cohesive force of Means in those brilliant investigations by a highly competitive and goal-oriented group of younger physicians. Much of his genius lay in his ability to nurture the creative enterprise of the staff. He believed in and encouraged the "fecundity of aggregation." (Means often used this phrase which Walter Cannon attributed to Josiah Royce and quoted in his book *The Way of an Investigator*.)

The ward, as part of the Medical Service, was under Means' general supervision. In the preface to his history he wrote: "The policy that I followed was to invest in investigators of high promise and then to give them as much freedom of inquiry as possible." That policy was sensed by those who had the privilege of working on Ward 4, where intellectual freedom led to innovation.

Another outstanding contribution Means made to the American teaching hospital was the specialty unit. Departments of cardiology, arthritis, endocrinology, and others developed under his tutelage, but the first of these, and the one closest to his heart, was the Thyroid Clinic. The origins of this clinic can be traced to his early interest in respiration and to his studies on metabolism. Soon after the metabolic laboratory began, case discussions were being held before a small group that soon attracted students.

The clinic and the laboratory were under the charge of a staff person, but Means continued far beyond his retirement to play a participatory role. It was the center of his intellectual academic life. Nothing interfered with his attendance at its weekly sessions. For years his wit and perception provided the spark that kept the clinic alive; it was a sounding board for new ideas, the birthplace of countless research projects, and a center of learning and teaching. Its graduates have made major contributions to medical science in this country and abroad.

Each spring Howard Means joined the growing migration of eager teachers of medicine to Atlantic City where the results of their studies and treatment of disease were revealed. He became president in 1942 of their senior organization, the Association of American Physicians, and received its highest honor, the Kober Medal, in 1964. Three years earlier he had written a history of its first 75 years, tracing the mainstream of the development of academic medicine through the accomplishments of its members. It is a remarkable record of the achievements of American medicine.

As an educator Professor Means taught generations of medical students on the wards of the MGH. He guided the Medical Service during those years of prodigious change in medicine when the great transition from bedside art to scientific discipline took place, and when therapy became for the first time rational and measurably effective.

A series of extraordinary events stemmed from a colloquium in Vanderbilt Hall on November 12, 1936, when the president of MIT, Karl T. Compton, lectured on "What Physics Can Do for Biology and Medicine." The portion dealing with radioactive isotopes had been prepared by Professor Robley D. Evans. Compton related the startling news that Enrico Fermi and his co-workers reported they had irradiated all available elements with neutrons and produced one radioisotope of iodine. Instantly Means and others from the Thyroid Clinic recognized the great potential of such a tool as a tracer of physiologic events. This was based on the well-known avidity the thyroid holds for iodine. Excitement ran high and, as Evans wrote, "A mutual kinetic force thrust their leader

Means toward Compton." He hurried to the platform to propose a cooperative venture between MIT and the MGH to explore the physiologic use of radioiodine. A collaborative effort was soon developed in conferences between Means and Evans. Soon Evans produced Fermi's I^{128} with a half-life of only 25 minutes. Use of this tool by Evans, Roberts, and Saul Hertz (head of the Thyroid Clinic) proved that rabbits concentrated the isotope only in the thyroid. The next move was obvious, but the short half-life was a deterrent until the world's first cyclotron built exclusively for biologic and medical use began operation at MIT on November 1, 1940. Its first product of radioiodine (I^{130}) had a half-life of 12 hours, and the first patient was taken to MIT for treatment on January 31, 1941, where Hertz administered a "radioactive cocktail."

Further experience with radioactive iodine in the Thyroid Clinic, directed by Means, culminated in reports at the meeting of the American Medical Association in June 1946 that a single effective dose could replace hazardous surgery and even destroy the whole gland. Surgeons felt threatened, but the bud of nuclear energy had burst into flower, and a surge of isotopes to research laboratories throughout the world soon produced blooms of new knowledge in the fields of biology, physiology, and medicine.

Howard Means was also concerned with the interaction between patient and physician. His booklet *The Amenities of Ward Rounds* stressed the importance of the dignity and rights of the patient and the behavioral attitudes of the physician. Recognizing the role of social factors in human disease, he extended the Social Service Department at MGH. In his speech on the occasion of the fiftieth anniversary of the founding of medical social service at the hospital, in 1955, he said, "I would like to stress that the Medical Social Worker, because of her intimate knowledge of the patient's whole family background, is one of the most important integrating persons in the whole medical care team." His broad interest in the social, ethical, and emotional content of the patient was highlighted by his foreword to *The Ethical Basis of Medical Practice* by Willard L. Sperry, then dean of the Harvard Divinity School. Means wrote:

It is a source of gratification to me that a question asked by an intern on a ward of the MGH should have set off the chain reaction which has led to the production of this book. Dean Sperry has advanced our thinking in an area which vitally concerns the doctor, but in which the doctor not infrequently feels somewhat lost. Dean Sperry has at least clearly identified the problems, and that is the first step toward solving them.

In his presidential address to the American College of Physicians in 1938 he charged the American Medical Association with ultraconservative postures that he considered contrary to a wider and better distribution of medical service. He became a strong proponent of group practice and medical insurance at a time when these concepts were bitterly opposed. In 1953 the preface of his book *Doctors, People and Government* began with the statement: "The American people are entitled to the best medical service which science and art permit, and which they can afford to buy. They are entitled to get it at the lowest price consistent with high quality, or to have it given to them if they cannot pay. . . . The health of the citizen is his concern, but it is also his neighbor's. . . . The affairs of medicine, therefore, are the affairs of the people no less than of the medical profession." Two of his articles written for the *Atlantic Monthly*—"England's

Public Medicine: The Facts" (March 1950) and "The Doctors' Lobby" (October 1950)—won him the Sidney Hillman Award in 1951.

Howard Means had a lifelong interest in international medicine. In 1950 the possibility arose of a team of medical investigators going to study endemic goiter in the province of Mendoza in western Argentina. The plan received his enthusiastic backing, and he was able to generate the fiscal resources to make the expedition a success. (See also pages 136–138, Thyroid Unit.)

Means was a master English stylist. He wrote prodigiously and produced more than 200 scientific publications and eight books. He accomplished this with an economy of effort because he was able to write or dictate in a style that required little, if any, revision; it came forth whole, complete, and finished. In 1934 he published *Diseases of the Thyroid,* a masterpiece of medical writing and a most important contribution to clinical medicine. In it there is not a single ambiguous sentence, fuzzy concept, or wandering reflexive pronoun. The remarkable thing is that the science is all there too. The same can be said for the second edition published in 1948. He also published his Thayer lectures on the thyroid as a monograph and wrote a tribute to his father, who was one of the pioneers of aviation.

To his many friends, Howard Means was a dynamic intellectual with great humor, responsive to his environment and especially sensitive to color and form. These latter qualities are evident in the watercolors he painted during vacations in many lands but with greatest feeling for Maine. Each year he chose a watercolor to reproduce as a Christmas card, and he insisted on addressing the cards himself. They went to former members of the house staff and fellows as well as old and new friends both here and abroad. In 1943 the subject was a drawing of a room in the Treadwell Library. The card carried a special greeting to all those on active war service and was signed by more than 30 members of the "MGH family on the home front."

Means anticipated with excitement his travels on medical affairs to Europe, South America, and the Far East. In 1955 he served as visiting physician at St. Luke's Hospital in Tokyo; 1956 found him at St. Bartholomew's Hospital in London for a month acting as temporary director of the full-time Medical Unit. In 1960 he was made an honorary member of the Royal Society of Medicine.

After his retirement from teaching responsibilities in 1951 Means demonstrated his "deepest conviction that for happiness it is necessary to have a line of work one loves and to continue at it as long as the Lord will let him" by returning to MIT to take an active part in student health care for six years. Once he took special pride in a night's vigil with a young man ill with severe pneumonia. He regarded these years at MIT as a broadening and thrilling experience because of the opportunity it afforded him to mingle with engineers of all kinds, basic scientists, and scholars in the humanities. It was during these years and for some time thereafter that he found time to lecture and to write as well as to serve as a member of the National Advisory Council of the Public Health Service.

Writing for his 55th Harvard College Class Report he summed up the thinking of his later years: "My philosophy is that at our time of life we will do best by working at something we find rewarding, and by using our feet as much as possible for locomotion. I believe that man's only hope of survival is to stop despoiling his planet, and to learn to control his numbers."

Once, in leaving one of us in nominal charge while he went on a summer holiday, he said, "You know, you have to keep this place in a constant state of intellectual ferment." That comment described his own life which was one of constant creative intellectual activity.

With the assistance of *Carol Means*

11. Walter Bauer

LLOYD H. SMITH, JR., AND DANIEL D. FEDERMAN

Among the more interesting philosophical speculations that recur in literature is the question of whether men create history by the sum of their acts of free will or whether the innate momentum of historic events creates men. No history of the MGH of the past generation would be complete without an analysis of Walter Bauer's impact upon an institution in change. Many would concur that no other individual played such a pivotal role in guiding the future direction of the hospital, in part because of the importance of the Medical Service per se but mostly because of his forcefulness as a leader. In considerable measure Bauer was a product of the MGH and the Harvard Medical School to which he devoted his entire career (with loyalties in that sequence). Furthermore, his own gifts of leadership were uniquely needed at the time when he assumed the position of Jackson Professor of Clinical Medicine and chief of the Medical Services in 1951; the man seemed to match the occasion. Yet the qualities that Bauer brought to his position and that attracted others to him were not the by-product of Boston medicine in his era. Rather, they were deeply rooted in his person in a mix of emotion, culture, values, judgment, sensitivity, resolution, and energy, which defies separation into component parts.

Who was Walter Bauer? By what steps did he reach the Jackson Professorship?

Walter Bauer was born June 7, 1898, in Crystal Falls, Michigan. He received the B.S. degree in 1920 and the M.D. degree in 1922 from the University of Michigan. After internship and residency at Long Island College Hospital in Brooklyn, New York, Bauer came to the MGH in 1924 as chief resident in Medicine and was associated with the hospital ever after. In 1926 he was appointed a research fellow in Medicine at the Harvard Medical School, and in 1927–1928 he worked in the laboratory of Sir Henry Dale in England. At Harvard Bauer was an instructor in medicine from 1927 to 1928, faculty instructor and tutor from 1929 to 1932, assistant professor from 1932 to 1936, and associate professor of medicine from 1936 to 1951. He was elected to the American Society for Clinical Investigation and the Association of American Physicians (of which he served as president in 1959).

At MGH Bauer was a charter member of the illustrious Ward 4 team—which included Joseph Aub, Fuller Albright, and Oliver Cope—that initiated metabolic studies of hyperparathyroidism, lead intoxication, and hyperthyroidism. In the early 1930s he turned to the study of arthritis and the rheumatic diseases, the focus of his research and teaching for the next 20 years. He headed the Robert W. Lovett Memorial Unit for the Study of Crippling Diseases and played a large role in developing academic awareness of the chronic diseases and of the patients who have them. Bauer served as a physician at the MGH from 1936 to 1951. In 1951 he was chosen to succeed James Howard Means as Jackson Professor at the Medical School and chief of Medical Services at MGH.

In 1951 the department of medicine at the MGH was one of the most highly regarded in the United States for its excellence in patient care, clinical teaching, and research. James Howard Means, who retired from the position of chief after

28 years, had been surrounded by a talented group of colleagues that included Bauer (rheumatology), Paul White (cardiology), Chester Jones (gastroenterology), Joseph Aub (oncology), and Fuller Albright (endocrinology). In addition to these leaders in their respective disciplines, there were many others of national stature, especially in clinical research and patient care. Over this Hanseatic League of specialty units Means presided benignly and with a loose hand, secure in the knowledge of MGH preeminence. His distinguished colleagues, who were mostly of his generation or within 15 years of his age, greatly respected Means as a physician and as a laissez faire administrator. He appointed John B. Stanbury to run the Thyroid Clinic and Unit but otherwise had made no major appointments in the department within the prior decade. Although skilled and devoted clinicians filled patient care and teaching responsibilities, there were no organized units or divisions with assigned space for research and postdoctoral training in chest medicine, infectious disease, metabolism, hematology, or allergy-immunology. To the house staff Means in his later years was a rather remote figure who was an excellent and entertaining attending physician on the Bulfinch wards for approximately two months each year but with whom there were otherwise very few encounters. The service was largely administered by the chief medical residents, admirable and amphoteric physicians who belonged partly to the rabble and partly to the establishment. Nevertheless there was excellent esprit throughout the Medical Service and a strong collegial spirit among the house staff.

Walter Bauer catapulted into this comparatively tranquil scene in 1951. Already a powerful and popular figure on the Medical Service through his leadership of the Arthritis Unit, Bauer quickly shifted his intense focus of attention to patient care and training programs and concentrated his efforts on those responsibilities until his terminal illness 12 years later. It is difficult to trace the events of those tumultuous years in temporal sequence. Perhaps it would be most useful to comment briefly on Bauer's impact on the MGH under several separate headings.

The Teaching Program.
Means had been detached, but Bauer was totally and personally involved in virtually all phases of the teaching program. This began with the medical students who were assigned to the MGH for their clinical clerkship experience: Every Friday afternoon he met with the students and the chief medical resident in a session that quickly came to be known as "the Bauer Hour." Actually this was a symposium of about two hours at which each student was required to present a talk and lead a discussion on some nontechnical problem in medicine, such as euthanasia, telling the truth to the patient, the cost of health care, etc. In these sessions Bauer anticipated the problems medicine would grapple with many years later; he taught fledgling physicians to maintain a constant awareness of the needs of sick people. Guests were often invited and discussions were spirited, with Bauer deeply involved and probing in his comments and candor. He became very interested in individual students and often met with them to discuss their problems. He personally presided over grading sessions to ensure that all facets of performance were judiciously balanced in the final evaluation.

Walter Bauer's greatest interest lay in the careers of the younger physicians at the MGH—the members of the medical house staff and the new staff physicians whom he personally chose. The medical house staff was Bauer's particular pride and concern until the day of his death. Despite his many responsibilities, he found time to be remarkably conversant with each of the diverse and talented physicians who served under him during 12 years, until his increasing respiratory insufficiency led to his incapacitation. He came to know his residents intimately, especially those who spent two or more years in the Bulfinch. He had an astonishing capacity to break through the concentric shells of reticence that impede personal interactions in order to reach the person's core feelings. His judgments were sometimes hasty and occasionally harsh; more often they were accurate and recognized as such by those being judged. None doubted the sincerity of Bauer's interest in him as physician and as human being, even when in disagreement with his conclusions.

Much of Bauer's information about his residents was gained on the fly, by chance encounters at meals, in the corridors, or during weekly "Allen Street Rounds," named for the euphemism describing the former location of the morgue. By means of these reviews of deaths and complications he maintained a broad grasp of current patient care problems on the service and in so doing learned much about his house staff as well. He met with each member of the house staff repeatedly to discuss performance and future plans, and he was tireless in promoting these plans. Most fortunate were those who, by the luck of assignment, worked with Bauer as an attending physician. His devotion to all aspects of patient care was authentic and intense, and he was able to transmit that feeling to all patients on an open Bulfinch ward. He visited his Bulfinch patients seven days a week and demanded a similar commitment from his house staff team. When his mood swung toward elation, his exuberance knew almost no bounds, and many who read these pages will recall complete evening ward rounds and midnight telephone calls to check on the progress of a seriously ill patient.

Walter Bauer was especially close to his chief residents who worked with him in a preceptor relationship. The responsibilities of this position were major ones, and during the fifties the chief residents were on call, sleeping in "the Moseley flats" three or four nights each week. The following individuals were chief residents under Bauer:

1951	Isaac M. Taylor	Professor of Medicine, and former Dean, University of North Carolina School of Medicine
1952	Evan Calkins	Professor and Chairman of Medicine, SUNY, Buffalo
1953	Morton N. Swartz	Professor of Medicine, HMS Chief, Infectious Disease Unit, MGH
1954	Frederick C. Goetz	Professor of Medicine, University of Minnesota School of Medicine
1955	Richard A. Field	Associate Clinical Professor of Medicine, HMS
1956	Lloyd H. Smith, Jr.	Professor and Chairman, Department of Medicine, University of California, San Francisco
1957	Stephen M. Krane	Professor of Medicine, HMS Chief, Arthritis Unit, MGH

1958	John H. Knowles	Former General Director, MGH, and President, Rockefeller Foundation (deceased, 1979)
1959	Donald B. Martin	Professor of Medicine, University of Pennsylvania School of Medicine
1960	Ralph C. Williams	Professor and Chairman, Department of Medicine, University of New Mexico School of Medicine
1961	K. Frank Austen	Professor of Medicine, HMS Chief of Medicine, Robert Breck Brigham Hospital
1962	Mitchell T. Rabkin	General Director, Beth Israel Hospital
1963	Hibbard E. Williams	Dean, School of Medicine, University of California, Davis

It was not only the chief residents who shared a sense of special affinity with Walter Bauer. It was his genius to know and deeply influence many other members of a remarkable house staff, which included a Nobel laureate (Edelman), a Pulitzer Prize winner (Mack), other departmental chairmen (Federman, Thier, Tisdale, Vagelos, Rasmussen, Wyngaarden), and prominent academic figures in medicine at Harvard and throughout the nation.

The Academic Program. Although the MGH was an eminent center for medical research and training in 1951 when Walter Bauer was appointed chief, change was in the air. A new national commitment to research was about to begin, and Bauer's response to that opportunity through reconstitution of the specialty divisions was his most enduring legacy to the MGH. His vision of this new academic program was spelled out in detail in his presidential address to the Association of American Physicians (1959) and in an address to the Karolinska Institute (1960) entitled "The Responsibility of the University Hospital in the Synthesis of Medicine, Science and Learning" and published as a Special Article in the *New England Journal of Medicine*. In the article he wrote: "The onward rush of progress has brought us to a point of unprecedented difficulty. We must now answer the question: How can medicine care for the sick in the highest humanitarian tradition and at the same time bring to the clinic the full weight and authority of modern science?" In the addresses he developed his theme that "scientific rigor and traditional humanitarianism are complementary aspects of medicine." Others spoke or wrote in a similar vein, but Bauer put theory into practice in ways that were both bold and disquieting to his more traditional associates. As opportunities occurred, he appointed new chiefs to the specialty units, choosing young people well trained in science and clinical medicine but often with little or no training in the subspecialty. He was confident of his hunches and was willing to take chances which could charitably be called imaginative extrapolation or, uncharitably, wild gambling. Over a comparatively few years ten chiefs of units were appointed; John Stanbury remained as chief of the Thyroid Unit, but his approach to medical research was entirely consistent with that being developed in other units.

The appointment of Kurt Isselbacher as chief of Gastroenterology can be cited as a case history of Bauer's approach. An honor graduate of Harvard Medical School, Kurt came to the MGH in 1950 as a medical intern and remained for two additional years in the residency. He then went to the National Institutes of Health where he was associated with Gordon Tomkins and Herman Kalckar. Among other important research contributions, he first demonstrated the enzyme defect of galactosemia in red cell hemolysates. Even at that stage of postdoctoral training he was invited by Bauer to return to the MGH to develop a new division of gastroenterology. In 1956 he returned to Boston and spent an additional laboratory year. The following year, seven years after graduating from medical school and with no formal specialty training, he was appointed to succeed the illustrious Chester M. Jones. Isselbacher went on to become Mallinckrodt Professor at the Harvard Medical School, president of the Association of American Physicians and of the American Gastroenterological Association, and the leader of a whole era of American academic gastroenterology.

Bauer's pattern of appointment, repeated in a number of instances, led to consternation in the MGH and more generally in the Harvard Medical School. Among the young people so appointed, however, it was a special time of intense excitement and high creativity which is difficult now to recapture. All were aware of participating in an era when a great institution was undergoing a rapid transformation, and they felt a special sense of loyalty to Walter Bauer who had a clear vision of the future and the courage to act upon that vision. When one of the authors (Smith) was so appointed, Bauer announced his decision in the following way: "I believe that you've got the ability to make a go of it in academic medicine. During the next five years I'm going to be rooting for you and helping you in every possible way. If you don't make it, I'm going to kick you out of here!" This kind of sporting proposition held great attraction, particularly since one knew that Bauer meant every word of it, despite the quick grin at the end. Laboratories expanded; research and training grants vastly increased; and a new generation of physician-scientists were attracted who were able to understand and collaborate with the Fritz Lipmanns, Herman Kalckars, and Paul Zamecniks who brought fundamental science to the setting of a teaching hospital. Always, however, Bauer hammered away at the theme of continuity between science and patient care, and everyone was expected to take his turn as a Bulfinch attending physician and in student and house staff teaching. Many of those chosen are still in key positions at the MGH and the Harvard medical community.

One evening in the early seventies, three chairmen of American departments of medicine were having dinner together. All had been house officers and two had been chief residents under Walter Bauer. They began reminiscing about "W.B." and his impact upon them. Each of the professors admitted that Bauer's continuing influence took many forms but that the principal one was moral example. When confronted with an ethical dilemma, each of the men realized he was likely to ask himself "What would W.B. want me to do?" Then he would find that the problem would sort itself out rather easily.

Walter Bauer had a remarkable impact upon the lives and professional careers of many young men and women, and through them upon the MGH and American medicine at large. Impact is used advisedly since those who were the recipients of this attention would agree that it was an active process from which few emerged unaltered. It is difficult to describe the forces of personality and intellect that made him unique in his time as a leader in the setting of the intermingling of science and medicine. Those who did not know him will remain unconvinced by a simple recitation of his traits and accomplishments, for both were flawed and incomplete. Those who knew him well will miss the chemistry of their own interaction, the evoked response that was the true source of his power. Evocation is intensely private. There are certain conventional categories in which an evaluation of a leader in academic medicine could normally be segregated. As we shall see, they do not suffice for our purpose.

Was Walter Bauer a great clinician? He was a highly effective physician but not a brilliant clinical scholar. His interest in the welfare of his patients was profound and even obsessive, encompassing all aspects of disability broadly defined. This empathy was instantly transmitted to his patients who were devoted to him. Through broad experience and intuitive insight he was especially skilled in the care of the chronically ill, never becoming discouraged or abandoning his patient. Intensity of commitment was the core of his philosophy of medical care, and he imprinted this upon those who were fortunate enough to work with him. He was not, on the other hand, an exceptional scholar in clinical medicine. Bauer did not read broadly in medicine and its relevant sciences but largely relied upon his associates on the MGH staff and house staff from whom he skillfully extracted information with Socratic rigor. He bragged to his visitors that the MGH residents collectively constituted his "walking library."

Was Walter Bauer a great teacher? Strangely enough, this magnetic man was a drab speaker, poorly organized and at a loss for the felicitous phrase or expression. His most widely quoted speeches were in considerable measure ghostwritten by younger associates. He was frustrated by this relative disability and spoke of it openly. His ideas erupted with creative energy but were inchoate and amorphous in public exposition. In a formal talk he was therefore unexceptional, although occasionally the sheer power of his conviction would break through with compelling force. In sharp contrast, Bauer was extraordinarily effective as a teacher in small groups or at the bedside. Few can forget the qualities of honesty and commitment that illuminated those specific episodes. Not merely the details of biomedical science but one's whole philosophy was subject to probing attack. It was an exhilarating experience to participate in these encounters, which remain strongly imprinted in memory when more facile and conventional instruction is long forgotten. If education is defined as "what you have left when you have forgotten the facts," Bauer was a remarkable teacher who would not allow one the comfort of opinion without the discomfort of thought. The settings were informal but suffused by a creative tension since one's best was always in demand. Usually there was a sharp focus on all aspects of the patient's problems with little attention to the intricacies of roundsmanship. The result was more than the transfer of knowledge; it was the sharing of an ideal.

Was Walter Bauer a creative scientist and clinical investigator? He received superior early training in medical science with Sir Henry Dale and Joseph C. Aub. As a pioneer in establishing rheumatology as a specialty discipline, he published many articles of lasting value that described major syndromes and the natural history of rheumatic disorders. He was elected to the major scientific societies and received national and international respect for his accomplishments. But when weighed against Fuller Albright or Paul Zamecnik, Bauer was not unusually gifted as a scientist. In personal contributions to medical science he was perhaps less distinguished than his contemporaries who were chiefs of service at the other Harvard teaching hospitals. Against this reservation, however, must be weighed his intuitive grasp of the role of science in the future of medical investigation. This insight seems obvious now when the triumph of the new biology is everywhere apparent, but it was revolutionary 30 years ago when the leitmotif of clinical investigation was that of inspired amateurism. Bauer had a profound conviction that the only rational approach to the conquest of disease was through the systematic development of the biologic sciences and that the wave of the future lay in this integration which must occur within the individual, the division, the department, and the institution. Along with other men of vision he was instrumental in imprinting this philosophy upon the MGH a generation ago. Its implementation was his major legacy. As a result the MGH was among the first of the great teaching hospitals to develop a rigorous program of fundamental biologic science. That program, always precarious to maintain in a hospital setting, is still the ultimate source of the institution's strength as a center of scholarship.

Was Walter Bauer a cultivated and learned man? This is difficult to evaluate in conventional terms since the context of our association was almost exclusively the cauldron of an institution in change, the MGH of the 1950s, which dominated his attention. We heard little from Walter Bauer of art, music, literature, or history, and one had the impression, perhaps erroneous, that they did not rank high in his turbulent career. He spoke admiringly of his friend Dickinson Richards, with whom he shared his year in England, and contrasted his own background with Richards' broad erudition and cultural advantages. With a grin he said, "If my forebears had remained in Germany, I'd be the best Goddamned cobbler in Württemberg!" Bauer was at ease with individuals of diverse backgrounds because his interest in them was authentic rather than socially contrived, and few can resist that ultimate flattery. He was erudite in human affairs but this understanding was derived from the synthesis of personal experience rather than distilled from the published works of other men.

No portrait of Walter Bauer can be considered candid which does not touch upon his mood swings. Bauer seemed endowed with most human traits in extra measure. This clearly pertained to the "cyclothymic fluctuations" that not infrequently carried him from exhilaration to depression. When "up" he radiated energy and ideas; every house officer of that era has personal stories of midnight ward rounds and other reflections of a buoyancy that could not be contained and spilled over into everything about him. When the weather of his mind became inclement, it was only through personal discipline that he could meet the daily challenges of his considerable patient care, teaching, and administrative responsibilities. Life with Bauer was therefore further enlivened by a certain unpredictability based on these successive phases of temperament.

Was Walter Bauer an effective leader? His qualities as a leader of men were so exceptional as not to require the modifications expressed in other arbitrary categories touched upon above. Leadership is based on attributes that are not difficult to perceive but that defy precise definition. Bauer had a matchless capacity to judge both the motivation and the potential in those around him and to transmit that judgment with a penetrating and sometimes painful honesty. In that capacity, exercised with intuitive skill and exquisite timing, he permanently influenced the lives and the careers of a generation of his younger colleagues. In the process he enlarged his environment, and those who shared it with him were enhanced and expanded in spirit and scope. His greatest quality of leadership was therefore to see into and touch the lives of others in ways denied to other more brilliant men.

Secondly, Walter Bauer had a clear vision of the future directions of science in medicine and of scientific medicine as patient care one step removed. He saw this trend earlier than most of his contemporaries in American medicine and immediately set about to further its achievement. Finally, Bauer had the courage to match his convictions and was willing or even eager to bet that he was right. He took breathtaking chances in the major decisions and appointments that permanently altered the Medical Service at the MGH and placed it in the vanguard of the new scientific medicine. These elements of leadership, combined with a high seriousness, attracted men to him and created an aura of excitement which is hard to recapture. Many who are now in positions of responsibility look upon their interaction with Walter Bauer during this turbulent period of change at the MGH as the most important influence on their subsequent careers.

12. *Alexander Leaf*

SAMUEL O. THIER

Alex Leaf was born in Yokohama, Japan, while his parents were fleeing from Russia. He grew up on the West Coast and attended the University of Washington before beginning his trek eastward to the University of Michigan School of Medicine. After graduation from medical school, he did an internship at the MGH but regressed to the Midwest to take a residency at the Mayo Clinic. He subsequently returned to the MGH for a fellowship and spent fruitful sabbatical time studying with Hans H. Ussing and Hans A. Krebs. His early research into the physiology of salt and water balance led to a number of highly original observations. For example, it was Leaf who first described the syndrome of inappropriate secretion of antidiuretic hormone by producing the syndrome in himself and his colleagues. What is now known as the Schwartz-Bartter syndrome was, in fact, originally described and defined physiologically by Alex Leaf. One of his most important contributions was the development of the toad bladder as a model for epithelial transport; that model became the basis for more than two decades of fruitful research. Few would have guessed that the transport capabilities of the toad bladder could be so great as to carry a full grown man to the Jackson Professorship.

In 1966, at the height of his investigative career, Leaf was appointed the James Jackson Professor and chairman of the Department of Medicine at the MGH. Many commentaries on leaders in academic medicine begin with apologies indicating that, though the person was not a great investigator or a great clinician, he or she was nonetheless a great leader. In reviewing Alex Leaf's career at the MGH, no such apologies are in order. Leaf is a truly outstanding investigator of international stature; he is also an absolutely first-rate clinician. And at the end of 15 years as chief of Medicine at the MGH, he turned over to his successor a department that was still one of the very best in the country. That fact deserves further elaboration. Leaf received from his predecessor a department that was considered by most people to be one of the very best in the United States. Given a run-down department or a new department, it is easy to build and to show growth; what is far more difficult is to take a truly great department and maintain that greatness during a time of enormous change. Leaf, given little room to improve upon the quality of his department, nonetheless added, remodeled, channeled evolutionary trends, and maintained its excellence. One needs only to review the decline of many renowned departments in as short a period of time to appreciate what he accomplished.

Aside from receiving the prestigious title, the beginning of Leaf's tenure was not terribly auspicious. In fact, he arrived for his first day as chief of Medicine when I arrived for my first day as his chief resident. Unfortunately, Leaf had not been given the correct key to his office, and neither of us got off to a flying start. Fortunately, he did pick up steam, and the department moved along with him. During the next 15 years, which brought enormous changes in medical education, in the social fabric of our communities, in the attitudes of students and faculty, and in the support for academic departments of medicine, Leaf placed his own stamp on a great department. He supported innovative directions ranging from evaluation of intensive care to the development of a primary care track in his residency program. He helped to foster the growth of a group practice, outreach clinics, and ultimately the construction of new facilities for inpatients as well as outpatients. A strengthening of the clinical educational programs, an increase in their flexibility, and the creation of new clinical facilities and services are important activities for any chairman of medicine, and particularly so for one noted for his deep commitment to basic science. During the same period of time, Alex protected the strongest sections of his department and recruited exciting new people to strengthen others. It is particularly worth noting that he recruited the individual who 15 years later was felt by the faculty to be the best person to become his successor.

As Leaf's first chief resident, I cannot help noting with some pride that, of the 15 chief residents he recruited, all remain committed to academic medicine. Members of this cohort of chief residents now work as deans, hospital administrators, department chairmen, and most important, academic scholars. The department of medicine at the MGH has always taken pride in noting the accomplishments of its chief residents. Though most of Leaf's recent chief residents remain somewhat embryonic academicians, they show every promise of continuing a great tradition.

It must be noted that Leaf was not exclusively committed to activities at the MGH. He was also a well known and active traveler, a person greatly interested in the very aged. I can still remember the fuss that was created by the report in the *National Geographic* of his studies on aging. He pointed out to me wryly that nothing he had ever done scientifically had ever created half the excitement of his studies on aging. Nor did he fail to see the humor in the situation when one of the old individuals he interviewed in Russia identified himself as being 104 years old on Leaf's first visit and some two or three years later described himself as 112 years old. Leaf's travels to distant places became near-legendary. The legend was not known, however, to a new secretary who stopped a man from entering Leaf's office, telling him that Dr. Leaf was overseas. The somewhat bemused visitor indicated that he *was* Dr. Leaf.

Leaf's laboratory served as the training ground for numerous leaders in investigative renal physiology. True to his own qualities, he continued to evolve and moved from the chairmanship of Medicine into exciting studies on the clinical aspects and cell biology of acute renal failure. His research contributions have been recognized time and again; he has been elected to virtually every prestigious academic society in his field and has served as an officer of several.

A brief review of Leaf's academic career and his accomplishments as chief of Medicine fails to highlight the man. He is a person deeply concerned about his fellow beings. He worried about his students and his house staff and would quietly follow up on their personal problems without ever intruding. In fact, his genuine interest in others was so often hidden by his quiet and shy manner that there were those who mistakenly judged him to be distant and aloof. A friend writing to me about Leaf noted, "What was believed by some to be aloofness was really a shyness which kept people from getting to know him well, their distinct loss." I, for one, had the opportunity to get to know him well, and it was certainly my distinct gain.

13. Eminent Physicians

Paul Dudley White

"By birth and family tradition Dr. White was a true product of New England," wrote his good friend and colleague, Edward F. Bland. "He was born in Boston, educated at Harvard, and served internship and residencies at the Massachusetts General Hospital. He was the son of a dedicated family doctor and the eldest of four children. A younger sister died at the age of twelve of acute rheumatic fever. Her untimely death and the admiration he felt for his father influenced his choice of medicine for a career.

"He graduated from the Harvard Medical School in 1911, serving first in Pediatrics as the second intern on this service, newly established at the MGH. The next two years he spent on the Medical Service under Dr. Roger I. Lee. Together they devised a new technique for the determination of blood coagulation time, a procedure still in use and known as the Lee-White method." (Of this work White remarked, "It was my only contribution to hematology.")

"Thereafter," Bland continued, "circumstances led to a year at University College Hospital in London where Thomas Lewis was mapping the action currents of the heart with a new device, the string galvanometer of Einthoven. It was here that he met and admired Sir James Mackenzie and became acquainted with his assistant, John Parkinson, with whom 20 years later he and Louis Wolff described the W-P-W syndrome.

"In 1914 he returned to the MGH with one of the earliest electrocardiographs in the country, a cumbersome and tricky affair requiring frequent adjustments, glass photographic plates, a darkroom, and sponge electrodes in pots of saline. Despite its idiosyncrasies this instrument remained in use and served well for 20 years."

Recalling those years in his charming autobiography *My Life and Medicine* White wrote: "I felt like a lonely adventurer entering an unexplored and unknown country, planning to spend my life in a new and yet unrecognized specialty limited to the heart and blood vessels, both normal and diseased. . . . My former medical school teachers or hospital chiefs would warn me that I was entering an insignificant special field and would never be heard from again. Even the nurses would advise me not to study such a difficult part of the body as the circulation, which was customarily relegated to a few back pages of the medical textbooks. . . . In the autumn of 1914, I set up my new electrocardiographic laboratory in a small closet in the basement of the Skin Ward, which I was given 'because there was no other place for it.' " White's laboratory was destined to lead the peripatetic life of most MGH units. Within a few years it graduated upstairs to the old apothecary shop on the ground floor of Bulfinch; from there it returned to the basement awaiting more ample quarters in the Bulfinch east wing.

Whenever White recalled the early days he invoked the name of Richard Cabot whose investigations of the causes of heart disease and emphasis on prevention rather than diagnosis and treatment impressed him deeply. Cabot's teaching did much to shape White's medical attitudes. The influence of Cabot could be detected in White's crusade to prevent heart disease, in the long follow-up studies of patients, and in his sensitivity to the physiologic individuality of people.

The First World War interrupted White's research. He served first with the Harvard unit of the British Expeditionary force near Boulogne; then, after the United States joined the war, he helped organize MGH Base Hospital No. 6 near Bordeaux. In 1919 he headed a Red Cross typhus control mission in Greece, a service for which the Greek government awarded him a decoration. But White found few rewards in military duties, "the few hours of the excitement of heroism and the drama of victory being outnumbered a hundred-thousand-fold by the millions of tragedies of wounds, illness and death of the young people of the many countries involved, and especially by the utter boredom and futility of this technique of settling disputes, a relic of the caveman." As this observation suggests, the war had made him a committed pacifist.

White returned to the MGH in the fall of 1919 and resumed his investigations of the heart and circulation. In 1920 he was appointed the first chief of the Outpatient Department, a position he held until 1925. Bland believes that the decades of the twenties and thirties were "perhaps the most active and productive of his full and useful life. During this period he organized the cardiac unit at the hospital, he established the electrocardiograph as a useful tool for diagnosis and for clinical investigation, and he began to attract young men to the new field of cardiology. . . . [In 1924] he helped form the American Heart Association, served as its first treasurer, and presided at the birth of a new specialty. Possibly his greatest contribution during this period was his book *Heart Disease*, published in 1931, which reflects eloquently his wide experience, his academic diligence, and the clarity of his thought and expression."

Also in 1924 Paul White married Ina Reid, a member of the Social Service Department at the MGH, whom he had met when she was a student at Smith College. They enjoyed a long, companionable relationship; she contributed to his manuscripts, shared his pleasures and his convictions on moral issues, and accompanied him on many of his travels. She was also a devoted mother to their two adopted children, Penelope and Alexander.

The pace of White's professional life quickened in the thirties. "Not only were we (one or two research fellows and myself) in the heart unit at MGH intensively involved in our clinical researches in cardiology," White explained, "but we were also very active in our teaching, for which our ward and dispensary patients volunteered as subjects. I had developed a busy private practice in addition, affording me much more material to teach with, especially in a long follow-up. . . . Our teaching in the field became much more involved with postgraduate students than with undergraduates, who were not expected to enter specialized fields before graduation. Now and then, however, a fourth-year student would join us for a term or two and this custom grew as cardiology gradually became, during the thirties, a more recognized specialty."

White also led a short summer course for graduates for about a decade. The principal social event was a picnic at his country house in the town of Harvard. The day began with a softball game in the pasture—and there was a keg of beer beside third base. During one of those games, White stole home to tie the score. In reaching the plate, he collided with both batter and catcher and broke his leg—a matter of high spirits rather than fierceness of competition.

The MGH heart unit attracted increasing numbers of students and researchers, many of them from abroad. White was a gifted teacher, admired and beloved by his students. He and his colleagues in the unit produced books, numerous scientific papers, and articles for the lay public; among the latter was White's 1937 article on "Walking and Cycling" in which he pointed out the beneficial effects of exercise on the heart and general health, long before exercise became fashionable. When the *Encyclopaedia Britannica* required an authoritative and comprehensible article on the heart and heart disease for the 1939 edition, its editors appealed to Paul White.

White was asked to deliver the Ether Day address at MGH in 1936. (It was a greater-than-usual honor since the hospital was celebrating its 125th anniversary that year.) White made an excellent speech outlining the development of cardiology at the MGH. "The keynotes have not been love of medicine, love of mankind and hard work, though we do ourselves confess to them," he observed. "Essential though these things are they were part of the life of the doctors here one hundred years ago when so little was known about heart disease. Nor has the motive been the utilization of brilliant minds, though I do agree that we have gained much in that respect from Frederick Shattuck and Richard Cabot. The answer is simple and obvious. *More and more time has been devoted to the study of heart disease by more and more persons.* When that happens we are bound to make rapid progress in an undeveloped field. We would be stupid indeed if we did not."

White produced a prodigious quantity of research, and it is difficult to single out elements of his work. Henry K. Beecher and Mark Altschule, writing in *Medicine At Harvard,* said of *Diseases of the Heart,* which White wrote with Bland in 1933, "It brought precision to a field that had long been largely a collection of clinical impressions." White's most distinguished contributions, perhaps, grew out of observations carefully accumulated over years. He followed his patients with the tenacity of a terrier, and if one died, White wanted to know why. Benjamin Castleman recalled that White once persuaded a widow to have her husband's body exhumed so he could verify the cause of death.

In 1931 White and Bland initiated a long-term follow-up study of 500 patients with angina pectoris and 200 with coronary thrombosis. Their findings, published 20 years later, showed that, contrary to customary expectations, people with coronary disease often survived several years. The study provided statistical confirmation of the optimistic view that White had developed through clinical experience. In 1937 White collaborated with R. Earle Glendy and Samuel Levine in the publication of a paper on "Coronary Heart Disease in Youth," a comparison of 100 patients under 40 with 300 patients over 80; a multidisciplinary study of myocardial infarction under the age of 40 appeared in 1954. These and other studies instigated by White helped demonstrate that atherosclerosis was not necessarily a natural consequence of aging, thereby signalling possible preventive measures.

Pacifist though he was, White volunteered for active duty when the United States entered the Second World War. "This war we accepted without reservation as a very necessary crusade against a cruel dictator. . . . A science for peace was still nonexistent." His services were accepted in a civilian capacity, and he became chairman of a special committee on cardiovascular disease established by the National Research Council to review the standards for the armed services. He also organized and headed a regional committee to examine men who had been rejected by local draft boards for cardiovascular defects, many of whom his group found fit for active duty.

White spent three postwar years at the MGH and then relinquished his directorship of the Cardiac Laboratory and Clinics along with his professorship in order to serve as the first director of the National Heart Institute of the U.S. Public Health Service. In the few months immediately following his retirement he had a delightful illusion of freedom, of time perhaps to read those books he had set aside in favor of medicine. "For over thirty years I had been a sort of prisoner in the hospital, spending most of the days and sometimes the nights, on duties concerned with the care of patients, on clinical research, and on the teaching of residents and interns. I now had a private office about a mile from the hospital . . . and during those first few months I walked the streets and paths along the Charles River Basin to and from the hospital with great enjoyment."

The sense of freedom soon faded, however. As executive director of the National Advisory Heart Council, White "*was* the Council," said Theodore Cooper. White saw the inherent dangers in mixing politics with medicine and worked to ensure the integrity of the National Heart Institute. He testified before congressional committees on behalf of funds for medical education and research, sometimes appearing with prominent patients in support of his testimony. The chronicle of his accomplishments in "retirement" would fill pages; they can be summarized by saying that having pursued one career as healer, researcher, and educator, White dedicated his later energies to broad humanitarian objectives.

Leaving aside for the moment the matter of White's role as a physician to President Eisenhower, one notes that during the fifties and sixties the doctor became an international traveler, combining the two prevailing passions of his life, medicine and world peace. As president of the International Society of Cardiology he succeeded in forming a subcommittee to study the effects of temperature on circulation under the joint leadership of an Egyptian and an Israeli—no mean achievement at the time. In 1961 he became the first American member of the Soviet Academy of Medical Sciences. His work was to help countries develop the means to combat heart disease; his covert mission was peace. Typically, White failed to mention in his autobiography that he had been nominated for the Nobel Peace Prize in 1970. That same year, with the Vietnam war in high gear, he invented the word *irenology,* meaning the science of peace—noting that, though man had institutions to teach the science of war, he had no colleges or ministries for peace.

Paul Dudley White was one of the most honored physicians of this century. No fewer than 13 universities bestowed on him honorary degrees; six governments, including his own, decorated him; professional societies here and abroad heaped awards upon him. Beyond these formal tributes, he achieved a somewhat dubious distinction: He became a genuine celebrity.

Through research and teaching, White had established a splendid reputation as a cardiologist by the 1930s. Yet, though known and respected by his peers, mention of his name outside medical circles would have elicited blank stares. The public spotlight fell upon him suddenly in 1955 when he was called to Denver to consult in the management of President Eisenhower's first heart attack. Although a team of physicians, including two excellent Army cardiologists, was already attending the president, White was asked to be spokesman for the group.

His professional eminence and his seniority made him the logical candidate for that role perhaps, but the selection was a political, not a medical, decision. The nation needed reassurance. (The president had been stricken on a Saturday; on Monday the stock market recorded its greatest decline since 1929.) White's presence was indeed reassuring: He radiated competence and calm and issued precise, clear explanations of the president's condition. Looking back at the first press conference years later, White noted that his opening statement "was later broadcast throughout the country and I suppose did more than any previous efforts to inform the public about the disease that had become the great American epidemic."

Unlike John Knowles—the only other MGH personality of this era to acquire comparable, if not identical, public recognition—White did not have a propensity for speaking in headlines, nor did he cut a rakish figure. He was, rather, the quintessential doctor: wise, avuncular, and gentle. Castleman, who knew White as both colleague and patient, said simply, "He was a lovable person who would never say no to anyone." And there was his manner, at once assured and unassuming, and his ability to communicate human concern. The glare of publicity made White uneasy. "I accommodated myself slowly and with difficulty," he acknowledged, "emerging from the relatively quiet life of a practicing physician and teacher of medicine." Though never entirely comfortable with being approached by strangers, he learned to appreciate the usefulness of fame in promoting the causes of medicine and world peace.

"Time was kind to Dr. White," Bland concluded. "As the years advanced he took in stride a little angina and even a small infarct, but his continued good health and vigor remained an inspiration to all. In 1971, at the age of 85, he went with the first group of American physicians to mainland China and the following year welcomed his Chinese hosts to the U.S.A. He viewed this exchange of visits with great satisfaction, for in these later years it was his hope that somehow physicians in many lands united by international associations and dedicated to the saving of lives might likewise help save a troubled world. These thoughts were in his mind, as were the plans for a new book, when the end came, peacefully, in the eighty-eighth year of his age."

Chester Morse Jones

PERRY J. CULVER

Chester Morse Jones was born in Portland, Maine, in 1891, and grew up in Newton, Massachusetts. He left among his papers an autobiographic fragment, written in 1944, in which he described his early years as follows:

After graduation from the Newton High School, I took a routine academic course at Williams College, graduating in 1913, and then proceeded to go into the investment business without any thought of entering any profession. I chalked up a complete failure as a salesman, and thought it wise to choose something that did not involve business in any form. I did not feel good enough to be a minister, or crooked enough to be a lawyer, so arbitrarily decided to go into medicine. This necessitated making up premedical prerequisites, a lot of which was done through the University of Chicago Correspondence School. With this as a background I entered the Harvard Medical School in 1915 and graduated in 1919.

The Medical School, of course, was a rather distracted and harrowing experience after the first two years because of the acceleration during the First World War. Along with several others in my class, I started an internship without the benefit of any fourth year medicine and received my degree some months after the war internship, making up several months' school work. The internship was at the Massachusetts General Hospital on the old East Medical Service. My one war experience consisted in work at Halifax during the disaster [an explosion, December 6, 1917, of ammunition ships in the harbor, that caused 1,600 deaths], as part of the MGH Unit, while I was a third year student, and subsequently covering the needs of the Harvard Regiment along with 12 other members of my class. . . .

With this very inadequate and haphazard medical training, I then started to settle down to the job of obtaining a proper medical education. I was fortunate enough to be assigned to work under Dr. George Minot at his laboratory at the MGH on the rate of formation of bile pigments in the various anemias and biliary tract conditions. Stemming from this by pure chance, I edged into the gastrointestinal field via the duodenal tube, and devoted a large measure of my interest to the digestive tract and biliary disorders from then on. In addition, I carried out numerous studies on pancreatic enzymes, and started seriously to observe and study the mechanism of pain arising from various levels of the gastrointestinal tract.

In 1924 I was awarded the Moseley Travelling Fellowship to study in Europe, and after going through some of the English and Scandinavian clinics, I settled at the University of Strasbourg under Professor Leon Blum.

In 1925 Jones returned to the MGH where he spent the greater part of his professional life in both research and practice on various broad problems of alimentary function. He ascended the academic ladder to become clinical professor of medicine at Harvard.

Jones was one of the pioneer gastroenterologists in the United States, yet he abhorred the term *gastroenterology* when used to define a subspecialty. He believed very strongly that a complete physician must be well trained in all fields of internal medicine and be able to diagnose and treat all internal medical diseases while placing special emphasis upon the diseases of the gastrointestinal tract.

Jones, together with Leland McKittrick, the surgeon, and Erich Lindemann, the psychiatrist, founded the first Gastrointestinal Clinic in the Outpatient Department at the MGH in 1924. This clinic was supported by the Social Service and the Dietary departments, and its patients received comprehensive advice and care. Meanwhile, within the hospital Jones' thorough understanding of surgical procedures won him the respect of the general surgeons who often consulted him before operating; his knowledge of surgery also enabled him to explain procedures and complications to his patients with great understanding.

Jones was a master of the art of history taking and an expert at physical examination. All the students and residents who came within his purview were drilled over and over until they could take an excellent history with attention to even the most minute details. In fact, Jones sometimes said that the difference between a consultant and a regular physician was simply that the consultant tried to get an absolutely precise history, engaging in extensive discussion with the patient in order to understand the patient's description of particular symptoms.

Jones was a demanding teacher, expecting the greatest output from himself and little less from the students and young doctors who worked with him. There was no fellowship training. The young physicians who helped Jones care for his private patients experienced a preceptorship that was much more intense than any fellowship could possibly be. Alexander Leaf, who had Jones as his first Visit on Bulfinch 2 when he arrived at the MGH as a "very green intern" in 1944, recalled: "I was enormously impressed by his broad clinical knowledge and his detailed information about each patient on our service. Rounds in those days started at 10 A.M. and often went on until 2:30 or 3:00 P.M., with Jones fascinated by each patient we presented to him."

In addition to his ability to stimulate young physicians, Jones had a remarkably creative imagination which led him to develop hypotheses for research projects after observing a curious phenomenon in only a few patients. His laboratory was known as "Dr. Jones' Lab," and the succession of people who worked with him in the care of his patients and in clinical research were called the "Jones' Boys." He constantly questioned his "boys" as to what the answers to questions might be and how they could be discovered in the laboratory and by clinical observation on the wards. By 1980 standards Jones' laboratory was most modest. In general there were one or two technicians, occasionally three or four when several projects were underway at the same time. Funding for research was miniscule; Jones obtained a few grants over the years, but much of the research in the laboratory was supported by his own patient income. In addition to all the clinical and laboratory tests on his own private patients, a number of important research projects were undertaken in Jones' laboratory over the years.

Following his interest in bile pigments, Jones became interested in the localization of pain in the gastrointestinal tract. By inserting balloons at various levels and observing the neurologic pathway for pain referral, he studied digestive tract pain and published a remarkable and still valid text on the subject. In the late thirties, in conjunction with several other investigators including a psychiatrist, Jones carried out many studies on mucous colitis. He coined the term *rectal blush* to describe the coloring of the mucosa when patients were emotionally upset. He also became interested in the appearance of the mucosa of the stomach in pernicious anemia when the rigid gastroscope was introduced; together with Dr. Edward Benedict, he recorded observations on the mucosa in anemic patients and also spoke of the value of the use of the gastroscope.

During the war years Jones turned his attention to the cause and management of peptic ulcer, including the vagotomy operation and the production of pepsin. He was also concerned about wound healing and from 1939 to 1942 studied the concentration of vitamin C in the body fluids of animals and humans and determined the rate of healing according to the amount of vitamin C present. This was an important discovery. In the late forties when needle biopsy of the liver became available, Jones directed studies of the effects of various types of nutrition, including vitamins and other supplements, and of bed rest on the course of subacute and chronic hepatitis. Somewhat later he guided an investigation of the effects of anesthesia on liver disease. Further studies on pain in the lower esophagus and in the duodenum and common bile duct were carried out, and the neurologic pathways were discovered in 1949. The effect of anticolonergic on motility of the gastrointestinal tract with the use of barium radiography studies was another project of interest to him.

Immediately following World War II Jones and the "Jones' Boys" used the resources of Ward 4 to carry out a number of studies on malnutrition and intestinal absorption. Various tests for malabsorption and maldigestion were modified or developed in the Jones Lab: fat and nitrogen balance studies, d-xylose absorption tests, microscopic examination of the stool to determine pancreatic insufficiency by the presence of undigested muscle fibers and unsplit fats. Jones and his teams studied patients with postgastrectomy steatorrhea, celiac disease or nontropical sprue, and those with pancreatic insufficiency, among others. Various supplements were administered to improve the intestinal absorption of fat. Antibiotics were given to patients with blind loop syndrome and small bowel diverticula with malabsorption to determine the effect of reduction of bacteria upon intestinal absorption of nutrients. Also during this era a large study was conducted in cooperation with the Fatigue Laboratory of Harvard University of the effects of vitamin supplements on a series of chronic diseases including ulcerative colitis, ileitis, arthritis, and liver disease.

For several years beginning in 1950 Jones conducted a fourth-year elective for one month in gastroenterology for ten students from the senior class of the Harvard Medical School; it was an exciting experience for both Jones and his "boys." The students who participated in this course are now among the leaders in internal medicine and gastroenterology throughout the United States. It was one more manifestation of the creativity and greatness of Jones as a teacher and a stimulator.

In the closing remarks of his presidential address to the American College of Physicians, he exhorted the new fellows and members of the College to present to the public, "by example and precept, the image of what Plato described as 'the true Physician'—a healer of the sick and not a maker of money; and the image of that individual described by Chaucer in a ringing phrase as one who would 'gladly learn and gladly teach.' The price of teaching is not small," Jones said, "but the rewards are great and these include in the end greater learning."

Fuller Albright

Fuller Albright was born in January in the last year of the nineteenth century. His childhood and youth were passed in that period of peace, prosperity, and general optimism that came to an end with the outbreak of World War I. His father was an industrialist, art patron, and philanthropist. His mother, a Fuller from Lancaster, Massachusetts, embodied the finest traditions of New England culture. It was a large, happy, and close-knit family in which parents and children spent much of their lives together—whether at the great house in Buffalo, on long summer vacations at the family camp in the Adirondacks, during winter holidays at Jekyll Island, Georgia, or on the Grand Tour of Europe.

It was a family characterized by a strong sense of humor, and no child growing up in it was in danger of developing an attitude of self-importance. Nor were the close family ties confining. It was a hospitable household with a constant flow of visitors. However, when he entered Harvard College at the age of 17, young Albright was possessed of a naiveté which was unusual even in those days and an appearance which was positively cherubic! that look of boyish innocence somehow stayed with him always. He also displayed a natural ebullience and gregariousness which enabled him to fit easily into the society of a Harvard undergraduate in the Boston community. In the Delphic Club at Harvard he established friendships that he cherished all his life.

He graduated from college in three years and entered Harvard Medical School in the fall of 1920. It was when he started to see patients that his long-range goals began to take form. At this time striking advances in medical research were being reported: James Howard Means returned from a medical meeting to announce the dramatic discovery of insulin, and biochemistry was beginning to furnish new insights into the functioning of the body. Albright's natural curiosity was stimulated by the possibilities of applying the new discoveries to the study of disease. It was whetted too by the emotional experience of observing at first hand what insulin could do for a patient near death from uncontrolled diabetes. Throughout his later career his investigations were apt to be linked to the puzzles his own patients presented to him rather than to abstract problems of biochemistry.

After an internship in medicine at the MGH, he spent a year of research with Joseph C. Aub whose studies in lead poisoning meshed closely with Albright's burgeoning interest in the metabolism of calcium. In this happy environment in the company of Aub, Means, and Walter Bauer, his latent talent began to blossom and clearly indicated the career that he should follow. Then came a year as assistant resident at Johns Hopkins under Warfield Longcope where he struck up an acquaintance with John E. Howard who shared his interest in endocrinology. They became fast friends and for years were in almost constant communication, trying out new ideas on each other. Often when such ideas reached fruition, neither of them knew whose it was in the first place—nor cared. Before returning to Boston Albright spent a year in Vienna with the pathologist Jacob Erdheim, who proved to be an inspiring preceptor and whom he continued to quote for many years.

The remainder of Albright's professional life was spent in research, teaching, and practice at the MGH. It was an extraordinarily productive career which brought forth new concepts in endocrinology and delineated a number of hitherto unrecognized diseases. During this period he had associated with him in his laboratory a succession of young investigators who became leaders in the field of endocrinology in this country and abroad.

In 1932 he was married to Claire Birge of New York in what proved to be a supremely happy match. Claire was a superb hostess, and their household provided warm hospitality to hosts of students and visitors from all parts of the world. They had two sons.

Albright's friend and colleague Howard wrote of him: "He had an amazing capacity for collecting facts from all sorts of disciplines and attempting to correlate them into homogenous patterns, with the idea of developing imaginative hypotheses which could be put to experimental test. There was simply no end to his thirst for knowledge. This was all carried out with a gentle and humble manner so that students were infatuated with him and fellows flocked to his door from all over the world. Fuller was interested in people, and nearly all his investigative efforts stemmed from clinical problems that he had met at the bedside or in outpatients. It should perhaps be said here that no small part of the success of Albright's efforts was provided by Means, who gave him his wholehearted support with funds and the use of Ward 4 (Metabolism Unit) to permit unhampered scope for the investigative flights of fancy which constantly emanated from his brain."

Albright's clinical investigations were highly original and far-reaching. His name is associated with the early clinical description of hyperparathyroidism and with the distinction between overactivity of all parathyroid tissue and the effect of adenoma of a single parathyroid gland. He called attention to the association of hyperparathyroidism with kidney stones, and on the basis of an extensive study carried out in his Stone Clinic, he laid the foundation for modern diagnosis and treatment of this condition. In his laboratory was developed a method of measuring gonadotropins in the urine which made it possible to characterize various types of amenorrhea as well as disorders of testicular function. In 1937 he described a condition that has come to be known as Albright's syndrome, the distinguishing features of which are precocious puberty in girls, cystic bone disease, and brownish pigmentation of the skin. More than half a dozen other original descriptions of disease might with equal propriety have borne his name: He pointed out the role of steatorrhea in depleting the body of fat-soluble vitamins; he first described renal tubular acidosis and its effective treatment with alkali; he called attention to the occurrence of thinning of the bones in women following menopause; he was among the first to use estrogen to inhibit ovulation in women and progesterone to correct the metropathia caused by estrogens; he unravelled the pathogenesis of Cushing's syndrome and sounded the first warnings of the harmful side effects of steroids on the tissues.

A total of 118 scientific papers bear his name, and his book *The Parathyroid Glands and Metabolic Bone Disease,* published in 1948, is still a prime source of information on the subject. He was the recipient of honors and awards from universities and learned societies all over the world. He was president of the American Society for Clinical Investigations in 1943–1944 and of the Association for the Study of Internal Secretions (later called the Endocrine Society) in 1946–1947.

In 1935, at the height of his productivity, the early signs of Parkinson's disease made their appearance. John Howard recalled, "It was when we were sharing a room together at Atlantic City and both lying on the bed polishing talks for the next day's meetings that Fuller suddenly turned to me and said: 'You've been looking at my thumb; do you think I am getting Parkinson's disease?' I had indeed been observing the first hints of pill-rolling movements but denied the thought of Parkinson's." The symptoms progressed gradually but relentlessly for nearly two decades; by 1940, for example, he was no longer writing in patients' charts. This long period was one of almost feverish activity for him, as if he were trying to outstrip the inexorable advance of his disease. He maintained, nevertheless, a sublime indifference to his disability and managed to communicate complex ideas with extraordinary lucidity. Finally in 1956 he underwent the newly devised surgical treatment for Parkinson's disease, although he was advised that he was a poor candidate for the operation; it left him worse off than before. The remainder of his life was spent in helpless invalidism, mitigated only by a clouding of the sensorium and the devoted care of nurses and attendants at the MGH.

In 1955 Harvard awarded Fuller Albright the honorary degree of Doctor of Science with the following citation: "Brilliant investigator in the complex field of nutrition and metabolism, your keen mind and enormous courage are a credit to this University and to Medicine."

His tastes were simple. He was never so happy as when casting a trout fly in an Adirondack lake, unless it was when talking shop with a colleague. He loved a good game of bridge. He had a good eye for color and form, but no ear at all for music. He and his wife Claire were both fond of travel and did a good deal of it in this country, in Europe, and in South America. His dress reflected his lack of self-consciousness: Who can forget the old tweed jacket, the baggy trousers, and the jaunty bow tie?

One of Dr. Albright's best remembered characteristics was the twinkle in his eye, which was a manifestation of his unconquerable *joie de vivre* and a slightly amused outlook on the human condition. He carried his sense of humor into his medical writings and even into his lectures with his simple line diagrams, a rare accomplishment indeed, which added immensely to his effectiveness and popularity.

In a tribute to Albright published in 1962, one of his young collaborators wrote as follows:

What about the personality of this remarkable investigator under whose luminous common sense so many knotty problems suddenly seemed simple? He never discussed personalities. His private life was uneventfully happy. He married Claire Birge and lived happily thereafter in a serene and comfortable home where friends from all over the world were received. What about his heroic battles with his tragic disease? Was it, after all, heroism which made him refuse to stop doing what he liked to do or was it just more of his famous common sense? His indifference to pity was the indifference of a profoundly serene and happy man to public opinion of any kind. Perhaps Claire's role was more heroic; certainly it was brilliant. Charming, vivacious and full of enthusiasm she appeared perfectly carefree as she added to her domestic duties the jobs of chauffeur, secretary and finally nurse and shouldered all the burdens of the man of the house while appearing to depend on her husband. Although he never was made to feel dependent on his wife, Fuller could not have continued to work productively without her. Perhaps they were both heroes, but they were certainly not martyrs. Martyrs are never so widely loved and respected in their own time.

Adapted from a Memorial Minute, *Harvard University Gazette,* Vol. LXVI, No. 19, Jan. 29, 1971, with the assistance of *Eleanor B. Pyle*

14. The Medical Services, 1965–1980

ALEXANDER LEAF

No history of the Medical Services would be complete without some comments on its growth in the past 15 years. Success during this period has been measured in terms of research funds attracted to the department, and money means more salaries for more staff. But more good staff of the quality that the MGH attracts means more successful exciting research, which means more research money and more staff. Thus growth occurs almost exponentially, although we all realize that funding will not increase indefinitely to support all the worthy projects we can conceive. From 1966 to 1980 the number of Medical Service staff appointees increased from 140 to 288. The number of house staff increased from 36 to 66, and the number of clinical and research fellows increased from 116 to 133 (this number came close to 200 during several of the recent intervening years).

This increase in staff results from the many new things physicians can do for their patients and the perception at the MGH that we must be prepared and able to provide everything that modern technology and practice can offer to those who seek our care. The doubling of the numbers of the house staff with a constant number of Medical Service beds reflects in part the increased levels of illness of our patients; we keep them alive longer, and this requires more intensive care which is labor intensive of physicians, nurses, and all other health workers. As a celebration of the move of the Medical Services to the Bigelow Building I was able to point out that the doubling of the house staff that occurred during my years as chief was not accompanied by an increase in the number of medical beds but, rather, was associated with a similar doubling of the medical staff. I therefore argued that a major function of the house staff was to care for the staff—which has at least a small grain of truth.

Medicine, unlike Surgery which included within its residency programs all the training required for passing the surgical specialty boards, depended on fellowships for subspecialty training. We felt quite virtuous because this relieved the hospital of the costs of subspecialty training in cardiology, pulmonary diseases, nephrology, etc. However, in the past ten years it became evident that clinical training grants in subspecialties would dry up, as it had become clear that we were already training too many subspecialists when the country needed generalists and primary physicians. Yet at the same time it was clear that for the convenience of running the hospital we needed a cadre of clinical fellows to respond to the subspecialty needs of patients and to assist the subspecialty consultants with their clinical loads and teaching. These fellows, obviously, are invaluable and exciting to have around. Thus I estimated the number of full-time equivalent clinical fellows needed for the subspecialty services, and Charles Sanders funded 22 positions under the rubric of essential medical residents.

One can appreciate the effect on medical practice and on increasing costs of medical care generally, and the potential danger to the referral of patients to the

MGH and other teaching hospitals, as our excellent subspecialty trainees move out into the community and are fully competent to manage the clinical problems that previously came to us. Several university hospitals have found empty beds and insufficient patients to maintain their clinical teaching functions as a result of the growth in numbers of qualified subspecialists in their communities. Although I tried hard to reduce subspecialty training opportunities, I succeeded only in decreasing the 22 positions to 18. I was resisted totally by the unit chiefs in all attempts to diminish their numbers of clinical fellows; my admonitions to train only those required for replacement in time fell on deaf ears. And, of course, the financial rewards—as well as the real or imagined intellectual satisfaction— of being a certified medical subspecialist bring ever-increasing numbers of prime applicants for training to our subspecialty units.

The days of unrestrained growth and unlimited resources now belong to the past. There will follow a period of retrenchment. Less support for research will mean austerity and some reduction in research activities. The availability of funds differs among branches of medicine. It is likely that more monies will continue to be available for cancer and heart research than for research on infectious diseases or arthritis. Thus oncology or cardiac units may remain large, with adequate research opportunities, while excellent investigators in other fields may have to close their laboratories for lack of funds. The imbalances already present within the Medical Services may even be intensified by the general but uneven reduction in federal funding. More of the faculty will have to be supported by clinical income; this will subtract more time from academic and scholarly efforts which, in turn, will erode the ability to compete for the dwindling research dollars.

The Medical Services are very vulnerable fiscally. In 1978–1979, for example, the total cost of professional salaries was $9,659,646, of which $1,550,688 was for salaries and fringe benefits for medical residents (64) and essential clinical fellows (18). Subtracting the house staff salaries leaves only 18 percent of professional salaries on "hard monies"; 52 percent comes from research grants. As federal research funds become scarce, there will have to be an increased dependence on clinical earnings to support the staff, and some of the research activities may have to be curtailed.

The Move to the Bigelow Building. In 1944 when I came to the MGH as an intern, the Medical Services consisted of four open wards in the original Bulfinch Building; in addition B-3 on the third floor accommodated our intensive care beds shared by the four ward teams. Bulfinch 4 consisted of the ten clinical research beds and was restricted to research admissions. The 87 medical beds served the teaching unit for the Medical Services, though Bauer had succeeded in securing the understanding that every bed in the Baker and Phillips House occupied by a medical patient was also a "teaching bed."

When the Medicare legislation was passed in 1967 guaranteeing payment for semiprivate hospital accommodations for all Medicare patients, it was evident that we would soon have difficulty keeping the Bulfinch beds filled. In no way could those large open wards be regarded as semiprivate accommodations. I measured the space and drew up plans to divide the wards into two-bed, double-occupancy rooms. We would have lost three beds on each ward in so doing, but an even greater problem was the stipulation that semiprivate accommodations include a window in each room. There was no way to accomplish this. Chopping through the 4- to 6-foot thick granite walls of the Bulfinch was prohibited, and painting window scenes on a wall in each room was unacceptable.

In fact, occupancy in the Bulfinch did diminish, and I began to agitate for new semiprivate medical facilities. Since John Knowles had had the Gray Building constructed with the shell of the tower ready to house later needs, this seemed the natural place in which to relocate the Medical Services. Architectural assistance was obtained, and a Determination of Need certificate procured. I had thought that we might accommodate the four wards of the Bulfinch on two floors and accomplish major economies in nurses' stations and service facilities. But the architects found that it would be necessary to cantilever the two floors in order to accommodate the beds. This was too much for the administration and trustees who, having just raised the money for the shell, would now have to tear out the walls. Thus we were assigned two extra floors, and the final arrangement on four floors provided a spacious excellent facility for the Medical Services.

Another foible related to restrictions on hospital construction to contain costs was that the number of beds was limited to exactly the number we had in the Bulfinch Building. However, there was no restriction on the space that the beds could occupy. Thus I succeeded in moving the beds from 14,000 square feet in Bulfinch to 44,000 square feet in the Bigelow Building!

Although the architects had experience in hospital construction, the questions of what facilities would be in the rooms, how many isolation rooms would be created, and all the details of the service areas were decisions I was expected to make. Actually I shared this responsibility with Dan Federman who seemed to have a knack for designing the service, just as he reveals a knack for virtually everything he does. Nevertheless when the construction was completed I feared that the first occupancy of the new quarters might disclose some horrendous oversight on our part and a major expensive deficiency would have to be corrected. For this reason I was able to contain my impatience to move the Medical Services to the Bigelow when it was decided that the Surgical Services would be the first occupants of our new home for a few months while White 6 and 7 were refurbished. If any flaws were to be uncovered, let them be found and corrected by the Surgical Services so that all would be perfect when we moved in.

The year we moved out of the Bulfinch to the Bigelow Building was a traumatic one for the house staff. Their conservatism invariably astounds me, but that they became contentious and almost rebellious over the move from antiquated and dismal facilities to the modern hospital accommodations of the Bigelow really boggled my mind. Nevertheless, many hours were spent listening to their complaints and reproaches that we were changing things in their training of which they had not been apprised before they started their residencies—a charge they invariably invoked when any change was introduced in their program. The house staff felt so threatened by the move that they literally destroyed Arnold Weinberg's ability to serve as assistant chief of service. It took all George Thibault's and my diplomacy to calm them down. Needless to say, once the move was accomplished, they would not have returned to life in the Bulfinch again for anything.

It is true that we made one major alteration in deployment of the house staff in moving to the Bigelow. In the Bulfinch Building we had all four teams follow their own very sick patients when they were moved to the intensive care beds on Bulfinch 3. This was the time-honored mode of practice, but often when one very sick patient on Bulfinch 3 demanded the attention of the resident during an evening and night, the patients on the lower floors, who were not so desperately ill, were virtually ignored. This led some of the staff, such as Stephen Goldfinger and Homayoun Kazemi, to advise that we have a separate team for the intensive care unit. I thought we should try this arrangement on Bigelow 8; we could always go back to the old system if the new one didn't seem to work satisfactorily.

That medical residents should fear trying something different at their age is worrisome to me. Change will always be with us, and when change is thoughtfully introduced to improve a situation, how can rational adults be so conservative as to refuse even to give change a try? I first sensed this degree of conservatism in the Bulfinch; we had our residents on every other night, and they were often exhausted with no time to read or think. I wanted to change to one night in three to give them two free nights for every one they had to work. I discussed my plan with them expecting no resistance. To my astonishment they held meetings of their own and spoke out against the change—for the best altruistic reasons. They argued that being on every other night they got to know their patients well, but if they missed two nights with their patients, they would lose touch. Furthermore, with a third resident on each team to cover one of the nights, they would have to communicate to two persons rather than one, and surely things would get fouled up by such redundancy. We took a vote, and the residents voted down my proposal. The next year I decided to divide the East and West services as a controlled experiment. On the West Service two residents would rotate nights on call in the traditional manner, while on the East a third house officer was assigned to share the rotation and everyone had two free nights out of every three. After one year the entire house staff had been exposed to both systems and, of course, that time they voted for my proposal.

Working with some of the brightest, most highly motivated, and often nicest young people anywhere is one of the greatest pleasures of being chief of Medicine, but this one character flaw, of extreme resistance to change, in such an exceptional group astonishes me. It cropped up over and over again in successive generations of house staff.

When we finally made the move to the Bigelow floors there were actually a few tears shed the night before. The transition was made remarkably smoothly, and I've never heard from anyone a wish to return to the Bulfinch. After 160 years, it was time for a change.

Personal Reflections on the Medical Services.

On January 1, 1966, it was with a feeling of great humility, but with pride and dedication, that I moved into Bauer's office on Bulfinch 1 and assumed the direction of what was then recognized as the leading Department of Medicine in the country. On May 1, 1981, I moved out of the Medical Services office on Bigelow 6 to make room for my successor with mixed feelings of pleasure and concern. The pleasure came from knowing that my successor, John Potts, was one of my protégés and exactly the right person to carry on—my own choice, if it had been up to me. The pleasure was also in the knowledge that after $15\frac{1}{3}$ years, I turned over to him what was still the premier Department of Medicine in the country and a staff of excellent physicians, teachers, and investigators that he would enjoy working with, even as I had. The flow of outstanding medical residents and fellows through the department and the opportunity to structure for them the best possible training experiences that the resources of the MGH provide were singular privileges and sources of satisfaction.

The concerns related to the difficult times ahead, with reduction in funding for our vast academic activities and even for clinical services that we regard as important. The combination of fiscal reductions and increased bureaucratic regulations has the potential for stifling much of what has been precious to me at the MGH. To me the MGH has always been a place where young, meritorious physicians were given every opportunity to train and grow in stature as clinicians, teachers, and scientists. We kept a few of the successful ones when the opportunity, space, and funding made this possible. Others moved to positions of distinction at other major academic institutions, and we were nearly as proud of them as of those who remained with us. It has been a time of exciting growth and unlimited horizons for dreams and accomplishments.

But just at a time when the new biology promises to yield its greatest rewards, doubts about the worth of science are widespread in the public and in government. The almighty dollar is being worshipped increasingly inside and outside medicine. We are now big business, and the privilege of being a bit remote from the marketplace with time to think big thoughts and pursue them in clinical and laboratory studies is being eroded. Whether we can ever recover the simple, undisturbed state with the respect, esteem, and support of our fellow citizens seems unlikely. The very technological imperative that we have helped create carries us with it into bigger, more complex, and more expensive functional organization in which interdependence increasingly replaces personal freedom.

These are new times. There is no turning back. The real and potential problems of world overpopulation, threat of nuclear war, pollution of the environment, too rapid consumption of our resources, demands of the Third World for its share of the world's produce, inflation, unemployment in the United States, increased materialism, and crime are all part of the present social fabric in which the future of medicine is enmeshed and will influence the life of every physician as well as medical centers—even the greatest such as the MGH. Now more than ever do we have to clarify our principles and exemplify all that is best in the long tradition of medicine to serve humanity.

15. The Medical Units

The partitioning of the Medical Services into subspecialty units, which began several decades ago, continued throughout the period under review as the department grew and the number of disciplines relevant to its operation proliferated. Several volumes might be filled with the work of the MGH medical units over the past quarter century; of necessity only the major activities have been described in this volume. The subjects of outpatient and community care have received a more detailed examination than others, a discussion appropriate to their role in the development of the hospital as a whole.

The Chief's View

ALEXANDER LEAF

By the time this writer took over as chief of Medicine in 1966 the unit system was well established. Dr. Bauer had formally enunciated the view that Medicine at the MGH would be divided into units representing each of the medical subspecialties, and these units taken together would constitute the guts of the Medical Services, embellished by clinical colleagues engaged in the full-time practice of clinical medicine. Of course, before Bauer, subspecialties had developed in several areas of medicine. Dr. Means recognized a thyroid unit, which he headed; a cardiac unit, directed by P. D. White; a gastrointestinal unit, headed by Chester Jones; an endocrine unit, directed by Fuller Albright; and an arthritis unit, headed by Bauer. There were other key physicians regarded as consultants in new subspecialty areas: Helen Pittman in pulmonary diseases, Wyman Richardson in hematology, Richard Field in diabetes, and Robert Sterling Palmer in hypertension, while I provided an embryonic renal, fluid, and electrolyte consultative service.

With Bauer the concept came to full fruition and, unlike Means, who seemed content to have a few very distinguished units leading in their research activities, Bauer's view was that each subspecialty of medicine should be represented by a unit in which clinical teaching and research activities would be combined and each would be the best of its kind. In 1966 there were 12 subspecialty units in medicine; at the end of my chairmanship there were 23.

Bauer's imprint on the unit system is evident despite many changes. He had realized that, though we would seek the most outstanding persons as unit chiefs, one individual would not encompass all the activities necessary to develop strong clinical and investigative subspecialties. His goal was to acquire a physician-scientist—as he called us—to head up the unit and let that individual recruit or recommend other colleagues who would flesh out the clinical services, teaching, and research activities. He advised that, given two topnotch physicians, one with proven research interest and the other with strengths as clinician and teacher, always select the one with research accomplishments as your unit chief. The physician with research accomplishments will attract and pick good clinical colleagues for his unit, while the clinician-teacher will not appreciate the need for, or be able to attract and develop, the research activities within the unit, which Bauer felt was the core of the unit system. The excitement created by an active research program is what attracts the bright young student, resident, or fellow and perpetuates excellence in the system. On a couple of occasions when I failed to follow his advice and selected a clinician-teacher as head of a unit, the system failed and the Medical Service was saddled with a mediocre unit. This attitude of Bauer's, which I share, does not demean the great importance of the clinician to the functioning of the service. It only confronts the reality that stagnation is avoided and intellectual excitement is created and sustained by the atmosphere of good research, and that the person responsible for the health of the unit must understand and nurture good research—a very difficult task for one who doesn't himself engage in and get his kicks from research: a simple fact of life.

Allergy Unit

ALEXANDER LEAF

The MGH Allergy Unit was founded in 1919 by Francis M. Rackemann who directed it until 1948. Walter S. Burrage was in charge until 1956, and Robert L. Berg was the unit's full time chief from 1956 to 1958. Looking back upon those two years, Berg reflected, "In the mid-fifties there were few links between the findings in the laboratory and the practice of allergy. An interesting similarity was to be found, indeed, among the specialties of allergy, dermatology, and psychiatry, where clinical practice had little relationship to the broaching of new frontiers in research, while each had developed a clinical style that required the patient to return at frequent intervals.

"In 1956 Walter Bauer suggested I should take on the unit as Burrage retired. Rackemann and Burrage continued active work in the clinic and as beneficent advisors to the program. Rackemann would still invite the allergy group to his combined clinical office and study at his Beacon Street home in the evening for discussion of research and clinical issues.

"Subsequently, Sidney Leskowitz created a new laboratory unit for the investigation of basic immunologic phenomena. . . . That brief interlude of two years was an eye-opener for me in the sense of seeing two superb clinicians, Rackemann and Burrage, provide care for hundreds of private and clinic patients with warmth, tolerance, and good humor. They managed, meanwhile, to keep happy and enthusiastic a group of part-time faculty who respected them mightily."

Following Berg's departure, Bauer brought in Francis Cabot Lowell from Boston University in June 1959. Lowell functioned as a classical allergist with his homemade brews of allergens used to desensitize patients with sneezes, running noses, and dermal and gastrointestinal allergies. A few drug trials of anti-allergens for pharmaceutical firms constituted the research efforts of the unit.

Nevertheless, the unit cared for a large number of ambulatory patients in the Allergy Clinic whom they were desensitizing or treating with various medications. Asthmatic patients treated primarily with corticosteroids were included in their large outpatient population, and patients were also seen in consultation on the ward services. Initially many respiratory problems such as emphysema and asthma were brought to the Allergy Unit; then the Pulmonary Unit became more active clinically, and they, too, now see many of these patients, both atopic and nonatopic. Otherwise, however, the allergy group had little visibility within the hospital.

When Lowell retired in 1976, Leaf appointed Kurt Bloch as chief of a new unit of clinical immunology and allergy. With the rapid development of immunology as a basic medical science, many insights into human disease became apparent. Both deficiencies and overactivity of the immune system can cause human disease, and methods of measuring immune system activity were being introduced. Bloch, with a background in rheumatology on the Medical Services, had proven himself to be not only interested in and capable of applying the new immunology to the patient population of the MGH but also a master teacher of the new discipline. Diagnosis and treatment of patients have been greatly strengthened by the facilities of the Clinical Immunology Unit. Since allergies result from aberrations of reactivity of the immune system, it seemed reasonable to combine allergy and clinical immunology.

Bloch's unit has worked closely with the Pulmonary Unit in its management of asthma and has shared fellows in clinical training programs. With the strengths of the Pathology Department in immunology, close relationships have developed with that department, although occasional jurisdictional disputes have surfaced regarding teaching roles and territory with respect to certain clinical immunologic tests. Overall, redefinition of this unit has been salutary, and Bloch has provided dedicated leadership.

With the assistance of *Robert L. Berg*

Arthritis Unit

STEPHEN M. KRANE

The Robert W. Lovett Memorial Group for the Study of Diseases Causing Deformities—named after the orthopedic surgeon who had cared for President Franklin D. Roosevelt—was established jointly at the Harvard Medical School and the MGH. It was under the active leadership of Walter Bauer from 1930 until he became Jackson Professor in 1951. Bauer initially emphasized pathology as the major scientific discipline of the group. This provided the background for careful, detailed, long-term observations of patients with rheumatic and other skeletal diseases. With Granville Bennett, L. R. Morrison, and later Peter Kulka, definitive descriptions of the articular and extraarticular pathology of rheumatoid arthritis were forthcoming. Other work led to important observations on the composition of synovial fluid and the alterations that occurred in it in disease. The clinical observations of this group brought order from chaos and improved understanding of the major rheumatic disorders such as rheumatoid arthritis, osteoarthritis, gout, and infectious arthritis.

The Lovett Group became one of the world centers for training and attracted individuals from all over. Bauer organized a broad program of research and made his viewpoint strongly felt—namely, that it was important for scientists and clinicians to work side by side, and, moreover, that it was necessary to have some individuals who combined research and clinical practice—his "physician-scientists." He thought that the mysteries of the rheumatic diseases would be solved by the study of connective tissue macromolecules, and he recruited young scientists interested in collagen, mucopolysaccharides (as they were then known), and glycoproteins to work with him while helping and encouraging them to establish their own independence. These young scientists who were brought into the group to direct their own laboratories included Jerome Gross, Roger W. Jeanloz, and Karl Schmid. Bauer was able to bring in money, and the group flourished.

When Bauer became Jackson Professor in 1951, he had less time to devote to directing the group, although he still played an active role clinically, in conferences, and in recruitment. He maintained a large practice with the assistance of such people as J. W. Zeller and William Clark. Clark was an important force in the clinical activities of the unit before he left for Western Reserve.

In the mid-fifties Evan Calkins was appointed chief of the Lovett Group. He had been Bauer's first full-time resident. By that time the group had a big clinical load. Marian Ropes and Charles Short, as clinicians, won an international reputation for the Lovett Group in the care of patients with rheumatic disease, and both were recognized by their colleagues in being elected to the presidency of the American Rheumatism Association. In addition to the outpatient service, there were the so-called state beds. Patients with rheumatic diseases could be kept on the wards for up to six months, supported by the state. These beds disappeared when the state swung its support to the new Lemuel Shattuck Hospital, and with them went the luxury of studying and taking care of a relatively large number of patients with chronic disease in a general hospital devoted primarily to the care of people with acute illness.

Calkins pursued his interest in amyloidosis and later brought in a clinical and research fellow, Alan S. Cohen, who became very involved in the amyloid project. His studies on the fine structure of amyloid in tissues showed that it was a fibrous protein and that it could be extracted from tissue in relatively pure form, thus making possible its biochemical characterization. Cohen became director of rheumatology at Boston University and then chief of the B.U. Division at the Boston City Hospital. He continues his work on amyloidosis and maintains a strong research program. Jeanloz, meanwhile, had built up his laboratory and attracted a number of excellent people in carbohydrate chemistry.

When in 1961 Calkins was lured away to Buffalo to become chairman of the Department of Medicine there, Bauer agonized over his replacement. Finally he appointed Stephen Krane, who had been one of his chief residents and a postdoctoral research fellow with Carl Cori at Washington University in St. Louis. At the time Krane was working in the Endocrine Unit on collagen and the process of bone mineralization, collaborating with Melvin Glimcher, then a promising young orthopedist-scientist.* Krane became head of the clinical unit of the Lovett Group. Within a few years the group came to be composed of three laboratories: Gross was head of the Developmental Biology Laboratory, Jeanloz head of the Carbohydrate Research Laboratory, and Krane head of the Arthritis Unit. (Schmid had moved to Boston University.)

Gross had come to the MGH after working with F. O. Schmitt at MIT. He

*The material on Stephen Krane was written by John Mills.—Eds.

believed that the secret of rheumatic fever might be found in the biology of collagen and set out to explore that protein. He made major advances in the study of its ultrastructure and then in understanding its biosynthesis and fibrillogenesis. In the late fifties he was teamed with a young British pathologist, Charles Levene; together they made pioneering observations on lathyrism which set the stage for an understanding of the molecular structure of collagen. A few years later (1962), with Charles Lapiere, Gross discovered the animal collagenases and described their mechanism of action, opening up a new field of biologic research. Many talented investigators went through his laboratory and on to positions of leadership.

Jeanloz concentrated on exacting chemistry, proving the structure of the complex carbohydrates by meticulous synthesis. His work provided the basis for the elucidation of the structure of the glycoproteins on the cell surface. Some of the properties of malignant cells can be ascribed to those molecules. The efforts of many able scientists in Jeanloz' laboratory led to the understanding of the biosynthesis of these important cell constituents as well as other glycoproteins and complex polysaccharides.

Meanwhile, Krane was welcomed into the group. Ropes and Short were still active clinically and contributed generously of their time and experience. Of the Arthritis fellows, two of whom entered the training each year, a number were interested in both the clinic and the laboratory. Claude Bennett, a holdover from the Calkins era, started his important work on immunoglobulin structure at that time, collaborating with Edgar Haber. He predicted many of the genetic controls of immunoglobulin synthesis and went on to become, eventually, chairman of medicine at Alabama. John Mills stayed with the group studying lymphocyte interactions in tissue culture. He also developed an expertise in several clinical areas such as the vasculitides; he is now one of the ablest clinicians on the MGH staff. Dwight Robinson, who came to the MGH as an intern on the Surgical Service before turning to medicine, returned from the Biochemistry Department at Brandeis all fired up about enzyme mechanisms and protein structure. Later, with Lawrence Levine of Brandeis and Armen Tashjian at the Harvard Dental School, he began his research on prostaglandins and their role in inflammatory reactions. Robinson is considered one of the authorities on arachidonic acid metabolism as it relates to rheumatic diseases. Kurt Bloch, after several years of postdoctoral research in immunology with Zoltan Ovary at NYU, joined the unit to become director of the clinical laboratory that had been established by Dr. Ropes in the preceding decade. He subsequently became head of the Clinical Immunology and Allergy Unit, succeeding Francis Lowell, but still maintains ties with rheumatology.

After assuming the leadership of the Arthritis Unit in 1961, Krane continued his work on the mechanisms of ossification and bone disease assisted by a number of able clinical and research fellows including Charles Nagant, John Evanson, Graham Russell, and Edward Harris. A previously undescribed enzyme defect in collagen synthesis that was responsible for a familial form of bone disease was demonstrated. Important studies of bone metabolism in Paget's disease were undertaken and continue to the present time.

In 1973–1974, Krane was a visiting scientist at the Sir William Dunn School of Pathology at Oxford and on his return began studies of the control of inflammation and collagen breakdown in the rheumatoid joint. These, pursued with

Jean-Michael Dayer, led to investigation of the roles of lymphocytes and macrophages in the mechanism of inflammation. In recognition of this work, Krane was awarded the Heberden Medal in 1980.

The breadth of Krane's interest in biology is remarkable but is almost matched by his interest in those who work in biology. Journal Club meetings are enlivened by his vignettes offered at random of the authors of almost any paper submitted for discussion. His desk is legendary: Piled at least 18 inches high with journals, manuscripts, correspondence, and notebooks, one of the lower spots is used for writing on. Somewhat more orderly stacks of journals and files, the result of semiannual desk cleanups, stand about on chairs and tables. Above it all is a sign that reads, A NEAT DESK IS THE SIGN OF A SICK MIND.

The Arthritis Unit has changed in other ways over the past two decades. The state beds are gone and so is the affiliated rheumatology service at the Shattuck Hospital that was so ably run by Bob Pinals following his fellowship in the 1960s. Utilization review has altered the pattern of hospital stay along with the attitudes of staff and house staff. On the Bigelow service we cannot keep patients with rheumatoid arthritis for six months as we did on the Bulfinch wards. The house staff discharges patients as they deem necessary and are not subject to the powerful forces active in 1955. It is in part their loss, since they will probably not gain that feel for chronic illness that Bauer stressed and a generation of physicians learned from Marian Ropes. From the patient's perspective, however, long-term hospitalization is probably no longer especially valuable. A better understanding of inflammation promises new and better medical therapies for connective tissue diseases, and the success of surgical joint replacement has also altered the picture. Much of rheumatology is outpatient care.

An important role remains for rheumatology in an acute care hospital, however. Our relations with orthopedic surgery and endocrinology have been close, and we still have a major interest in the heritable, true connective-tissue disorders as well as in metabolic bone disease. In many respects we are unique among rheumatology groups in the country. Those in the laboratory still maintain clinical interests—another singular quality. Major contributions to the education of fellows are made by our full-time clinicians, Lawrence Miller and George Cohen, and by Martin Wohl of the Harvard University Health Service.

Walter Bauer trained many of the leaders in rheumatology in the thirties, forties, and fifties. In the sixties and seventies many of the laboratory investigators and clinicians who were associated with the Lovett Group also assumed positions of leadership elsewhere, taking with them some of the MGH traditions.

Cardiac Unit

EDGAR HABER

The Cardiac Unit was founded in 1914 by Paul Dudley White when he returned from a year's postgraduate study with Sir Thomas Lewis in London. His impact on the founding of the new discipline of cardiology is well documented in previous volumes of this history as well as in other chapters of this volume. Shortly after White was asked to be the first director of the National Heart Institute,

Edward Bland was appointed chief of the Cardiac Unit in 1949. Under his aegis the unit remained at the forefront of diagnosis and therapy.

In 1951, soon after Andre Cournand and Dickinson Richards had demonstrated the value of cardiac catheterization, a laboratory was built on a roof of the second floor of the White Building, and the first catheterizations were performed by Gordon Myers and Allan Friedlich. Gordon Scannell, a thoracic surgeon, helped in instituting the daring procedure of transthoracic left atrial catheterization. This provided more definitive diagnostic information, particularly with respect to mitral valve disease. As a result of the more precise information available from the cardiac catheter studies, Scannell was able to attack the stenotic mitral valve with confidence, and the era of intracardiac surgery at the MGH was born. During this period there were always two or three cardiac fellows training in the unit, supported by one of the earliest NIH training grants, which is now in its twenty-fourth year.

My own interest in cardiology developed while I was an intern at the MGH from 1956 to 1957. I was distressed by the frequency of sudden death in patients suffering from myocardial infarction and wondered what might be responsible. During nights and weekends, with the assistance of my wife-to-be, I constructed a device from spare parts that would activate an electrocardiograph machine when the rhythm of the heart changed. Working with Edwin Wheeler, a member of the Cardiac Unit, we discovered that inapparent arrhythmias were very common in patients who had recently endured a myocardial infarction. This was, in a sense, the beginning of monitoring and of the Coronary Care Unit.

New Directions. In July of 1958, after completing an assistant residency at the MGH, I began research training at the National Heart Institute. While in my third year there, in the laboratory of Christian Anfinsen, I was most surprised to receive a letter from Walter Bauer inviting me to return, after appropriate training, to be chief of Cardiology. It was both an exciting and frightening prospect, since I would be succeeding two leaders whose names were almost synonymous with the discipline of cardiology. After an additional year of residency in internal medicine at the MGH and a year of cardiology training with Aubrey Leatham in London, I set up a small laboratory under the wing of Herman Kalckar, began research, and prepared to assume my duties as chief of the Cardiac Unit in July of 1964.

The unit, as I found it, was comprised of a strong group of clinicians: Bland, Conger Williams, Friedlich, Myers, and Wheeler. Roman DeSanctis had just been appointed to the staff as the most junior member and was beginning to take over some of the duties of the catheterization laboratory from Myers and Friedlich. There were two fellows in training, no research laboratories, and no research grants.

A great windfall occurred that augured well for the future growth of the Cardiac Unit: The trustees of the Harold Whitworth Pierce Foundation donated the funds for a building to be situated between the Bulfinch and Edwards Research buildings, which was to contain a new cardiac catheterization laboratory as well as research laboratories. The new laboratories were opened in 1965, and Charles Sanders, who had been a fellow under Bland, returned from service in the armed forces to head the catheterization facility. It was now my mandate to enlarge the training program, not only to meet the needs of our expanded clinical work, but also to provide much needed academic cardiologists to staff the growing cardiac units of medical schools around the nation and the world. The training grant that dated back to White's era was enlarged with enthusiastic NIH support.

It was my intent to create a well-balanced unit that, beyond retaining the strength in clinical practice and training traditional at the MGH, would add a strong investigative program which would not only enhance the ongoing clinical diagnosis and treatment, but also make an impact on cardiologic practice around the world. Both clinical and basic research were to be promoted, which meant not only laboratories studying animal preparations, cells, and molecules, but also the most modern clinical investigative facilities. In the building of this enterprise both external agencies such as the NIH and the American Heart Association and the sympathetic view of the hospital administration were the keys.

A cornerstone of the success of both clinical research and patient care activities is the remarkable spirit of cooperation that exists between the cardiac medical and surgical units. It began with Scannell, who was very close to cardiac clinicians in the early days, and was much augmented by the arrival of W. Gerald Austen as chief of Cardiac Surgery. The fact that, when the Cardiac Unit wrote a textbook, the surgeons carried equal weight and Austen was a coeditor, is representative of this rapport. Innumerable joint research projects were launched, and Austen's operative skills, as well as those of the younger associates whom he attracted, made the MGH a magnet for patients with cardiac disease. Upon this strong base a clinical cardiology training program was built that now attracts more than 200 applicants each year for five vacancies.

Myocardial Infarction Research Unit and the Ischemia SCOR Grant.

A signal example of cooperation between the NIH and the MGH was the founding of the intensive study area of the Myocardial Infarction Research Unit (MIRU). This contract, initially under the leadership of Sanders, provided the beginning of a strong interest by the unit in coronary artery disease research. The NIH provided the research funds for the purchase of equipment and for the salaries of research personnel, while the MGH gave that ever-scarce commodity, space. The successor to the MIRU is the Specialized Center for Research in Ischemic Heart Disease, a multimillion-dollar grant broadly aimed at the solution to a problem that affects most Americans. I am principal investigator of this grant with Austen, now chief of Surgery, as co-principal. This instrument, while seemingly aimed at a single disease process, had the effect of bringing considerable diversity to the unit. I promoted collaboration with the Peter Bent Brigham's cardiology division (which figures strongly in the grant) and promoted basic science investigation. As an example of the latter, the work of Ban An Khaw in the innovative use of antibodies as cardiac imaging agents has been supported by SCOR for many years.

In order to study acutely ill patients suffering from myocardial infarction, highly specialized facilities were needed. Again the MGH came through by establishing the Cardiac Catheterization Laboratory on Gray 3A. This is a combined research and clinical facility under the direction of Herman Gold and Robert Leinbach, which allows bold intervention in myocardial infarct patients with optimal safety as well as with maximum gain of new information. This facility and its predecessor, the Intensive Study Area, have yielded major advances in the understanding and treatment of the sequellae of myocardial infarction. Perhaps the finding that had the greatest impact was the realization that skilled operators could perform cardiac catheterization and coronary angiography on patients almost immediately after coronary occlusion without significant morbidity or mortality. Important findings from these studies include a clear understanding of the relationship of the fraction of the ventricular mass infarcted and prognosis in cardiogenic shock; the development of the intra-aortic balloon pump, a device that allows patients with low cardiac output to be maintained until some definitive therapy can be applied or recovery from surgical trauma occurs; and the implementation of streptokinase to open thrombosed coronary arteries in acute myocardial infarction.

The Fellowship Training Program. From the conception of the
Cardiac Unit, education has been a central priority. Over the past 16 years, the number of postdoctoral fellows in training has grown from three to 37. The clinical training program, under the direction of Peter Yurchak since 1971 (himself a trainee in the first group to complete training under my aegis), aims to produce well-rounded academic cardiologists prepared to lead clinical and research efforts in medical schools. Ten to 13 individuals are engaged in this part of the program at any one time. Our graduates can be found in major cardiac divisions in this country and abroad and lead these enterprises at a handful of institutions that are recognized as being at the top of American medicine. In Paul White's tradition, we continue to be interested in training cardiac leaders in other countries.

More than two-thirds of the fellows in training are not here to learn the fundamentals of clinical cardiology; rather, they have been attracted by the research that is being carried out in the many divisions of the Cardiac Unit and have come to work in our laboratories for two to three years. Among this group one can find not only cardiologists but also individuals with basic science training who have doctoral degrees in chemistry or immunology as well as physicians from other disciplines such as surgery and nephrology. They go on to distinguished careers in teaching and/or research.

Catheterization Laboratories. Invasive cardiac diagnostic tests have
undergone remarkable growth and evolution. As detailed above, a major change occurred in 1965 when the unit obtained its own facilities. The number of procedures done annually has grown gradually from about 100 to 2,419 in 1981. There are many reasons for this substantial increase. It is self-evident that the clinical demand for cardiac care at the MGH would grow with the reputation of its physicians and surgeons, but the magnitude of the change can only be explained by an evolution of the practice of cardiology itself. When Sanders first assumed direction of the laboratory in 1965, valvular heart disease was the major diagnostic indication for catheterization. At that time cardiac surgery had just begun to achieve success with valve replacement, and not only mitral stenosis but stenosis and regurgitation of any cardiac valve could be attacked. The number of patients with valvular heart disease was limited, however. Rheumatic fever has been far less prevalent since the widespread use of penicillin, and the number of congenital lesions has remained relatively constant. The advent of coronary

artery surgery entirely changed the pool of clinically appropriate patients. An almost limitless number of patients clamored for diagnosis and symptomatic relief. Adding to these demands were two further areas of activity that developed in the catheterization laboratories. By virtue of Warren Harthorne's interest in pacemakers, the MGH became a major center for the care of patients with asystolic episodes and bradyarrhythmias. He soon accumulated vast clinical experience and became one of the world's leaders in this field, as indicated by his election as first president of the Pacemaker Society. In 1974 Harthorne assumed the directorship of the Pacemaker Laboratory.

The second area of intense activity revolves around the diagnosis and treatment of the dangerous ventricular dysrhythmias. It became apparent that empirical treatment with the increasing number of antiarrhythmic drugs available did not ensure success and that failure was at times first manifested by sudden death. Provocative electrophysiologic trials, in which the heart was stimulated electrically by a catheter electrode within its chambers, proved a more reliable method for determining the efficacy of a given pharmacologic regimen. Jeremy Ruskin was appointed director of the electrophysiology laboratory in 1977 and soon attracted great numbers of referrals for diagnosis and for the establishment of sound treatment programs.

Additional demands on this laboratory in the future will come from therapeutic interventions in coronary artery disease. Peter Block, who has been director of the catheterization laboratory since 1974, has implemented the technique of percutaneous coronary artery dilatation at the MGH. This method allows the opening of narrowed coronary arteries by the introduction of a balloon at the end of a catheter. When applicable, the technique relieves a major symptom of coronary artery disease, angina pectoris, without the need for coronary bypass surgery.

Coronary Care Unit. Even though one of the first cardiac monitors was devised and used at the MGH in 1957 and the frequency of cardiac arrhythmias in myocardial infarction documented, it was not until 1971 that a six-bed Coronary Care Unit was built on Phillips House 2. Its first director was Roman DeSanctis, who was later ably assisted by Adolph Hutter. In 1981, with the assumption of additional administrative responsibilities by DeSanctis as director of clinical cardiology, Hutter assumed the directorship of this unit. More than 2,000 patients have been treated, and a wealth of information has emerged from clinical studies that have influenced coronary care throughout the world. With the opening of the Jackson Building and the Bigelow Service, ten additional coronary care beds became available under the supervision of George Thibault.

ECG Laboratory. Paul White's original electrocardiograph was a cumbersome and fixed piece of equipment. Today electrocardiograms are remotely transmitted by telephone lines to a central computer that stores the data, both the electrical signals themselves and the patient's identification and diagnosis, on magnetic discs from which they may be instantly recalled. A single disc may store 100,000 cardiograms. Yurchak, who has been director of the ECG laboratory since 1976, shepherded the installation of this modern system.

Not all electrocardiographic findings wait for the technician to appear at the bedside. Transient disturbances are often of great importance in making a diagnosis. Hasan Garan has undertaken supervision of a service that places a small boxlike device on a patient's belt and permits him to carry on his normal pursuits at home or in the work place. At the end of 12 or 24 hours, he returns a tape to the laboratory, and all his rhythm disturbances during that period may be discerned.

Echocardiographic Laboratory.

The use of sonar to detect enemy submarines dates to World War II; its application in medicine is more recent. Intracardiac diagnosis may be effected by analysis of reflected sound waves without invading the patient in any way. Gordon Myers and Robert Lees introduced this technique and founded the Non-invasive Diagnostic Laboratory in 1968. In 1980 we were happy to be able to attract Arthur Weyman, a leading figure in this field, as director. He brought with him methods that allow observation of a moving display of the structures inside the heart and in many cases eliminate the need for invasive diagnostic procedures. Newborn infants can now go to the operating room, the surgeon secure as to the diagnosis, without the very real risk of cardiac catheterization.

Pediatric Cardiology.

The Cardiac Unit at the MGH has been unusual among cardiology divisions in that pediatrics has long been incorporated as an integral part of training, research, and patient care activities. Perhaps the reason is the availability of individuals with interest in both children and adults from the very beginning. Paul Dudley White had a long-standing interest in congenital heart disease, and his younger associate, Friedlich, studied under Helen Taussig at Johns Hopkins and returned to the MGH with considerable competence in this field. He was a primary consultant to the pediatric service for many years. In 1965 Allan Goldblatt, who had trained in pediatric cardiology with Alex Nadas at the Children's Hospital Medical Center in Boston and with Eugene Braunwald at the NIH in cardiovascular research, joined the unit. He held the unusual position of being simultaneously an appointee of the medical and pediatric services. In 1974 he was joined by Richard Liberthson, who had training and interest as both an adult and pediatric cardiologist with a strong interest in the structure and natural history of congenital lesions of the heart. The presence of this strong division in the unit is of great importance to our trainees, who become well aware of the origins of adult congenital lesions and the transition in which children's problems gradually blend into those of adults.

Hypertension.

The clinical treatment of hypertension has had both a varied history and affiliation at the MGH. In the late 1930s and early 1940s Reginald Smithwick attracted international interest with his new operation, bilateral lumbar sympathectomy, designed to cure hypertension. After a brief flurry of optimism, it became apparent that for most patients the beneficial results were very transient. Hypertension moved from the surgical to the medical realm when useful drugs for its treatment first became available. Lot Page assumed direction of the Hypertension Clinic while Bauer was chief of Medicine. Page was not only an astute clinician but also a perceptive clinical investigator. In the mid-sixties he and I collaborated on the first assay for plasma renin activity and began to examine the role of renin in hypertension. After he left to assume the post of chief of Medicine at the Newton-Wellesley Hospital, Jan Koch-Weser ran both the Clinical Pharmacology Unit and the Hypertension Clinic—a direct extension of his interests in the pharmacology of cardiovascular drugs. When he left to head the research division of Merrill Drugs in France, the mandate fell to the Cardiac Unit. A young clinician and investigator, Eve Slater, had developed a strong interest in research in the renin-angiotensin system and also undertook the care of hypertensive patients. Randall Zusman has now replaced Slater who moved to Merck, Sharp and Dohme as head of their hypertension drug development section.

Nuclear Imaging. The first nuclear test in medicine had been developed by Earle Chapman and his collaborators at MIT. They produced radioactive iodine at the MIT cyclotron and used its uptake in the thyroid to make the diagnosis of either over- or underactivity of that organ. With the advent of Gerald Pohost as director of nuclear imaging in the Cardiac Unit in 1976, new techniques such as thallium imaging for myocardial ischemia were developed; these had a major impact around the world. Electrocardiographic exercise testing, always considered an imprecise method for predicting the presence of coronary artery disease, was enhanced in its value by the simultaneous application of an exercise thallium scan. Timothy Guiney took an active role in the marriage of these techniques when he became director of the exercise laboratory in 1975. Cardiac nuclear tests began to be performed very frequently and, together with echocardiography, significantly diminished the number of invasive cardiac tests required.

Nuclear Magnetic Resonance. In 1977 Pohost traveled to England to examine the new concept of nuclear magnetic resonance applied to imaging of the living body. He discovered that a physicist in Nottingham was making remarkable progress in what promised to be a powerful method for studying the chemistry of organs (particularly the heart) without invading the patient. X-radiation, with its inherent dangers to genes, was not used. Indeed, there were no known biologic effects of the magnetic fields that were intrinsic to the method. Pohost prevailed upon this physicist, Waldo Hinshaw, to come to the MGH and pursue his research in a clinical setting most conducive to the rapid application of the technology to problems in medical practice. With the help of Juan Taveras, chief of Radiology, Hinshaw set up shop in the sub-basement of the MGH, and one of the two existing clinical nuclear imaging laboratories in the world was born. The venture also represented one of the earliest moves by the MGH to garner industrial support for unfettered research: The Technicare division of Johnson & Johnson handsomely funded this project in its initiation. While still an experimental tool, nuclear magnetic resonance imaging promises to reveal the organs of the human body in great detail without the use of ionizing radiation and to offer as a major dividend an insight into the chemistry of living tissue.

Physiology Research. A major underpinning of clinical cardiology is an understanding of the physiology of the circulation. John Powell came to the clinical fellowship program with prior research training in cardiovascular physiology under the noted investigator, Stanley Sarnoff. After he completed clinical training in cardiology (1972), I encouraged him to develop a laboratory devoted to the physiology of the heart which would be both a vehicle for teaching the basic science of everyday practice to clinical trainees and a testing ground for concepts later to be applied to clinical research. It has been eminently successful in both spheres. Many of the division's trainees who cut their teeth in research, particularly in the area of ischemic heart disease, under Powell's guidance and investigations, have gained national recognition.

Cellular and Molecular Research Laboratory.

At the time that I was appointed chief of the Cardiac Unit, cardiology research largely reflected the concerns of cardiac practice. The way that patients could be helped was to intervene in problems related to diminished cardiac output, impaired blood flow through the cardiac valves, and occlusion of the coronary arteries. Clinicians felt the greatest affinity for research in the area of physiology that dealt most immediately with the concepts that directly underlay clinical problems. Yet the detailed mechanisms whereby the circulation is controlled involve hormones, neurotransmitters, and receptors; the distortion of valves as a consequence of rheumatic heart disease is best explained as a perversion of the immunologic mechanism; the occlusion of coronary arteries is fundamentally the product of an error in metabolism. Thus I elected to emphasize fundamental research in this section of the Cardiac Unit, taking a longer view of the evolution of the field. It was necessary to help patients in the best manner presently available and, therefore, clinical and physiologic research needed emphasis; but the underlying problems of cardiac disease would never be solved until their fundamental mechanisms were uncovered.

My training with Anfinsen at the NIH was in the field of protein chemistry. The problem examined during my time in Bethesda was the origin of the three-dimensional structure of proteins. Since the information contained in DNA was only linear, how was the structure of proteins, which are complex three-dimensional objects, specified? We showed that all the information that determined the arrangement of a protein molecule in space was contained in the linear sequence of amino acids and thus could be determined by the sequence of bases in DNA. The first problem that I attacked on returning to the MGH was an analogous question concerning the structure of the antibody molecule. Antibodies manifest millions of different specificities for the complementary antigen. How is antibody specificity determined? Is it imprinted on a malleable protein as Linus Pauling had hypothesized, or is it the result of the linear translation of a DNA sequence to an amino acid sequence in an antibody molecule? I showed that the three-dimensional structure of an antibody could be destroyed and that, if the amino acid sequence was preserved, it would re-form spontaneously in the absence of antigen. Thus all the information came from the gene, and all the millions of specificities mean millions of different amino acid sequences. I was convinced that this protean system would prove a powerful tool in cardiovascular research.

We set about using antibodies to measure the hypertensive hormone renin in human plasma; to measure the concentration of important cardiovascular drugs such as the digitalis glycosides; to help in the isolation of renin and the alpha- and beta-adrenergic receptors; and as very specific agents in the reversal of digitalis intoxication in man, in the localization and imaging of myocardial infarcts, and in the demonstration of the physiologic and pathophysiologic role of renin. The excitement of contemplating the development of antibodies as the basis of a new pharmacology has not diminished in this laboratory.

The Cardiac Unit Today. The Cardiac Unit today is comprised of 42 staff physicians and scientists, 37 clinical or research fellows, and 153 administrative and technical personnel. Its major functions include clinical care, laboratory service, teaching, and research.

The primary care of cardiac patients as well as consultation throughout the hospital is a major mandate of the unit. It has direct supervisory responsibility for the coronary care units and the intensive care area in the Baker Building. The following laboratories are engaged in direct patient service: ECG, Diagnostic Cardiac Catheterization, Non-invasive Diagnostic, Echocardiographic, Electrophysiology, Nuclear Imaging, Cardiac Immunodiagnostic, and Cardiac Rehabilitation laboratories.

Training is a major function of the Cardiac Unit. Harvard medical students rotate through the unit as do house staff from the Medical Service. A formal training program aimed at educating academic cardiologists is supported in part by a training grant from the NIH. There are 37 fellows in training in both clinical cardiology and applied and fundamental research. The design of the training program allows individuals to attain clinical competence while also mastering a research discipline. Research may be carried out in any of the divisions of the Cardiac Unit, including fundamental research in the Cellular and Molecular Research Laboratory.

The breadth of research interest is considerable. Subjects covered include clinical studies of heart failure; the natural history of congenital heart disease; evaluation of cardiac disease utilizing nuclear imaging; evaluation of cardiac pathophysiology utilizing ultrasound; the renin-angiotensin system as a physiologic and pathophysiologic regulatory mechanism; interactions among angiotensin, renins, and prostaglandin; the pathophysiology of acute myocardial infarction and intervention in the early hours of this process; the structure and function of the antibody combining site; antibodies (particularly monoclonal antibodies) as diagnostic and therapeutic reagents; the natural history of adult cardiovascular disease; the genesis of cardiac dysrhythmias through basic and applied electrophysiologic studies; physiologic and pathophysiologic changes in myocardial ischemia; the structure and function of the alpha- and beta-receptors and associated adenylate cyclase systems.

The younger staff investigators of the Cardiac Unit have been recognized by prestigious training awards. Seven current staff individuals hold Established Investigatorships of the American Heart Association (far more than any other division in the nation), and two staff members hold Young or Clinical Investigatorships of the NIH.

The unit has obtained research grants from the NIH, the American Heart Association, the Education Foundation of America, and the National Aeronautics and Space Administration as well as from several industrial corporations and foundations. There are presently 35 active grants including a program project grant and a specialized center of research of the National Heart, Lung and Blood Institute.

Clinical Pharmacology Unit

ALEXANDER LEAF

When Otto Krayer, then professor and chairman of the Pharmacology Department, proposed the development of a unit of clinical pharmacology, it seemed that were such to survive in our busy clinical setting it should encompass some clinical subspecialty of medicine as well. Since management of hypertension was accomplished almost entirely by drug therapy and because the control of blood pressure was critical in many key physiologic systems and was affected by numerous humoral and neural influences, it seemed natural to fuse a new clinical pharmacology activity with an old clinical need. Jan Koch-Weser was thus appointed chief of a combined unit. He gave good leadership to this combination, and he gained national prominence in the field of clinical pharmacology for his scholarly accomplishments in several successful early clinical trials. However, a conservative Department of Pharmacology did not regard his studies to be of a sufficiently basic nature—despite the Department's insistence that they were trying to develop clinical pharmacology at the Harvard Medical School—to merit a permanent appointment, and Koch-Weser accepted an important position in the pharmaceutical industry.

After his departure I appointed his industrious and knowledgeable young associate, David Greenblatt, as chief of the unit; hypertension management became an administratively distinct activity under the direction of Eve Slater. Greenblatt had extensive experience with mood-modifying drugs, having collaborated closely with psychiatrists at the Massachusetts Mental Health Center. Laboratories for the Clinical Pharmacology Unit were located in Temporary Building 2, and the status of the unit in the hospital was not high, despite the very good service and research performed by Greenblatt and his fellows. He inherited the same doubts about clinical pharmacology on the part of the Department of Pharmacology at the Harvard Medical School that had plagued his predecessor, and it was clear that he would not receive departmental recognition. In the late seventies, when he was offered a full professorship at Tufts Medical School to run their clinical pharmacology activities, I reluctantly but realistically had to advise him to seize the opportunity. There being no space to house a Clinical Pharmacology Unit, I regretfully closed that chapter, and the Medical Services has not had such a unit since Greenblatt's departure.

Computer Science Laboratory

OCTO BARNETT

"One development during Dr. Robert Ebert's short tenure as Chief of Medicine," notes Alexander Leaf, "was the recruitment of Dr. Octo Barnett to establish a Laboratory of Computer Science (LCS). Barnett came with a background of training in cardiology as well as a period of training in Seattle in medical uses and applications of computer science. Initially it was not entirely clear to the rest of us just what Barnett was to accomplish. However, there was a general feeling that somehow the enormous information transmittal problems involved in the practice of medicine in a large hospital might be simplified, and the availability of data upon which medical practice is based might be improved, by the computer. The wisdom of Ebert's initiative is clearly evident by the accomplishments of Barnett, chief of the LCS, and his colleagues.

"It took some time before their first contribution had significant impact upon the practices in the hospital. This was the reporting and computerization of the chemistry laboratory results; that whole operation from the delivery of samples to the lab, the logging in of the identification of each sample into a computer, and the subsequent test results on each sample with laboratory printouts on the clinical floors has markedly accelerated and improved the reliability of the laboratory reporting. In some areas of the hospital the turn-around time from drawing of blood sample to the report is less than an hour."

From its beginning the LCS focused its efforts on developing and implementing time-sharing remote-access computer systems to improve medical information processing. From 1963 to 1968 the laboratory and a consulting firm, Bolt, Beranek and Newman, pioneered in this development. The MGH was the first to deploy such a system in hospital practice. By today's standards the system was very primitive; it had only a limited functional capability with many failures each week. Nevertheless, the promise of computer technology was clearly recognized, and the MGH maintained its commitment to its introduction and deployment in the hospital. Twenty years after it was organized, the LCS had a staff of over 40 professionals, including physicians, engineers, nurses, programmers, computer operators, and electronic technicians, and 14 computers which supported almost 400 terminals throughout the hospital.

Given the broad mission of improving the flow of medical information, the LCS over time developed specific objectives to (1) develop a computer-based information system to supplement and eventually replace the manual medical record; (2) design and implement a hospital communication system to process all doctors' orders and facilitate reporting from ancillary units; (3) exploit the computer database for research in quality assurance, utilization review, and health care planning; (4) supplement classic medical education with computer-based simulations of patient encounters; and (5) develop collaborative arrangements with other clinical investigators and provide experimental design and statistical and information-processing support. The laboratory launched a number of projects designed to meet these objectives; though space permits only a partial listing and description, even the abbreviated account demonstrates the enormous impact of computer technology on the hospital.

MUMPS. The development of the Massachusetts General Hospital Utility Multi-Programming System, affectionately known by the trademark acronym of MUMPS, began in the LCS in the mid-sixties and became the keystone of all application programming. This language was—and, to a large extent, still is—unique in terms of its power in data management for a time-sharing system that can be implemented on relatively small computers. The MUMPS language has had an international impact: It is now being supported by six different computer manufacturers in the United States and Europe and is being used by over 500 institutions, both medical and industrial, on five continents. Several commercial companies have been founded to market and support computer services based on application programs first developed in this laboratory. MUMPS is one of the few computer languages created with an active effort toward standardization to promote sharing and transferability. The LCS continues to develop MUMPS to take advantage of advances in computer technology.

MGH Computer-Based Information Systems. During the sixties the dominant model of a computer-based information system for a hospital took the form of a large central computer facility supporting a variety of activities. One of the early contributions of the MGH laboratory was to challenge this "total system" view by advocating and demonstrating the effectiveness of an incremental modular approach to the development of medical information systems. The LCS chose to identify well-defined areas of information processing that have a high priority within the hospital and then to develop computer-based modules specifically designed to meet the needs of staff members who use the information. The laboratory started by developing information systems for the clinical laboratories—notably chemistry and bacteriology—and the radiology scheduling and file control system. These systems have been in continuous 24-hour-a-day operation since the late 1960s. The same strategy was subsequently extended to the development of systems for the Hematology Laboratory, the Blood Bank, the Pathology Department, the Pharmacy, the Tumor Clinic, the Neuromedical Intensive Care Unit, the Anticoagulation Clinic, the Anesthesiology Acute Care Laboratory, the Department of Radiation Therapy, the EEG Laboratory, and a number of smaller laboratories in the hospital. In addition, the LCS developed an information system to support the data needs of the Utilization Review Committee. All these systems are programmed in MUMPS and are supported on computers located in the laboratory and funded by the MGH budget.

A striking advantage of this modular approach is that it can be implemented using relatively small computer systems with low start-up costs. Furthermore, it is possible to evaluate each system and to justify continuing support from the hospital budget. Willingness of the user to assume financial responsibility for the continued operation of a system has proven to be a valid measurement of that system's operational usefulness.

Quality Assurance. The predominant philosophy of the laboratory is that computer-based information systems not only improve the data processing functions of the institution by making information more available and better organized but also raise the level of patient care by facilitating programs of quality assurance. Consequently, three key characteristics guide all our developments: First, information is recorded in a specified fashion using a defined vocabulary; second, the computer systems provide integrated data management for administrative, financial, and patient care needs so that all pertinent data about the patient care process are recorded and available in a common information system; and third, the systems have the capability to monitor automatically and continuously all information they receive according to protocols specified by the hospital staff. For example, in the Chemistry Laboratory system, if the value of a patient's laboratory test changes over time at a greater rate than specified in a protocol, then the laboratory technician is notified to check for a possible test error. In the Bacteriology system, a very sophisticated monitoring device checks for changes in the sensitivity of certain organisms to various antibiotics. This trend monitoring is used routinely by the Infectious Disease Unit to guide the selection of antibiotics for MGH patients. In the Radiology system, there is automatic monitoring of the scheduling of new x-ray examinations and immediate feedback if the particular x-ray requested has been taken in the recent past; this automated surveillance has decreased overutilization of radiologic examinations by approximately 10 percent.

An example of a promising approach to providing a database that can be used to audit and improve patient care is the project developed to support the MGH Utilization Review Committee. In the early seventies it became clear that the federal government and third-party insurers would require the MGH to review the necessity for continuing hospitalization of its patients, a complicated administrative procedure. Federal regulations required the development of an information system that could be used to record data and prepare necessary reports. In designing this system, the LCS took a long-term view and created the capability to obtain a high quality database consisting of all the important medical problems causing admission of the patient and associated with the continuing patient stay. This information offers the opportunity for the first time to characterize the MGH patient population in terms of what diseases are confronted, what surgical procedures are performed, the complications of hospitalization, the length of patient hospitalization, etc. Eventually this data will be merged with information from other reporting systems to provide a truly comprehensive database of MGH patient care activities.

COSTAR. A major research activity in the LCS has been the development of a computer-based ambulatory record system known by the acronym COSTAR. Begun in 1967 as a collaborative effort with the administration and physicians of the Harvard Community Health Plan, this system has evolved from a simple index of the patient's problems, medications, and laboratory results to a comprehensive medical information system that has completely replaced the manual record at HCHP. As it passed through stages of refinement, COSTAR became a more generalized system that now includes not only medical record support but also scheduling and accounting information. The system is now commercially available and in use throughout the United States as well as in several foreign countries.

One example of an exciting application of computer technology to the improvement of patient care is the laboratory's collaboration with the MGH Primary Care Unit in using the database provided by COSTAR. Because COSTAR contains medical data on all the unit's patients in coded form, it is possible to identify patients with a particular set of diagnoses or patients who have received any group of specific medications. For instance, COSTAR has been used to characterize the degree of control of blood pressure in hypertensive patients and to identify high-risk patients to receive flu vaccinations.

Nurses and physicians collect data for COSTAR by recording the information about each visit on an "encounter" form which is then entered into the computer system by clerical personnel. The centralized database is always accessible for entering or dispensing information from remote locations through computer terminals. Any part of the patient's medical record may be displayed on cathode-ray-tube terminals (a television-like screen with a keyboard), and single or multiple copies may be rapidly produced on printers.

The laboratory is now developing a powerful retrieval language to allow the naive user access to any part of the database. This "Medical Query Language" has an enormously exciting potential to provide a relatively simple and inexpensive technique for carrying out any type of search or tabulation request on the database without incurring the costs and delays of the creation of a special program by a computer programmer.

Computer-Based Simulations for Medical Education.

Computer-based medical education offers unique advantages over traditional methods: an emphasis on problem solving rather than factual recall; a responsive and interactive learning situation in which a variety of reproducible clinical cases can be presented; the elimination of many restrictions of location and time by the availability of convenient computer access from home, office, or hospital; and a potential for reduced educational costs through repeated use and widespread circulation of the program library.

The LCS began the development of computer simulations to teach and assess clinical problem-solving skills in 1969. In 1972 the laboratory began an experimental computer-assisted instruction network to assess the feasibility of—and interest in—interinstitutional sharing of computer-based health science educational resources. The MGH became the first host institution on this national network. Since then, over 100,000 hours of computer-based medical education have been provided to 60,000 network users at 150 institutions throughout the United States and in foreign countries. The primary audience has been medical students and physicians. In 1981 approximately 50 medical schools and hospitals had contracts with LCS for access to the network.

Computer-based patient simulations offer an exciting and effective supplement to classic medical education methods. The programs developed at the MGH are influencing the evolution of computer-based instruction in medicine.

Collaborative Research Efforts.

In the mid-seventies, in response to numerous requests for consultation and collaboration in research design, data collection, statistics, and data analysis, we developed and began the support of a general purpose data management system, MEDINFO, which is currently used by a number of MGH research units in support of clinical investigation. MEDINFO allows a study to be created, updated, and analyzed by an investigator or project assistant without the need for professional programming support. The investigator can create a file for the storage of information, enter data into the file, manipulate and change data, print selected record summaries, carry out tabulations and cross-tabulations, and use standard statistical procedures. The laboratory's major collaborator in this area is the Medical Practices Evaluation Unit. The LCS provides all data processing support for the comprehensive data set collected on all patients in the medical intensive care units. (See page 131 for a description of this research project.)

Overall, it is difficult to overstate the importance of information in a modern teaching hospital, whether for clinical care or research. The old methods for processing and communicating information in hospitals proved to be inadequate to meet the challenges of modern medicine: the explosion of the knowledge base; the introduction of hundreds of new diagnostic tests, medications, and therapeutic procedures; the complicated accounting procedures; the requirements of regulatory agencies; the proliferation of specially trained personnel dealing with one individual patient; and the necessity for ensuring accountability to providers and institutions.

The effective practice of medicine and the efficient administration of a hospital became increasingly difficult because of the limitations of the manual processing of information. One could almost claim that, if the computer had not been invented for other reasons, it would have been necessary to develop such a tool to support the information-processing needs of medical care.

Diabetes Unit

ALEXANDER LEAF

In the earlier years of the period covered by this volume, the Diabetes Unit was under the direction of Richard Field. A stellar resident and chief resident, he had been sent by Bauer to Carl Cori in St. Louis for biochemical training and then brought back to head the unit. Once there he started some interesting metabolic studies on the sorbitol pathway and peripheral neuropathy in the diabetic. Collaborative studies with the neurosurgical and ophthalmology services were also in progress to observe the effect of hypophysectomy on the retinopathy of diabetes as well as on the nephropathy; results indicated that benefits were marginal at best, and fortunately this very invasive therapeutic intervention has generally been abandoned.

Field's attention, however, gravitated increasingly toward clinical activities, and academic pursuits within the unit waned. A change in leadership therefore seemed in order, and Donald B. Martin was named chief of the Diabetes Unit in 1966. Martin had also been a medical resident and chief resident. He had gone to the laboratory of Roy Vagelos, then at Washington University, and in a short time was senior author of a very important paper which demonstrated the feedback regulation by citrate on the glycolytic pathway by its action to inhibit 1,-6 diphosphofructokinase. Martin had a very salutory influence on the academic growth of his unit as well as on its clinical and teaching role in the hospital. When he left the MGH in 1979, he left behind a strong investigative group of young academicians.

Joseph Avruch of that group was the natural choice for the new chief, and he was appointed to that position. Following a research fellowship at the MGH with Wollach in Herman Kalckar's laboratory, Avruch had been chief resident at Barnes Hospital. He has studied the biochemical events involved in the mechanism of action of insulin, and his work on the phosphorylation of enzyme proteins as a means of regulation of their enzyme activities is highly regarded. In the late seventies there was an opportunity to nominate Avruch as an investigator of the Howard Hughes Medical Institute, which has provided personal support for him and for his research. In the reorganization of the Hughes institute that occurred in 1978, an institute laboratory was created on Bulfinch 3 on the site of our old medical intensive care unit, for Joel Habener and his new Laboratory of Molecular Endocrinology and for Avruch.

Lee Witters, who came to the MGH as a clinical and research fellow in endocrinology, joined the Diabetes Unit and developed an independent but complementary research program to that of Avruch. He has succeeded in culturing isolated hepatocytes and studies the regulation of carbohydrate and fat metabolism in this in vitro preparation. Lloyd Axelrod participates in the unit's research program, examining the role of prostaglandins in metabolism. David Nathan, a recent addition to the unit, has been assigned responsibility for developing the Diabetes Clinic as a group practice, and his research has been on the use of insulin pumps to provide continuous insulin replacement to the diabetic. The most recent member of the unit, Perry Blackshear, brings considerable experience with the development of continuous infusion pumps for the administration of insulin to diabetics.

Endocrine Unit

JOHN T. POTTS, JR.

During the period preceding that covered in this volume, endocrinology at the MGH was associated most strongly with the name of Fuller Albright (see Chapter 13), who devoted more than a quarter of a century to endocrine research. Eleanor Dempsey, Albright's chief assistant for many years, summarized his contributions most simply and eloquently in these words:

His papers were written about many diverse syndromes and diseases. They solved many questions as to what was the cause, or what treatment should be used, for too many or too few hormones produced by the parathyroids, adrenals, ovaries, testes, or pituitary gland. When he started his research, . . . patients with these diseases were medical curiosities. No one knew how to treat or cure the patient with hypoparathyroidism or hyperparathyroidism, Addison's or Cushing's diseases, metropathia hemorrhagica or ovarian agenesis, Paget's disease or osteoporosis, the adrenogenital syndrome, and many others. Dr. Albright made many discoveries which, with the advent of new drugs, antibiotics, steroids, and with contributions from others, made the treatment of many of these diseases routine.

By 1956, however, illness had incapacitated Albright, and his work was over.

In 1958 Walter Bauer asked Lloyd H. Smith, Jr., to become chief of the Endocrine Unit—as Smith observed, "despite the fact that I had had no formal training in endocrinology." His background had been in general internal medicine supplemented by approximately four years of training in biochemistry at Harvard, the Public Health Research Institute in New York City, the Karolinska Institute in Stockholm, and finally one year in the Huntington Laboratories in association with Paul Zamecnik. Smith headed the Endocrine Unit for six years, a period that he describes as "a relatively brief interlude between the days of the classic endocrinology represented by the brilliant work of Fuller Albright and his associates and the new era of molecular endocrinology under John T. Potts, Jr., and his colleagues."

Concerning his own tenure Smith writes:

Fortunately, we were sustained by the assistance of Nan Forbes and Janet McArthur from the great days of the Albright laboratory, and by the invaluable help of Oliver Cope in disorders relating to calcium metabolism. In addition, it was possible to develop a close collaboration for patient care and teaching with the Thyroid Unit, under the direction of

John B. Stanbury, and the Diabetes Unit, under the direction of Richard Field. In these latter activities, we developed joint Endocrine Grand Rounds for which the responsibility was rotated. We also held joint consultative rounds which often included patients from the Children's Service, brought by John Crawford, and patients from Gynecology, brought by Janet McArthur. These collaborations were extraordinarily important in buffering the beginnings of the new Endocrine Unit.

In these early days, Stephen M. Krane was of extraordinary importance in bringing his scholarship to studies of bone and calcium metabolism. Soon thereafter, however, he left the Endocrine Unit to become chief of the Arthritis Unit. Dan Federman, even at that time, was everyone's favorite clinician and teacher. He developed his interest in sexual differentiation through early studies on chromosomal disorders. After my departure to become Chairman of the Department of Medicine at UC San Francisco, he succeeded me as Chief. Nan Forbes continued her interest in general endocrinology and served as a particularly useful link to the Albright days. She also made important observations, together with Eric Engel, of the association of chromosomal disorders and endocrine diseases. Bernard Kliman was recruited from the NIH to establish modern methods for the measurement of steroidal hormones using the techniques, then very novel, of gas chromatography and isotope dilution. Andrew Frantz came as a clinical fellow from Columbia; he was the first individual at the MGH to set up the Berson-Yalow techniques for immunoassay of peptide hormones. He and Mitchell Rabkin collaborated in early studies of growth hormone secretion. Donald B. Martin continued his studies of the mechanism of action of insulin and the intermediary metabolism of carbohydrates. My own interest tended toward the metabolic basis of genetic diseases. We completed studies demonstrating the enzyme defects associated with hereditary orotic aciduria. In continuation of the long interest in kidney stones, we became interested in oxalate metabolism and were able to demonstrate certain genetic defects in primary hyperoxaluria.

All of us in the unit took particular pride that within this short interval no less than three of our collaborators who began as laboratory assistants went on to receive doctoral degrees. . . . In addition, a number of interesting fellows from abroad graced the unit for varying periods of time. During the last year (1963–64), I was on sabbatical at Oxford with Sir Hans Krebs, and Dan Federman ran the unit in my absence. When I went directly from England to San Francisco, he became the unit chief.

The four years between the departure of Smith from the MGH and the arrival of John Potts and his colleagues from the NIH were a period of rapid change in the Endocrine Unit. Federman, presently dean for students and alumni at the Harvard Medical School, provided very effective leadership through 1967 when he assumed new duties as assistant chief of Medicine. Even after his departure from the unit, Federman continued his effective program of clinical teaching and clinical research in endocrinology. Bernard Kliman served as acting chief of the Endocrine Unit from 1967 to 1968. He, Frantz, and Rabkin pursued their strong programs of clinical research, and Federman, while continuing his wide-ranging clinical investigations into disorders of sexual maturation, published his highly regarded textbook on this subject.

In addition to two changes in chairmanship, several senior researchers left the unit during the sixties. Frantz returned to Presbyterian Hospital where he assumed a major leadership role in endocrinology. Rabkin left to become the general director of the Beth Israel Hospital in Boston, and Martin became chief of the MGH Diabetes Unit. Moreover, Eleanor Dempsey, who had been Albright's chief laboratory assistant, left to work with Alexander Leaf in the Renal Unit, and several of the clinical fellows departed. Thus the size of the endocrine research staff was considerably reduced for a short period of time.

In 1967, the year before the arrival of John Potts, both Forbes and McArthur were still on the Endocrine Unit research staff, although McArthur had already begun to spend more time in her growing role of leadership in the MGH Gynecology Service, where she initiated an extensive program of clinical investigation. Robert Neer joined the unit at this time as a clinical fellow and began his distinguished career in clinical investigation at the MGH.

In 1968 Potts accepted Leaf's offer to return to the hospital as chief of the Endocrine Unit; three of Potts' colleagues—Henry Keutmann, Leonard Deftos, and Hugh Niall—came with him to the MGH from the laboratory at the NIH. Potts had been a member of the MGH medical house staff as an intern and assistant resident from 1957 to 1959. He then accepted a position as a clinical and research fellow at the National Heart Institute in Bethesda in the laboratory of Christian Anfinsen, who at that time was conducting the pioneering studies in protein chemistry for which he later received the Nobel Prize (along with Stanford Moore and William Stein of the Rockefeller University).

Potts became interested in parathyroid disease when he was a medical student at the University of Pennsylvania; this attraction to the intricacies of calcium metabolism was greatly strengthened during his two years as a house officer at the MGH, with its tradition of studies by Cope, Bauer, Aub, and Albright, all of whom contributed so enormously to the definition of the pathophysiology of disorders of calcium and bone metabolism as well as to many other areas of research in endocrinology.

Having learned the technique of protein chemistry from Anfinsen, Potts in 1960 began eight years of collaboration at the NIH with Gerald Aurbach, who had developed the first successful technique for extraction of parathyroid hormone from parathyroid glands while working in the laboratory of Ted Astood in Boston. Aurbach and Potts combined their biologic and chemical training to accomplish the isolation and partial structural characterization of parathyroid hormone from bovine and human tissue. The complete structural characterization of bovine, human, and other forms of parathyroid hormone was not completed, however, until Potts and his colleagues returned to the MGH.

Many new currents of research in endocrinology developed between 1968 and 1975. General great advances in techniques—such as automated methods of protein sequence analysis, rapid techniques for synthesis of polypeptides by chemical methods, and rapid deployment of radioimmunoassays by improved and more sensitive techniques secondary to the pioneering work of Berson and Yalow—combined to provide a previously unimaginable impetus to basic research in the field. Peptide hormones from the pituitary, hypothalamus, parathyroid, thyroid, and other endocrine glands were isolated, structurally characterized, and synthesized during the decade of the seventies. As is characteristic for a period of such rapid advance in research, results, in turn, led to new clinical approaches both in understanding the pathophysiology of disease and in improved methods of treatment.

Niall, who had come to Potts' NIH laboratory from the laboratory of Pehr Edman in Australia, brought with him for its first use in the United States the automated technique for protein structural analysis developed by Edman. Niall directed the preparation of automated equipment that made possible the rapid structural analysis of parathyroid hormone and calcitonin. During the period at the NIH and then in Boston, Niall, Potts, and their colleagues determined the complete structure of ovine, bovine, porcine, and salmon calcitonin, and bovine and porcine parathyroid hormone. In the late seventies Keutmann described the complete structure of human parathyroid hormone.

Geoffrey Tregear, who had been a close colleague of Niall in Melbourne, came to the Endocrine Unit in 1969 and established a program of chemical synthesis using the technique of solid-phase peptide synthesis. In 1971 he and his group performed the chemical synthesis of the biologically active portion of parathyroid hormone and began a decade of studies in which the relationship between structure and biologic activity of this hormone was defined.

After Tregear had been working for several years in the Endocrine Unit, he was joined by Michael Rosenblatt, then a student at the Harvard Medical School. Rosenblatt took a year's leave-of-absence to work with Tregear and then rejoined the unit after completing his medical house staff training at the MGH. He thus initiated a continuous period of distinguished service to the Endocrine Unit as a clinician, teacher, and investigator, which culminated in his succeeding Potts as unit chief in 1981 when the latter became chief of the Medical Services. Rosenblatt delineated the structural basis of biologic activity of parathyroid hormone through synthesis of fragments and analogues of the hormone. His research spawned much basic and clinical research into the mode of action, metabolism, and assay of parathyroid hormone.

Deftos applied a number of immunoassays for calcitonin (which he developed at both the NIH and the MGH) to studies of the role of this peptide in human disease, such as in patients with medullary carcinoma, and in the comparative endocrinology of calcitonin in mammals and fish. He left the MGH to become chief of Endocrinology at the Veterans Administration Hospital in La Jolla, California.

In the middle of this very productive decade of research, Niall and Tregear returned to Australia to assume leadership posts in the Howard Florey Medical Institute in Melbourne, and Rosenblatt and Keutmann, along with Gino Segre, assumed responsibility as senior laboratory investigators, leading the group's expanding program of research on parathyroid hormone.

The collaboration between the Endocrine, Thyroid, and Diabetes units which began under Smith's chairmanship was augmented by Potts. Upon becoming chief of the unit in 1968, Potts began working closely with Martin, the newly appointed chief of the Diabetes Unit; Farahe Maloof, who had recently become chief of the Thyroid Unit; and with McArthur, who had developed programs in reproductive endocrinology, to develop a coordinated training program in reproductive endocrinology, thyroid, diabetes, and general endocrinology. This represented the first time in the history of the Department of Medicine at the MGH that these units operated a unified program for clinical care, for selection and training of clinical fellows, and for close coordination of research and scholarly activities.

Thus the Endocrine Unit flourished, with energetic growth in clinical programs and the development of strong programs in research which attracted many brilliant young investigators and clinicians, many of whom, after periods of initial training in the combined program, took up posts as junior faculty members in one of the four cooperating units. Outstanding trainees came from many centers in the United States, as well as from Great Britain, France, Australia, New Zealand, Japan, China, and other countries. Many who came from abroad returned to faculty positions in academic medical centers and research institutes in their home countries. Trainees from the United States assumed important leadership posts in clinical and research activities in medical centers throughout the country after completion of their training; others remained at the MGH to work in the Endocrine, Thyroid, Reproductive, and Diabetes units.

The decade of the seventies brought a great flowering of endocrinology at the MGH. The unit's activities at this time included programs of research involving thyroid hormone biosynthesis, the molecular biology and biosynthesis of parathyroid hormone, the chemical structure of pituitary and pancreatic peptides from a wide variety of human and animal species, and the photobiology and metabolism of vitamin D. The unit also conducted detailed investigations of the mechanism of action of insulin and studied the clinical significance and therapeutic potential of the hypothalamic-releasing hormones in reproductive endocrinology. By 1980 the clinical and research staff of the endocrine divisions had grown to include over 35 faculty members along with numerous technicians and postdoctoral trainees.

Robert Neer, presently director of the General Clinical Research Center (GCRC), the NIH-supported unit in the famous Mallinckrodt Ward 4, established extensive clinical programs in metabolic bone disease and in the endocrinology of calcium metabolism. As program director of the GCRC he coordinated clinical investigations in many areas of endocrinology. Joseph Avruch, who succeeded Martin as chief of the Diabetes Unit, led studies of insulin action. E. C. Ridgway, who, after a period of training in the Endocrine Unit, joined Maloof in the Thyroid Unit and later succeeded him as chief of that unit, continued the tradition of studies of thyroid hormone, both basic and clinical. William Crowley joined McArthur's group and established a broad program of clinical research in reproductive endocrinology. Joel Habener who, like many others, came to the MGH from the NIH, and Henry Kronenberg, an MGH house officer who also trained at the NIH, led a new program of research into hormone biosynthesis.

Under the leadership of Habener and Kronenberg, the late seventies witnessed the explosion of the new technology of recombinant DNA. Biosynthetic precursors for parathyroid hormone were discovered and characterized. The gene for parathyroid hormone from humans and several animal species was successfully isolated and structurally analyzed. Parathyroid hormone and several other polypeptide hormones were produced biosynthetically in bacteria and mammalian cells. These discoveries permitted a new level of understanding of the cell biology of endocrine tissue and the pathophysiology of endocrine disease.

Alexander Leaf documented the development of the Molecular Endocrinology Unit as follows:

The Molecular Endocrinology Unit was created *de novo* in 1978 largely through the recognition by John Potts that endocrinology was rapidly developing as a laboratory pursuit on the frontiers of modern molecular biology and that the new genetic and immunologic sciences and technology provided means of exploring hormonal synthesis and regulation on the molecular level. Furthermore, though the Endocrine Unit under Potts had pursued this approach in relation to understanding parathyroid hormone structure, biosynthesis, and functions, the techniques were applicable to other peptide hormones and neurotransmitters. Joel Habener had distinguished himself in this aspect of endocrinology and gained national recognition for his research. To stabilize Habener's position in the Medical Services, a Howard Hughes Investigatorship was obtained for him; and with a Howard Hughes Medical Institute Laboratory—built for him and for Joseph Avruch, our other Hughes investigator—we were able to create the Laboratory of Molecular Endocrinology with Habener as its chief in 1978 to serve all endocrine research at the basic level of his interests. William Cin of the Thyroid Unit has brought his interest in TSH biosynthesis to study with Habener, and others are doing the same.

By 1981 six cooperating units had been developed: the Molecular Endocrinology Laboratory headed by Habener; the Endocrine Genetics Unit headed by Kronenberg; the Reproductive Endocrine Group headed by Crowley; the Diabetes Unit headed by Avruch; the Thyroid Unit headed by Ridgway; and the Endocrine Unit headed by Rosenblatt.

The combined training program in endocrinology has grown in scope and stature, making the MGH a leading world center for clinical and research training in the field. Michael Holick established an outstanding clinical and laboratory program in vitamin D research, and Gilbert Daniels assumed leadership as the coordinator of the clinical training program from his base in the Thyroid Unit. The NIH supports eight trainee positions at the MGH per year, enabling young physicians to be trained in clinical endocrinology and to undertake several years of intensive research training in one of the six cooperating units.

The MGH traditions of investigations into the basic processes of endocrinology and metabolism have continued into the present decade. Powerful new research techniques promise to allow new insights into these processes and to provide improvements in clinical practices. Chemical synthesis of polypeptides, application of recombinant DNA techniques to the cloning, nucleotide-sequence analysis, and expression of endocrine genes have become commonplace. New approaches to the understanding of endocrine physiology and to the treatment of many endocrine-deficiency syndromes have been developed in the General Clinical Research Center and in the outpatient clinics of the cooperating endocrine units. Many radioimmunoassays and special isotope techniques have been developed which have permitted MGH clinicians to use in patient care all the most current measurement techniques for peptide and steroid hormones.

The annual publications of the cooperating groups in endocrinology cover a diversity of topics which range from molecular biology to endocrine physiology. Many new and important clinical papers have described metabolic defects in endocrine pathways important in disease and have aided the development of new approaches to the treatment of osteoporosis, precocious puberty, infertility, hypothyroidism, and malignancies associated with overproduction of peptide hormones.

The Endocrine Unit, now headed by Rosenblatt, continues to conduct an effective program of clinical care, research, and teaching. Extensive programs of collaboration with the Endocrine Surgery Unit headed by C. A. Wang, the Gynecology Service headed by James Nelson, and the Orthopedic Service headed by Henry Mankin have helped us to achieve excellence and breadth in clinical care and research consistent with the ever-changing focus of the mission of endocrinology and metabolism at the MGH.

> With contributions from *Eleanor Dempsey* and *Lloyd H. Smith, Jr.*

Gastrointestinal Unit

DANIEL S. ELLIS

The beginning and evolution of a discrete gastrointestinal unit at the MGH go back to the time of Dr. Means' chairmanship of the Medical Services. Chester

Jones had become interested in the then young specialty of gastroenterology and, as related in the section describing him as an individual (page 83), had provided leadership in establishing a gastrointestinal clinic in the outpatient department.

In the 1930s and 1940s, as a geographic full-time member of Means' service, Jones was *the* physician in the hospital whose medical opinion and advice were sought for patients with any important gastrointestinal problems arising within the hospital. His ability and skill in the care of these patients led to both a local and national reputation that put great demands on him to carry a large patient load. Because of his continuing interest in clinical research previously described and his large commitment to teaching both medical and postgraduate students, he was able to carry his patient load only by taking on promising young physicians in a preceptorship role who would help him with his practice. He was generous in his financial arrangements with these "associates," and he encouraged them to set aside time to carry out clinical studies under his guidance in addition to the time spent in developing their clinical practice of gastroenterology.

As time went on, from 1944 to about 1957, he was able to secure funds (from a few institutional grants but mostly from affluent friends, patients, and his own pocket) which enabled him to offer modest support to one, and later two, clinical research fellows a year who worked primarily in his laboratory with his technicians, Gladys Drummey and Anne Ryan, on research projects inspired and directed by him. These fellows also began to see gastrointestinal consultations on the teaching service. The demand for such consultations grew. In order to improve the quality of this consulting service and also to enhance the teaching of the clinical fellows, a weekly gastrointestinal rounds was established, conducted at first by Jones and later on a rotating basis by staff physicians who had done a clinical preceptorship with him. These rounds were attended by the fellows in the laboratory, members of the staff who had been trained by Jones, interested surgeons, supportive personnel from psychiatry, dietetics, and social service, and graduate and undergraduate students interested in gastroenterology. Regular journal club meetings were held for all those who cared to attend, and Jones, with his fellows and technicians, conducted a weekly session to review the research projects going on in the laboratory.

Out of this there evolved a discernible gastrointestinal unit that was strongly clinically oriented. Dan Ellis, Perry Culver, Warren Point, Ed Maynard, and later others who had been trained by Jones joined him on the staff and provided the clinical care of patients and the teaching needs in gastroenterology at the MGH in the early years of the group. Ben White, Wade Volwiler, Harrison Shull, and John Benson, all early members of the Gastrointestinal Unit, moved out of state to become outstanding clinical gastroenterologists or, in the cases of Volwiler and Benson, to accept chairmanships of departments in other teaching institutions. Thus, at the time of Jones' retirement there was a strong nucleus of physicians interested in, and trained in, clinical gastroenterology who would continue to supply the needs of patient care and clinical teaching in the specialty, and who would give this sort of support to the new chief of the unit as he developed a strong component in basic research.

Upon Jones' retirement Bauer wanted to have a stronger investigative activity in the Gastrointestinal Unit and made what seemed a rather bold move in selecting Kurt J. Isselbacher to succeed Jones, since at that time Isselbacher was just over 30 years of age and, although he had training in research and basic investigation, he was not a gastroenterologist. After a short clinical apprenticeship with Jones, Isselbacher was made chief of the unit. It is worthwhile making an anecdotal observation concerning Bauer's approach to this appointment. One Friday afternoon he visited Isselbacher in his laboratory and posed the question: "Which do you want to head up? Endocrinology or gastroenterology? Let me know your decision by Monday." Isselbacher agonized over this unexpected opportunity throughout the weekend and then told Bauer, "I think I would choose gastroenterology even though I have worked primarily in the area of metabolism, which would be closer to the field of endocrinology. However, the problem in suggesting gastroenterology is that I really don't know any." Without hesitation Bauer replied, "I am perfectly aware of that. But people aren't born gastroenterologists, so you will just have to learn to become one."

Isselbacher's appointment subsequently had Jones' support, and the results have been noteworthy. Isselbacher managed to retain the clinical strengths of the unit, the support of the practicing group, and at the same time to pioneer in the development of modern gastroenterology. Leaf, who observed the unit's evolution with satisfaction, noted, "Isselbacher has a marvelous ability to work at a basic biochemical and physiologic level but continuously develop clinical applications and insights of great importance from his basic studies."

A continuous stream of important findings has emerged from Isselbacher's laboratory, only a few of which will be cited here. Before returning to the MGH from a two-year period of research at the National Institutes of Health, Isselbacher described one of the first inborn errors of metabolism identified due to an enzyme defect, namely galactosemia. He identified the enzyme responsible and developed an enzymatic test which since that time is routinely employed in the screening of newborns, thus preventing the complications of galactosemia. The MGH unit's observations on intestinal structure and function included the identification of the pathways and mechanisms for normal fat absorption by the intestinal cell and the role of the intestinal cell in lactose intolerance.

Investigations of liver disease yielded elucidation of many of the metabolic effects of alcohol on the liver and unravelling the mechanisms whereby alcohol leads to a fatty liver. Isselbacher worked out the mechanisms for the impairment in galactose as well as glucose metabolism that occur with alcohol ingestion. At the clinical level, members of the unit were the first to demonstrate that the extrahepatic manifestations of acute and chronic hepatitis are due to circulating immune complexes. Most recently Jack Wands and Isselbacher have taken advantage of the advances in immunologic techniques and have developed a monoclonal antibody to the surface antigen of hepatitis B. This antigen is more sensitive than any of the current commercially available methods for detecting hepatitis B and will soon be used in hospital laboratories since the assay developed by Wands and Isselbacher will be commercially available.

During the course of studies on membrane alterations associated with malignancy, a discovery was made demonstrating the secretion by tumor cells of a unique enyzme—namely, galactosyltransferase. This involved not the normal galactosyltransferase, but an ioenzyme referred to by Isselbacher and his colleagues as galactosyltransferase II, or GT-II. Since then basic and clinical studies have resulted in the demonstration that GT-II is secreted by tumor cells, and when it appears in the bloodstream it can be used as a marker for malignancy. Various members of the gastrointestinal group over the past five years have contributed to the study of over 1,200 patients with documented gastrointestinal tumors, and the GT-II test has been positive in about 70 percent of them. Perhaps most important is the fact that the false positive values are only in the range of 1 or 2 percent. These observations are now leading to the development of a clinical test for GT-II which it is hoped will prove to be one of the more important tumor markers.

The Gastrointestinal Unit continues to attract excellent young physicians and physician-scientists who seek careers in academic gastroenterology. To a large extent they are drawn by the clinical program at the MGH but perhaps even more so by the basic and applied science that has been ongoing in the unit over the past 25 years.

> With the assistance of *Alexander Leaf* and *Kurt Isselbacher*.

Geriatrics Unit

ALEXANDER LEAF

It was not possible to watch the occupancy of the Medical Services over the past 15 to 20 years without noticing a marked change in the age of our patients. This relates to the "geriatric imperative." The proportion of the population in the age group of 70 and above has been increasing rapidly in the past decade. Older citizens are those most prone to illness which is often serious and affects many systems simultaneously. The fragility of the older patient makes him or her subject to chronic serious illnesses. In the past several years 40 to 60 percent of the patients on the Bigelow service were over 65.

It was also apparent that many of the teachings in medicine that apply to the vigorous 30- or 40-year-old patient are inappropriate for elderly, more fragile individuals. Nevertheless, the staff and resident staff managed them in a comparable way, irrespective of the differences of life expectancy, the number of other systems that might be afflicted by disease, and the general frailty of the older patient. Furthermore, differences in metabolism of drugs and of tolerance to the procedures seemed not to be adequately appreciated by the physicians on the Medical Services—or on other clinical services, either. Therefore, it seemed appropriate to develop a Geriatrics Unit within the Medical Services which would have the responsibility of bringing to the attention of the staff the medical differences between young and older patients to assure that the latter receive care that is optimal for their conditions.

In 1979 Tad Campion was appointed chief of the Clinical Geriatric Group. In order that he have the opportunity to see and manage the problems of the elderly within the acute care hospital, experience could be provided at the MGH, but it is probably as important for the development of a Geriatrics Unit that patients be followed in some more chronic facility. Fortunately, the Massachusetts Rehabilitation Hospital was willing to appoint Campion on a half-time basis as chief of their Geriatric Service.

It has not been easy for Campion to define his territory on the Medical Services, since many internists feel that they are quite competent in caring for the elderly in the same manner that they care for the middle-aged sick. However, he has set about developing a team including psychiatrists, social workers, nurses, physio-therapists, occupational therapists, dietitians, and internists to help with the problems of the elderly on the Bigelow Medical Service. Given his interest, the staff will in time recognize the benefits of having an individual with special geriatric medical competence to advise them in the care of their older patients.

The MGH neighborhood health center in Chelsea has also developed an interest in geriatric medicine. With a housing development for the elderly in the community, there are a number of patients requiring care who could be spared hospitalization by having that care provided to them on an ambulatory basis. Physicians in the neighborhood health centers have been cooperating with Campion so that there is now a program embracing the acute patients at the MGH, the longer-term hospitalized patients at the Massachusetts Rehabilitation Hospital, those who reside in their own homes in the community, and a special relationship with the Don Orion Nursing Home. Thus the resources are in place for the establishment of a strong geriatric program at the MGH in medicine. The only obstacles have been lack of staff interest and of the fiscal support needed to promote the teaching and research endeavors of the unit. These will surely develop with time and patience, since the idea is a good one and the need is great.

Hematology/Clinical Laboratories

WILLIAM S. BECK

One development of the past 25 years that very accurately symbolizes the advances of modern medicine was the establishment in 1957 of a new Hematology Unit in the Medical Service and a service laboratory that came to be known as the Clinical Laboratories. Before 1957 the great majority of laboratory services in hematology were performed by medical students and interns as part of their regular responsibilities in the care of patients. Indeed, the wise men of that day resolutely maintained that an essential part of the educational harvest of patient care came from performing blood counts and urinalyses with one's own hands. It was a time when the weary house officer would return to a dismal, crowded laboratory after his other work was finished.

In 1927 it was recognized that an important area of medicine had been too long neglected at the MGH, and a physician with considerable experience in hematology was put in charge of one technician in the Phillips House laboratory. The man was Francis T. Hunter, a recent graduate of the West Medical Service, who had worked in hematology with George Minot at the Collis P. Huntington Memorial Hospital. When the Baker Memorial unit opened its doors in 1930, Hunter and three technicians organized a new laboratory on the second floor, and its work increased rapidly. During the next ten years small laboratories were established in the Emergency Ward, in the Outpatient Department, in the White Building to cover the Surgical Services, and, finally, in the Vincent-Burnham Building.

Following Hunter's death in 1954, responsibility for the Baker Laboratory was given temporarily to Charles DuToit, director of the Chemistry Laboratory. Meanwhile, a search was launched for a new director by a committee made aware of rapid progress in the field of hematology by Walter Bauer who was interested in establishing such a unit within the Medical Service. The obvious solution was to combine the two missions—directorship of the Baker Laboratory and chief-ship of the new unit—in one man. This was done with the appointment of William S. Beck, whose experience has been mainly in hematology research, particularly its biochemical aspects.

Before the establishment of a formal hematology unit, the medical staff had to rely for expertise on the talents of members of the Medical Service who happened to have an interest in hematology but had no academic group to back them up and could offer no formal training program. Such individuals did a superb job in covering the hospital's need within existing limitations. Bernard M. Jacobson was one of the distinguished internists who in this way had made hematology a field of special interest and long served the hospital. With the establishment of the new unit in 1957, he became one of its most useful senior members. The Hematology Unit was thus initiated in tandem with the new service laboratory, the Clinical Laboratories. It was immediately evident that the laboratory was a valuable asset to the research and training programs of the unit because it was now possible for clinical and research fellows in training to work closely with laboratory technicians, to keep a wary eye on what was coming through the laboratory, and indeed to receive practical training in laboratory aspects of hematology. The field does, after all, have a uniquely important laboratory basis, and every good hematologist must be experienced and skilled in the laboratory side of the discipline.

One of the major decisions in the early sixties was to eliminate parasitology from the list of services offered by the Clinical Laboratories. As hematologists, we had always been rather amateurish in this field. The time had come to develop a truly professional effort in the area, particularly in view of the rising numbers of soldiers returning from Vietnam and other exotic climates. A separate new Parasitology Laboratory was established in 1963 as an adjunct to the Infectious Disease Unit.

Also during the sixties the major services persuaded the hospital administration to transfer the burden of laboratory work from their own overworked house staff to the Clinical Laboratories. One of the earliest to win such privileges was the Surgical Service, Dr. Churchill having eloquently convinced the administration that surgical house officers were too busy for such duties. Bauer held the line, but the Medical Service under his successor, Dr. Ebert, finally came into the fold, the last service to do so. Thus in 1966 professional technicians for the first time did a job that had traditionally been the cherished privilege of students and house officers on the Bulfinch service.

One of the striking features of modern hematology is its scientific sophistication and the development of a large number of test procedures. The performance of these tests requires equipment of the type found only in research laboratories and a type of research technician not usually found in hematology laboratories. Accordingly, the new Clinical Laboratories service was notable for the early establishment of two subdivisions called the Special Hematology Laboratory and the Special Clotting Laboratory. In the former were performed such tests as the serum vitamin B_{12} assay, the serum folate, leukocyte alkaline phosphatase, various red cell enzymes, hemoglobin electrophoresis—all typical of the procedures that make hematology the powerful discipline it is today. The same consideration led to the establishment of the Special Clotting Laboratory. Although routine screening-type clotting tests were performed in the Clinical Laboratories, modern clotting theory had yielded a long list of special tests that require a sophisticated scientific environment for their performance, including the various factor assays and, in later years, the platelet function tests. Physicians with expertise in the then arcane field of blood coagulation headed this laboratory.

The special laboratories were very special in one important sense: They had an enormous potential for furthering clinical research, and a good deal of new knowledge emerged, such as the development of methods for the assay of serum vitamin B_{12}, the leukocyte alkaline phosphatase, new methods for the assay of serum folate, and a large number of new procedures in the clotting field.

The Clinical Laboratories came to resemble the modern organization of this day with the opening of the Gray Building in 1969. The occupation of a modern facility on Gray 2 was accompanied by the closing of all the satellite laboratories except the one in the Emergency Ward. The main justification for discontinuing these satellites was the arrival of new equipment for performing blood counts—the large automated Coulter counters which now perform white counts, red counts, hemoglobins, and hematocrits with great rapidity and an accuracy never possible with manual methods. It made no sense to duplicate equipment of that type—and so an era ended. The Coulter counters tremendously enhanced the reliability and precision of laboratory reports, and in the early seventies the computerization of the Clinical Laboratories brought this efficiency to an even higher level. It became possible to issue prompt, accurate, and legible reports, to keep results of patients in a computerized file, to prepare all sorts of scientific and managerial statistics, and to maintain various kinds of surveillance over testing procedures so as to prevent error.

Meanwhile, with the support of NIH training grants, the Hematology Unit trained many able young people in clinical hematology and hematology research. One of them, John T. Truman, later became chief of a new Pediatric Hematology Unit. The research programs were largely in the field of vitamin B_{12} and folic acid metabolism and their role in DNA synthesis, and substantial discoveries emerged concerning these important vitamins. Distinguished research was also conducted in the area of blood coagulation.

In 1971 Leonard L. Ellman, a former medical house officer at the MGH who received his hematology training under Carl V. Moore in St. Louis, succeeded to the position of chief of the Hematology Unit, and in 1975 he assumed the directorship of the Clinical Laboratories. Ellman emphasized teaching medical students and house officers, and the clinical activities of the unit were increased. In 1977 when the Hematology Unit was combined with the Oncology Unit, then under Thomas P. Stossel, to form a new Hematology-Oncology Unit under his leadership, Ellman continued to run the Clinical Laboratories. The hyphenation of hematology and oncology was after the fashion being followed in a number of hospitals and medical schools throughout this country. There is certainly considerable overlap between the two fields, and it is a fact that today most young people desire exposure to both fields. Unfortunately there is widespread disagreement over whether the two fields ought to be brought together and, if so, how. As a result, a considerable amount of confusion has developed in the planning of training programs and certification examinations. Be that as it may, Stossel brought new scientific vigor into the area at the MGH. He is a distinguished investigator in the field of white cell physiology, and the new combined unit is thriving. (See page 336 for further discussion.)

Infectious Disease Unit

MORTON N. SWARTZ

The absence of a unit in infectious disease at the MGH in the immediate post-World-War-II years stemmed from the belief that the introduction of penicillin and other antimicrobial agents had effectively eliminated infectious diseases. This clearly had proved incorrect by the early fifties, and the special requirements for expertise in the use of antimicrobial agents provided the initial impetus for the formation of the unit in 1951. Thomas F. Paine was appointed to head the new unit. However, following his departure in 1953, no staff member of the Department of Medicine was assigned to this area. Finally, in 1956 Walter Bauer appointed Morton N. Swartz unit chief. Alexander Leaf has said of Swartz, "He is a clinician's clinician. He and Stephen Krane (chief of the Arthritis Unit) possess the most encyclopedic knowledge of medicine of any physicians I have known."

From the mid-to-late fifties the unit's responsibilities involved a consultative role in the care of patients in all hospital divisions, teaching activities for medical students and house staff, the building of a research program, and the development of an energetic and productive staff to fulfill the needs of the unit, the hospital, and the Harvard Medical School in the forthcoming decade. Whereas during its first five years the Infectious Disease Unit had only one member responsible for consulting on patients in the MGH, Baker Memorial, and Phillips House as well as in the Pediatric Service and the Massachusetts Eye and Ear Infirmary, the subsequent quarter century saw the staff expand to 12 physicians who answer consultations on over 3,000 patients annually. Since 1955 five former or current staff members or trainees in the MGH unit have gone on to become full professors on the Harvard faculty. They include K. F. Austen (chief of Medicine, Brigham and Women's Hospital), Bernard Fields (professor of microbiology and molecular genetics, HMS), Robert C. Moellering, Jr. (chairman, Department of Medicine, New England Deaconess Hospital), Arnold N. Weinberg (formerly chief of Medicine at Cambridge Hospital and currently director of the pathophysiology teaching program, HMS), and Morton N. Swartz (chief, MGH Infectious Disease Unit).

Due to the emergency nature of many infectious disease problems, one of the first concerns of the unit was to develop a capacity for prompt response to requests for consultation; that condition of readiness remains the prime consideration in the role of the unit. Achieving this capability required long hours, particularly during the unit's formative years when staff numbers were smaller. Thus the unit was prepared when presented with extraordinary circumstances such as the intrahospital outbreak of a *Salmonella* infection in 1956 and the major influenza virus pandemics of 1957 and 1968.

As time passed, it became apparent that the introduction of new antimicrobial agents had not eradicated infectious disease problems; in fact, the needs for special expertise increased in particular areas. For example, the development of Renal Transplant and Hemodialysis units in the sixties extended the opportunities for caring for formerly end-stage kidney disease patients. However, in the process of transplantation a variety of drugs must be employed, and their use sometimes renders the patient more susceptible to a number of unusual infections which require special skills for their eradication. Consequently, one member of the Infectious Disease Unit has been assigned to the Transplant Unit to optimize therapeutic results. Similarly, advances in ear, nose, and throat surgery posed new problems for infectious disease experts, and the unit now has a staff member functioning essentially full-time as a consultant to the Massachusetts Eye and Ear Infirmary.

The recognition of the importance of hospital-acquired infections coupled with the development of ever more complex instruments and procedures for diagnosis and treatment has necessitated increasingly careful surveillance within the MGH. Due to the size of the hospital and its numerous specialized services, a staff consisting of a member of the Infectious Disease Unit and several nurse-epidemiologists are now involved practically full-time in this activity and have contributed measurably to improved patient care.

The development of new therapeutic approaches in infectious diseases has been accompanied by newer diagnostic methods requiring expansion of laboratory facilities. Four different laboratories were developed during the past two decades to provide service functions in patient care: the Viral Diagnostic Laboratory, the Parasitology Laboratory, the Antibiotic Blood Level Laboratory (for monitoring the levels in the blood of potentially toxic antibiotics in order to minimize adverse side effects), and the laboratory for special tests (determination of serum bactericidal levels, determination of the susceptibility of fungi to various antifungal antibiotics, immunologic diagnosis of fungal infections).

Activities at the MGH have had national and worldwide impact in terms of demonstrating the significance of infectious disease divisions in the care of patients. This institution's unit was one of the first in this country dedicated to infectious disease problems in a general hospital. Formerly, those problems had been considered communicable diseases and segregated in so-called contagious disease hospitals. The emphasis on patient care established by this unit has served as a model and stimulated the development of comparable units in nearly all major teaching hospitals as well as large community hospitals in the United States. A very large number of publications from this unit dealing with the diagnosis and management of infectious disease problems appearing in a general hospital also have contributed to the wider improvement of patient care. Finally, many other institutions have benefited from the efforts of the MGH staff in defining problems that are broadly applicable in the care of hospitalized patients.

In perhaps the most celebrated instance, a collaborative study between members of the Infectious Disease Unit and the MGH Bacteriology Laboratory (Lawrence Kunz, director) of the occurrence of sporadic cases of infection with an unusual bacterial species (*Salmonella cubana*) had national consequences. Several patients at the hospital developed intestinal infections due to this organism at different times over the period of a year. Were it not for the excellent detective work of Dr. Kunz, his staff in the Bacteriology Laboratory, and members of the

Infectious Disease Unit, the common thread linking these unusual infections would never have been discerned. The vehicle, a dye stuff widely used in hospitals and in industry (as coloring for food, clothing, cosmetics, etc.) was incriminated as a result of the MGH detective work. The dye was subsequently withdrawn from the marketplace. Some time later, *The New Yorker* (September 4, 1971) featured an account of this brilliant investigation in an "Annals of Medicine" article by Berton Roueché.

In view of the large number of complex and innovative surgical procedures performed at the MGH, special expertise in infectious disease has been in ever greater demand. About half the consultations of the unit involve patients with problems in many of the general surgical and surgical subspecialty areas. The experiences of the unit staff in dealing with problems of infection within the central nervous system and with complications of open heart surgery have been adjuncts to advances in these two fields in particular.

The educational activities of the Infectious Disease Unit began in 1956 with a one-month teaching program for each of the 12 medical assistant residents. It was the first specialized rotation for house staff in any subspecialty unit on the MGH Medical Service. Electives for medical students began during the 1960s, and two HMS students received special clinical training in infectious disease for a period of one month throughout the year. The unit obtained a training grant from the NIH in 1962, and it has been in operation steadily since that time; 70 postdoctoral fellows have been trained under the program, and many of them have gone on to prestigious clinical or academic positions in this country and abroad.

In 1964 the Infectious Disease Unit introduced another teaching innovation when it began joint rounds with Louis Weinstein's similar unit at Tufts–New England Medical Center and Tufts Medical School. These rounds, which alternated between the two institutions on a weekly basis, provided teaching in differential diagnosis and management of problem cases in infectious disease. The format was unique in that a senior staff member from each institution was involved in discussing a particular patient. An attempt was made to allow one experienced clinician to discuss each case so that his thought processes might be evident and serve as a model for younger staff members and students. This approach proved so successful that it has been replicated innumerable times in the Boston academic community, involving all the subspecialties of medicine. The Infectious Disease Unit continues its program, but the focus of the exchange has shifted recently to the Brigham and Women's Hospital.

Like patient care and educational activities, the research program has expanded steadily since 1956. Major contributions by members of the unit have been made in the areas of DNA sequencing, the role of viruses (SV40 and murine leukemia viruses) in relation to tumor induction, the role of interferon in suppressing activation of viral infections during organ transplantation, the role of combination (synergistic) antibiotic therapy in the treatment of certain forms of infections of heart valves (endocarditis), and the development of a simplified, one-day program of treatment of urinary tract infections. In recent years laboratory research in this unit has led to the development of newer methods for diagnosing (by the demonstration of antibody) the occurrence of systemic fungus infections.

Much of the current research deals with the problem of antibiotic resistance and the role of resistance factors (extrachromosomal bits of DNA) in bacteria producing this resistance. Increased understanding of the role of such R-factors in antibiotic resistance in enterococci has led to improved approaches to the treatment of life-threatening infections due to these organisms.

(With a note by *Alexander Leaf*)

Massachusetts Eye and Ear Medical Unit

ALEXANDER LEAF

Over the years the MGH Medical Services had had an uneasy relationship with the Massachusetts Eye and Ear Infirmary. There was a constant need on their part for medical consultations to cover their patients. Many people who came to the eye service needed treatment of complications of diabetes; many others were older patients with cardiovascular diseases of varying degrees of severity. The MEEI ran a busy clinical service which required clinical support from the MGH. For years the Medical Services had maintained a coverage of the Eye and Ear Infirmary by senior residents who provided preoperative evaluations of the ability of MEEI patients to undergo surgical procedures and anesthesia. Consultative services were also provided for any medical problems that arose during the course of hospitalization of their patients, such as diabetic ketoacidosis, heart attacks, congestive heart failure, etc.

But the academic climate at the MEEI was distinctly different from that at the MGH, and medical residents did not appreciate this service because there was no instruction during rotations in the Eye and Ear Infirmary. MEEI physicians also depended upon consultative services from some of our full-time practitioners, although this again was an activity which the latter did not usually appreciate. When Richard Field left as head of the Diabetes Unit, he devoted a considerable portion of his time to consulting at the MEEI; but when he moved most of his activities to the Beth Israel Hospital, the Eye and Ear Infirmary again found itself short of medical consultative help.

In 1977 the MEEI chiefs of services visited Leaf to solicit the Medical Service's assistance; Leaf saw an opportunity to develop a really good service for them while strengthening the medical residency program. Lloyd Axelrod had recently completed his chief residency in medicine and joined the Diabetes Unit. Since his interests were primarily clinical and he was regarded as one of the better young clinical teachers on the Medical Services, he seemed an ideal person to head a strong unit of the Medical Services based in the MEEI. After extensive negotiations, and with the strong support of the two chiefs, Drs. Dohlman and Schuknecht, and others, Axelrod was appointed director of the MEEI Medical Unit. His role was to provide the medical coverage needed there while improving the teaching of MGH residents during their rotation in the infirmary; it was also agreed that he would help teach the residents in the MEEI how to care for the common medical problems that they would encounter in their specialty practices.

Aside from a few stormy sessions when certain members of the MEEI staff insisted that Axelrod's unit should be responsible for all the initial physicals and histories on patients admitted to the MEEI and a few other jurisdictional issues, there has been substantial improvement in MEEI-MGH relations. Axelrod continues to be one of our strong teachers. His presence in the MEEI with appointment on their staff assures that medical problems arising there will be effectively managed, avoiding possible embarrassment to the MEEI for poor medical management and to the MGH for failure to provide adequate medical coverage to a sister institution.

Medical Practices Evaluation Unit

ALEXANDER LEAF

In 1977 I created the Medical Practices Evaluation Unit which has been of special interest to me and to George Thibault, assistant director of the Medical Services, who was appointed chief of the new unit.

With the increasing technological advances in medical diagnosis and management, physicians are confronted with a broad spectrum of possible means of diagnosing and treating their patients. Most of these methods are useful but some are less useful or even, in some instances, positively harmful. Unless careful evaluations are made of new technologies and therapies as they are introduced, there is little hope of sorting out the useful from the useless or harmful. During his last year as president of the Milbank Foundation, Lee Burney, with Dean Ebert's backing, came to visit me and to offer support for the development of a clinical epidemiology unit within the Department of Medicine. At that time one of my major concerns was whether our Intensive Care Unit on Bigelow 8 was providing a useful medical resource for the patients treated there or whether it was simply a very expensive white elephant. There had been considerable controversy in the literature regarding the value of intensive care units, and it seemed important to determine whether our own was being put to appropriate use. I was therefore delighted when Burney offered to support an investigation that would involve including information on all patients who came into the Intensive Care Unit on a computer database and then a long-term follow-up to determine whether our interventions were helping or not.

I had with me in the Medical Services office Dr. Thibault, a former chief resident in Medicine who had completed his training in cardiology. As an excellent clinician and teacher as well as a very effective medical leader, all that he needed were some worthy academic accomplishments to become a very strong candidate for a major role in American academic medicine. Thibault took on the directorship of the Medical Practices Evaluation Unit and recruited Albert Mulley who serves as co-chief. Working very closely with our Laboratory of Computer Science, beginning in July 1978 they carefully logged the histories, physical findings, and laboratory findings on all patients admitted to the 18-bed intensive care unit on Bigelow 8. They also managed to obtain follow-up data on over 90 percent of the patients discharged from that unit.

This examination of the use of the expensive intensive care unit has been very illuminating. They found that the unit was used largely for monitoring patients who came into the hospital with a possible myocardial infarction. Patients were generally kept in the unit for three days while serial electrocardiograms, clinical course, and serum enzyme levels defined whether myocardial infarction had, or had not, occurred on that occasion. The cost of the three-day observation was approximately $2,400. The Medical Practices Evaluation team, by carefully examining the information on the patients, was able to distinguish a group for whom a determination could be made within 12 hours of admission to the intensive care unit and who could safely be discharged with little hazard of getting into serious difficulties on other floors of the Medical Services. The team has made other observations that led to more cost-effective and better medical management of patients admitted to the intensive care unit.

I view the activities of this unit as an example of what will be a much more general occurrence in the practice of medicine in the near future. Modern data processing techniques will make it possible to enter information on all our patients into comprehensive databases so that the clinical experiences of an institution—or of many institutions combined—can be brought to bear on the next patient who comes into the hospital rather than relying on individual anecdotal experience for the practice of medicine. The use of modern data processing capabilities will add enormously to the ability of the physician to classify a patient and to treat or manage that patient according to modalities that have proven most effective as indicated by data readily available in the computerized data bank.

The Medical Practices Evaluation Unit has served as a clinical epidemiology training unit within the Department of Medicine. We have been fortunate in acquiring support for the training of physicians in general medicine. Thibault and Mulley have had the benefit of most of the Kaiser Family Foundation fellows joining their unit to continue the evaluative studies in progress. If the activities of this unit move into other settings within the MGH and develop comparative databases—say in our Medical Ambulatory Clinics, in the neighborhood health centers, and elsewhere—it will eventually become one of the most important developments in the Medical Services; it is clearly a forerunner of major changes in the practice of medicine.

Pulmonary Unit

HOMAYOUN KAZEMI

The Pulmonary Unit as it existed in 1980 was the brainchild of Walter Bauer. As was his wont, Bauer chose a bright young medical resident, John H. Knowles, sent him to two preeminent respiratory physiologists (Hermann Rahn and Wallace Fenn in Rochester, New York) for training, and appointed him chief of a newly formed Pulmonary Unit in 1958. Prior to that time there were a number of prominent chest physicians on the staff but no organized unit as such. Knowles set about the task of developing a unit with the classic triple mission of patient care, teaching, and research.

John Knowles was an energetic, persuasive, and enthusiastic young physician, and he started with a bang. He began to measure oxygen consumption and quickly interested the endocrine and metabolic people in this work, particularly Fuller Albright who provided a laboratory for him next to the Metabolic Ward (Ward 4), where to this day the Pulmonary Unit remains. (The initial laboratory was enlarged and a new Cardiopulmonary Building built in 1964, but the nucleus of the unit continues to be the laboratory that Albright gave to Knowles in

1958.) Knowles wrote a book on pulmonary function in his first year as chief and was an effective teacher, good clinician, and able administrator; in 1962 he left the Pulmonary Unit to become general director of the hospital.

The unit struggled along without a chief for about two years. Following Bauer's death, Robert Ebert came to the MGH as chief of Medicine in 1964, and he assumed simultaneous responsibility for the unit on an interim basis. This was a critical time in its life, since the field of chest medicine was expanding rapidly: New techniques of diagnosis and management were being introduced into pulmonary medicine, new instruments were developed for respiratory support, and the whole field of pulmonary immunology and biochemistry was opening up. A new Cardiopulmonary Building was reaching completion, and a new instrument—unique in the annals of medicine—was being built for the Pulmonary Unit. This was a cyclotron to produce isotopes of oxygen, nitrogen, and carbon for studies of pulmonary pathophysiology and disease.

Dr. Ebert looked after the affairs of the unit at this critical time and in 1965 appointed K. Frank Austen as chief. As an immunologist, Austen added the dimension of studies of lung immunology, particularly the biochemical pathways in the lung in development of asthma, to physiologic studies of lung function in progress in the unit. Ebert became dean of the Harvard Medical School in 1965, and two years later Austen became physician-in-chief at the Robert Breck Brigham Hospital and moved across town, where he has continued his pioneering studies of immunology and asthma.

In 1967 Homayoun Kazemi was appointed chief of the Pulmonary Unit. He had finished his residency in medicine at the MGH in 1963, spent some time in the hospital's Cardiac Catheterization Laboratory, and then worked with John West on radioisotopes in pulmonary pathophysiology at the Hammersmith Hospital in London. Since 1965 he had been director of the Pulmonary Function Laboratory at the MGH.

Under Kazemi's direction the activities of the Pulmonary Unit have been multiple and varied. The addition of a cyclotron for production of radioisotopes has allowed for new and interesting studies of function of the lungs in health and disease. These activities have been undertaken in collaboration with Gordon Brownell of the Physics Research Laboratory. There have also been studies of lung transplantation and of the physiologic derangements that occur when a transplanted lung undergoes rejection. There is ongoing research on the behavior of blood vessels in the lung and the mechanisms responsible for constriction and narrowing of lung vessels and development of pulmonary hypertension in response to lowered oxygen tension. Investigators in the Pulmonary Unit were among the first to show that there were abnormalities in small airways and in gas exchange in the lungs of young, asymptomatic cigarette smokers even after only five years of smoking. Investigations of the complex problem of how the brain regulates the level of ventilation in the lung have shown how the metabolic activities of brain cells affect ventilation and how, when ventilation is inadequate and carbon dioxide concentration rises in the body, brain cells respond to this insult and protect their internal environment. An offshoot of these studies has been the research of Daniel Shannon in the diagnosis and prevention of sudden infant death syndrome (SIDS).

Members of the Pulmonary Unit, through the long-time efforts and in collaboration with Harriet Hardy, have investigated problems of beryllium toxicity on the lung; for ten years, 1968 to 1978, the U.S. Beryllium Case Registry was part of the MGH Pulmonary Unit. This interest in occupational disease has continued and expanded, culminating in the recent formation of a section on occupational medicine in the Pulmonary Unit, under the direction of Nancy Sprince and Christine Oliver. Lung immunology is a major part of the current research work, with emphasis on the function of lymphocytes in the lungs and development of various forms of interstitial lung disease when the immunologic function of lymphocytes is altered.

The Pulmonary Unit has the major responsibility for teaching pulmonary pathophysiology at Harvard and in the Harvard-MIT Program in Health Sciences and Technology. The clinical activities are extensive, and there are areas of significant interaction with the Children's Service, Anesthesiology, and Thoracic Surgery. Lastly, the unit has been a training ground for many specialists who now occupy positions in research, teaching, and patient care at other medical centers throughout the United States and overseas. Over 60 physicians and scientists have received their training in the unit since 1968.

The vision that Walter Bauer had for the unit when he appointed John Knowles as its first chief in 1958 has been the guiding principle, and its activities in research, teaching, and caring for patients continue to reflect that vision.

Renal Unit

ALEXANDER LEAF

It is difficult to specify a point in time when the Renal Unit came into being. When I returned to the MGH in 1949 with a National Research Council fellowship at the invitation of Means, I was not told where or how I was to work. Having long been an admirer of Fuller Albright, my personal medical hero, I arranged to be one of his fellows. Though the year was an excellent one for me, it led nowhere academically. Since Albright never assisted his fellows to find jobs when their time with him expired, I called on Means to explain my plight. He looked at me and said, "I never pay attention to anyone who comes to work with Albright. I had expected you to set up your own little laboratory when you arrived at MGH."

This was the first indication that any plans had been made for me. When I inquired if the space was still available, I was told that it was, and that day I moved my four rats to the fifth floor of the old Domestic Building. The elevator only went as far as the fourth floor, and stairs were the route to the top; but I had my own laboratory in the attic, and the fact that it was a bare little room of some 10 by 14 feet with no laboratory facilities—not even a sink—did not deter me. I brought up a heavy stone-topped table for my rat cages and was promptly in business with my assay for antidiuretic hormone. In a short time I had two research fellows: Audley Mamby, who now practices in Chicago, and Oliver Wrong, who is professor and chairman of the Department of Medicine at University College, London. Our studies involved the regulation of the concentration of body fluids and the renal excretion of water and sodium. Our chief working sites were Ward 4 for patient studies and the animal surgery rooms on Edwards 6.

In 1953 we moved to a single laboratory on Domestic 3; it was some 400 square feet and seemed most elegant with sinks, gas, air, and suction in the laboratory benches. E. P. Tuttle had joined us by then, and much of our research was conducted in association with Walter S. Kerr, Jr., whose adept surgery and sense of humor were both enormous assets.

In the fall of 1954 I went to Copenhagen to spend four marvelous months in the laboratory of Hans H. Ussing to learn biophysics of membrane transport activity; there I discovered that the urinary bladder of the toad could be used as a model for the study of sodium and water transport. In January 1955 I moved to Oxford and passed two happy and productive years in the biochemistry laboratories of Hans A. Krebs.

Shortly after my return to the MGH I was appointed chief of the new Cardiorenal Laboratories on the first floor of the Edwards Building. By this time we had a considerable informal consultative service on problems of fluid and electrolyte disturbances and kidney diseases. We were considered nephrologists—though that term had not yet come into use. The teaching of students and house staff in this nascent discipline was our responsibility, and I can still remember my first Grand Rounds when, discussing the management of chronic renal failure, I recommended a low protein diet and was openly challenged by Joseph Aub.

Our laboratory research centered largely around transport physiology in toad bladder and dog kidneys. We attracted numerous investigators who subsequently moved on to important positions in academia around the world, and we were equally successful in attracting funding to support our efforts.

In 1967 the unit moved to the superb laboratories that I had designed for it on Jackson 7, but my appointment as chief of Medicine in 1966 of necessity changed my relationship with the unit. By that time three distinct strongholds had developed within the enterprise: a clinical activity headed by Cecil H. Coggins, with Norman Lichtenstein and Nina Tolkoff-Rubin providing clinical consultation and teaching; a biochemical pharmacology research activity directed by Geoffrey W. G. Sharp who held a Ph.D. in pharmacology; and another research activity in transport biophysics with myself and Donald DiBona, a Ph.D. in biophysics, as central investigators. I participated in the clinical activities with a month as the renal consult, and my research activities were related to those of DiBona and biophysics of membrane transport. Coggins was acting chief of the unit throughout my $15\frac{1}{2}$ years as chief of Medicine, since I had always expected to return there after a reasonable stint as chief of service. The separation of the Renal Unit into three fiefdoms was not wise because it divorced the clinicians from the research and reduced the cross-fertilization that is the essence of a strong unit. With Sharp's departure to Tufts in the seventies, the unit's Laboratory of Biochemical Pharmacology was phased out, but when DiBona accepted a professorship at the University of Alabama, John Mills replaced him in the Laboratory of Renal Biophysics. Only with my return to the Renal Unit in May 1981 did I reassume the position as chief and formally abolish the subsections.

Hemodialysis Unit.

The Hemodialysis Unit was informally established as a necessary adjunct to the Surgical Transplant Service to sustain patients with end-stage renal failure while suitable donor kidneys were obtained and also for the management of the many patients with acute renal failure who may need this life-sustaining procedure to tide them through their periods of suppressed kidney function. George Baker and Lot Page initially supervised this activity, and Baker continued in this role after Page left to become chief of Medicine at the Newton-Wellesley Hospital. In view of Baker's other duties and practice demands, additional supervisory dialysis physicians were needed; Bud Back was added upon completion of his clinical fellowship in nephrology, but he accepted a position at the University of California Medical Center in San Diego. In 1974 Nina Tolkoff-Rubin was appointed to head the hemodialysis facility as a member of the Renal Unit. Rubin has provided coverage of this service and the teaching of house staff and renal fellows who divide their clinical year of training between the busy consult service and the dialysis facility.

Thyroid Unit

JOHN B. STANBURY AND EARLE M. CHAPMAN

James Howard Means, the founder of the Thyroid Clinic in 1920, continued his consuming interest in the enterprise for more than a decade after his retirement in 1951. In Washburn's history of the MGH Means mentioned "a recent and novel turn" involving a collaboration with the Physics Department at MIT and that Dr. Hertz, then head of the clinic, had made some progress in the study of the course of the radioactive iodine through the body. But Faxon's volume made scant reference to subsequent events that led to the development of this noninvasive, safe, and less expensive form of therapy for Graves' disease. Thus, it seems reasonable now to retrace the historic steps of this therapeutic advance between 1935 and 1955.

We have already seen in these pages (p. 66) Dr. Means hurrying toward the podium in Vanderbilt Hall on November 12, 1936, to propose the MIT-MGH partnership to explore the physiologic uses of radioactive iodine, as well as the first treatment of a patient in this fashion in 1941. This important contribution to medical diagnosis and treatment was slow to achieve full recognition; the beneficial effects were uncertain because the patients treated by Hertz in 1941–1942 were also treated with stable iodine which in itself has a favorable effect on the course of Graves' disease. But the doubt was resolved after Hertz left for active duty in the Navy, and a series of patients were treated by Earle Chapman and Robley Evans who defined the single effective dose of radioactive iodine used without any other therapy; they also produced hypothyroidism (myxedema) from over-treatment with a single large dose. The report of ten years' experience with radioactive iodine in 1955, by Chapman and Farahe Maloof, led to greater usage. A review of treated patients and controls, sponsored by the U.S. Public Health Service in 1968 and 1974, laid to rest the danger of increased incidence of leukemia and cancer of the thyroid following radioactive iodine therapy.

The account of this therapeutic mode has, however, catapulted us ahead of other events in the Thyroid Unit to which we must return. On January 1, 1949, Means appointed John B. Stanbury, who had just completed a term as chief resident, to head the unit. Under his guidance, weekly clinical sessions on Tuesdays became a meeting ground for MGH staff members from many specialties: Jacob Lerman, Oliver Cope, Edward Hamlin, John Raker, and George Nardi attended regularly along with Chapman and Maloof. Gardner Quarton, a psychiatrist, was on hand for a while; Gordon Brownell, a physicist from MIT, joined the group in 1951, followed shortly by Austin Vickery, the pathologist. These meetings were stimulating and lively as internist, pathologist, physicist, psychiatrist, and surgeon each made contributions to the analysis of patients' problems and their treatments. But with the passage of time and the changing nature of hospital practice, the sessions evolved into seminars for the presentation of current developments in special aspects of thyroidology.

An encounter with a patient in 1949 was to have long-lasting effects on the research activities of the Thyroid Unit. This patient was a severely retarded young woman with a huge goiter who was brought for care along with two similarly afflicted brothers. All three proved to have a disorder of the thyroid that resulted from an inherited error of thyroid metabolism: The defective metabolic step was in the forming of iodine into an organic compound in the cells of the thyroid. It was the first biochemical abnormality of the thyroid in the medical literature to be clearly identified.

Then, in 1955 Stanbury spent a sabbatical leave at the University of Leiden with Andries Querido who had been a research fellow in the Thyroid Unit in 1949. Stanbury, Querido, and his staff discovered a second inborn error of the thyroid, and Stanbury was later involved in similar discoveries elsewhere. Thus, over the years most of the inherited metabolic errors of the thyroid that have been described were first identified in the MGH. One by-product of these activities was the publication of a monograph on the inborn errors of human metabolism entitled *The Metabolic Basis of Inherited Disease,* edited by Stanbury and two former MGH fellows, J. B. Wyngaarden and D. S. Frederickson. The text, the standard one in its field, is now in its fifth edition.

Another portentous event in the history of the Thyroid Unit was an afternoon visit on a Tuesday early in 1950 by Hector Perinetti of Mendoza, Argentina. His vivid description of the huge goiters caused by iodine deficiency in the waters flowing from the nearby Andes led to a proposal for a joint study of endemic goiter in Mendoza province, where the disease had long been a problem of major public health concern. In the summer of 1951 Stanbury, Brownell, and Douglas S. Riggs—a pharmacologist and expert in iodine biochemistry from the Harvard Medical School—joined their Argentine colleagues for an intensive study of the iodide-deprived people. It was the first time that this important health problem of developing countries had been studied with modern scientific methods. The results were published as a monograph which generated great interest in Latin America, with the result that a stream of research fellows sought the Thyroid Unit for their postdoctoral training. Means once quipped that Henry Plummer of the Mayo Clinic put iodine on the map, but we can say that this expedition put South Americans into the MGH. In 1961 a request for assistance from the Pan American Health Organization led to the establishment of laboratories in a half dozen Latin American countries for the study of locally prevalent thyroid disorders.

Over the years the Thyroid Unit was host to many young clinicians and investigators in addition to the Latin Americans. Each participated in the ongoing research of the unit. Many investigations were made of the synthesis of thyroid hormones, the metabolism of hormone precursors, and the abnormalities in these processes that result in thyroid disease. Endemic cretinism and familial goiter became disorders of intense interest, and Leslie De Groot and George Riccabona published significant papers on these subjects. Laboratory progress was much enhanced by a complete renovation of the space in the Bulfinch basement in 1961, made possible by a grant from the NIH and the contributions of individuals.

In the spring of 1966 Stanbury left the Thyroid Unit to pursue activities at MIT, and Maloof became the new chief. His studies of the mechanism of action of the antithyroid drugs in preventing the utilization of iodine by the thyroid for hormone synthesis continued. Other studies within the unit included the structure, synthesis, and metabolism of the thyrotrophic hormone and an investigation of the pituitary hormone prolactin in relation to thyroid disease.

No account of the Thyroid Unit would be complete without acknowledgment of the long and devoted service of Ann Guardo. For many years, until her retirement in 1977, she shepherded the patients, kept the records, did the metabolism tests, and contributed in many ways to the smooth operation of a very busy clinic. Every research fellow—and there were many—remembers her with gratitude and affection.

During this quarter century the Thyroid Unit continued its tradition of bringing together clinicians of varied interests and backgrounds to foster an ever-growing competence in understanding and treating patients with thyroid disease. The laboratory research arm of the unit grew dramatically, providing increasingly sophisticated services for patient study and for exploring the innermost functions of the gland. The unit also served as a training base for postdoctoral fellows who came from all over the world to work and learn and share; most of them returned to their home institutions where they occupy positions of major academic responsibility. Thus integrated patient care, research, and learning continued to be the mission of the Thyroid Unit.

Ambulatory Care Division and Community Medicine

JOHN D. STOECKLE

World War II interrupted the Depression debates about care outside the hospital, but they were quickly taken up again in the postwar years by the public, the profession, and the staff of the MGH. Medical practice—its organization, financing, and the education for it—was to be reformed through group practice, national or comprehensive private health insurance, and patient-centered care and education, with the firm hope that access to care would soon be universal and treatment improved for everyone, particularly the poor. While these themes were discussed at the MGH, the topics were local ones: The reorganization of the outpatient department (OPD) and the staff's private practices were seriously reexamined for the first time in 70 years in a postwar climate that held promise for change.

Many of the hospital's private staff considered forming a group practice for a number of reasons. Returning from wartime experiences in military medicine, they were faced with the uncertain prospects of rebuilding their old solo practices, they wanted to continue their wartime "working together," and they were aware of the perquisites and tax benefits that salaried group work might offer. Daniel S. Ellis, Marshall K. Bartlett, Otto Aufranc, Daniel Holland, Edward F. Bland, Earle Chapman, Joseph S. Barr, Stanley Wyman, and others made up an informal group called the Associates which later became an official staff organization, the MGH Staff Associates.

The staff were not alone in their interests, for even earlier, from 1944 to 1947, the general director, Nathaniel W. Faxon, repeatedly mentioned "my one man's vision" of a doctors' office building. In Faxon's view, the issue was an expansion to improve accommodations for private ambulatory patients. Observing that 60 full-time staff members, of a total of 436, were already permitted to see a limited number of patients in their hospital offices, he argued, using an analogy to the hospital's expansion of beds: "It was obvious that the Hospital must solve the problem of providing as adequate care for the ambulatory patient, whether paying or charity, as it now did for all classes of the community as in-patients." His idea was echoed in 1947 by an Outpatient Committee report as well as an "office building" report by the King Committee that detailed the conditions of occupancy and fee schedules in a fashion that might, in effect, convert the office building into something of a group practice.

With a view much larger than a building plan, James Howard Means, in his book for laymen *Doctors, People, and Government,* advocated comprehensive private—though not national—health insurance and organized group practice. Similar positions were held by Allan Butler, then chief of the Children's Medical Service, who had already been active before the war in founding a short-lived prepaid group practice (The White Cross, 1937), as well as by organizations that promoted the ideas of national health insurance and group practice despite their lack of popularity with, and often opposition from, the rank and file of organized medicine including, not surprisingly, many of the MGH staff.

In 1951 the appointment as general director of Dean A. Clark, fresh from the successful operation of a prepaid group, the Health Insurance Plan (HIP) of New York, contained a promise that the trustees, if not the staff, might be open to exploring and developing new practice ventures while continuing their perennial struggle with the hospital deficit. After noting the deficit and the percentage of unoccupied beds, Clark would write in 1952: "One principal means of counteracting the trend will, it is hoped, be the establishment of an organized medical practice group, tentatively called the Massachusetts General Staff Associates."

Pragmatic as the hospital's intention might have seemed, it did not have wide appeal. It was Means who articulated the larger vision: "My suggestion is to join together a medical school, a teaching hospital, a comprehensive prepayment plan, a home care plan, and an organization of doctors for group practices on a salaried basis. Medical education and research should be conducted whenever possible in close relation to care of patients. Preventive services should be provided as well as curative. . . . To reach this goal, the divisive action of special loyalties must be mastered."

As Means noted, the politics of that vision would not be easy, and the trustees concentrated on incremental reform, a pace that acknowledged the conflict Means perceived.

After several years of discussion, the organizational issues relating to group practice finally became focused when in 1951 Walter Bauer accepted appointment as chief of Medicine with the understanding that the care of MGH out-patients would be improved and a new facility built. By this time inpatient care was already of high standard, though with separate facilities and staff. Only the OPD seemed out of place with a declining census, an inefficient, irregular oper-ation of morning sessions, limited resources, a persistent annual deficit, and a part-time staff whose voluntary ethic of free service was faltering as, everywhere else, professional work was paid. In the expansive postwar economy, many were skeptical whether the traditional OPD for the sick poor, or even a modernized one for everybody, was really necessary. Nearly everyone seemed on the way to becoming a paying patient and thus able to attend a private doctor's office, so that soon no one would use the clinic.

Bauer, however, was of a different mind. From his longitudinal clinic studies of arthritis patients in particular and his commitment to the care of chronic patients in general, he considered that organized long-term personal care was essential for the growing numbers of chronically ill. Moreover, at a time when university medical centers were developing referral teaching hospitals, not clinics, Bauer argued for the reorganization and modernization of the OPD on behalf of its patients; they had contributed to the excellence of the hospital in teaching and research but had not had their care in the OPD improved.

Yet that proposed reform would be difficult, for it involved more than expan-sion of the existing institution; rather it meant equality of treatment that only professional reorganization, about which there were many differences, could hope to accomplish. Much earlier, in an Ether Day Address in 1919, Richard C. Cabot had noted how the hospital consistently improved treatment through the increase of beds, successively providing for all classes of patients—although in separate facilities—first in the Bulfinch wards, then in the Phillips House, and finally in the Baker Memorial which had already been proposed by the time Cabot spoke. Faxon had made the same point in arguing for doctors' offices at the hospital.

The modern reform, however, was different. Two common, sometimes hid-den, expectations were held: one, that private and clinic practices might be in-tegrated in a hospital-based group practice; the other, that the private staff might form a private group practice, the advantages and principles of which were ar-ticulated in a policy resolution issued by the General Executive Committee in 1952 at the time of the formation of the MGH Staff Associates.

In August 1955 the GEC appointed a joint MGH-Massachusetts Eye and Ear Ambulatory Clinics Committee to make recommendations. The group had as its chairman Dana Farnsworth, an MGH physician and director of the Harvard University Health Services. Having reorganized college health services with full-time staff at Williams, MIT, and Harvard, Farnsworth was a strong supporter of group medical work; as a senior staff member who did not practice at the MGH, he could also view the issue with appropriate neutrality. After two years of deliberation the Farnsworth report recommended a new building for both clinic and private patients, but rejected any professional plan that would merge clinic and private practices. However, staff members viewed the report's *building* plan as a *professional* plan in which they would eventually become employees of the hospital and its clinical departments. Perceiving such prospects as the loss of traditional autonomy, the staff gave the recommendations less than full support. Some department chiefs were similarly hesitant. Edward Churchill, chief of the

Surgical Services, thought an MGH Clinic would erode the authority and power of the service chief. In addition, he felt the clinic might attract clinical researchers away from their academic tasks to more lucrative work as practitioners.

Hence "the divisive action of special loyalties" was not mastered. The trustees tabled the idea of a building as envisioned in the Farnsworth report. However, they did establish an Ambulatory Care Building Committee, chaired by Clark from 1959 to 1961, to plan for a clinic building alone; the site proposed for this alternative structure was on North Grove Street at the front of the hospital.

Like the proposals for a new facility with diverse practices and for an integrated private-clinic group, the notion of a private group practice also came to naught. The Staff Associates, even when they became a formal part of the hospital under the trustees, became less interested as they resumed their individual practices which were now busier than before the war. The group practice plan was not pursued.

Looking back, the reasons for failure were apparent. First, the private staff had achieved one major objective: practice accommodations on the hospital's grounds in the new Warren Building (1956), which had been enlarged to provide six additional floors with 75 offices for a doctors' office building. Many of the private staff had moved their Boston offices to private suites in the building, and somewhat later (ca. 1961), after the reconstruction of the West End near the hospital, others rented offices in and around the MGH. Second, rising personal incomes in the United States and expanding third-party payments assured the profession and the MGH staff of ample private as well as service or clinic-ward patients, eliminating uncertainties about rebuilding an individual practice or keeping the hospital full. Finally, the economic advantages of group practices (that could provide hospital salaries in lieu of fees for service and in turn the tax, insurance, and pension benefits of institutional employment) were realized by other forms of staff organization such as the Surgical Associates which was formed in 1960. This association, which acted as a common collection agency, did not alter the organization of office or hospital practice but did provide the benefits.

Not surprisingly, then, actions on behalf of group practice or a new building ceased while other priorities and a different climate emerged. By 1962 the hospital's main objective under the new general director, John Knowles, became the Gray Building, the construction of which would provide for new and better operating rooms, make possible the rehabilitation of some surgical wards, replace the old Bulfinch wards with semiprivate rooms and an intensive care unit, and add still more facilities for clinical research, laboratories, diagnostic radiology, and space medicine, all of which had grown beyond the expectations of the 1950s.

Modernization of the OPD.

While plans for a new ambulatory building and new practice organizations were suspended, other changes had begun which slowly modernized the administration, patient care, and financing of the OPD while enhancing its educational programs. Some of these changes represented distinctive departures in an institution that originally provided free care to the "indigent, deserving poor" through the voluntary duty of its staff.

Clark brought Michael White from the Health Insurance Plan of New York to help develop group practice and administer the OPD, where he was assisted by Ruth Farrisey, the OPD executive officer and head of ambulatory nursing.

White held his post until his retirement in 1962 when Henry Murphy, associate director who had recently organized the Emergency Ward, became administrator. The long-time OPD tradition of part-time voluntary service was broken when John D. Stoeckle was appointed chief of the Medical Clinic in 1954, becoming the first paid, full-time clinical staff member in the OPD; Stoeckle took over from Earle M. Chapman, who had held the post unpaid and part-time since the forties. The OPD was renamed the MGH Clinics to signal new efforts and remove the stigma of the past. The Committee on Clinics under Stoeckle's chairmanship became the forum for discussion and coordination of administrative and clinical practice among the several services.

Historically, clinic charges had been set at less than cost, automatically assuring a deficit. A new system of charges at cost was introduced, and patients were rated on their ability to pay, these being necessary steps to finance essential improvements, rising salary costs, diagnostic tests, and, eventually, physician services. Visit charges rose gradually from $1.50 to $3.00 in the fifties, to $10 in the sixties, to $30 to $40 in the seventies. The changes were so gradual and well buffered by third-party payments that patients' comparisons with the old 10¢ or 25¢ visit to the OPD were simply pleasant nostalgia. As the clinics began to charge at cost, the means test, which had been designed to exclude patients who could afford a private doctor, was abolished in 1961. Patients were thereafter admitted regardless of income while offered the option of selecting a physician from a private roster drawn up by the MGH Staff Associates. This policy ended more than half a century of conflict with private practice over the admission of paying patients—historically called "clinic abuse." By treating patients free who could have paid a private doctor's fee, the OPD had competed unfairly with physicians trying to build a practice when paying patients were scarce.

Still other changes followed with the growth of third-party payments. The clinics eventually ceased to rate patients in advance of medical attention, eliminating still another entrenched tradition, that of scaling clinic charges according to the patient's income. By 1974 differential charges for visits were introduced, and the clinics, in effect, adopted a mode of fee schedules similar to private practice. Also, in 1964 the clinics abandoned the practice of requiring patients to pay in advance of the visit.

The outpatient building, which had opened in 1904, went through successive alterations between 1951 and 1979 in an attempt to meet the rising expectations of public and staff. First there was a new paint job of various colors (1951), then new flooring and furnishings (1955), lowered ceilings (1963), and finally carpets, modern furnishings, and remodeled suites with the development of group practices (1972–1979). Most noteworthy, however, was the removal of wooden benches in 1960; installed in 1904, these antique symbols of charity care were wholly out of place in a practice struggling to modernize not only its facilities but also its relations with patients.

The long-term problem of ensuring immediate attention to walk-in patients while trying to develop and maintain appointment schedules was solved in part by admitting physicians who provided immediate advice and who could defer visits to a later date. Originally, one medical and one surgical resident each morning were located near the admitting offices in the clinics basement, a system developed in 1947; the area, called the dispensary clinic, served as a general practice for patients without appointments. This system evolved and was redefined as the Ambulatory Screening Clinic. The ASC moved to the first floor with four offices in 1972, expanded to eight examining offices in 1980, was put under the full-time direction of Richard Pingree in 1974, and was open 12 hours each day. Visits might total 80 to 100 per day. Initially staffed only by medical residents, the ASC began employing clinical fellows and regular staff for sessional work, for the first time paying these staff for such service functions that had traditionally been the prerogative, duty, and responsibility of residents.

Labeling a prescribed drug with its technical or chemical name, which is now so widely accepted, was begun in 1954 as a venture in patient education. The doctor's arcane habit of prescribing, and the patient's magical experience in receiving, bottles of unknown drugs by numbers (e.g., 88B, which contained but a quarter grain of phenobarbital) was gone forever—a precursor to the expansion of patient information that eventually included the package insert.

While no general group practice plan had emerged, pressures to experiment continued. In 1962 George Baker and Allan Sandler began to organize a small private medical group practice which eventually included Cyrus Briefer and Jan Koch-Weser. The practice was located in a suite of offices on the first floor of the clinics building. As a result, this old structure that was to have been replaced came to contain more than one form of practice, just as the Farnsworth report had recommended. Only once before at Cornell and at the MGH (1915) had a similar OPD "pay clinic" experiment been tried, and then with but transient success. From 1962 to 1970 these physicians took responsibility for much of the work of the hospital's Staff Clinic for employees. Sandler handled the care of members of Union Local 380 under a prepaid contract. The informal group continued until 1971 when Baker and Sandler moved to the Warren Building. Later, similar salaried attachments were made with Jerome Grossman and James Dineen for organizing and practicing in a diagnostic section of the clinic. Elsewhere, the pattern of salaried part- or full-time clinic chiefs in Orthopedics, Pediatrics, Psychiatry, and Surgery continued but did not expand.

Following a study of role dissatisfaction among clinic nurses and faced with limited prospects of attracting more full-time medical staff in 1961, the nursing staff (Ruth Farrisey, Anne Sweatt, and Barbara Noonan, with Dr. Stoeckle) rearranged nursing practice so that the nurse would see patients with chronic diseases on regular scheduled visits to her own office. Although similar programs had been organized outside of a medical practice, this was the first of such medical nurse-practitioner clinics within an outpatient practice and, as such, constituted a beginning of the trend towards interprofessional care and autonomy by nonphysician providers. In 1980 nurse practitioners in the MGH Ambulatory Care Division and its health centers numbered 41; in the medical group practice visits to nurse practitioners accounted for 15 percent of all medical visits.

The history of the OPD from the 1870s to the 1950s recorded the development of subspecialty clinics; between 1950 and 1980, however, relatively few new clinics emerged. In 1978 the Orthopedic Clinic developed the Sports Medicine Clinic. General Psychiatry evolved subspecialties in psychopharmacology, hypnosis, alcohol, and acute psychiatry but in the form of group practices rather than as clinics. Subspecialty group practices of pediatrics followed divisions established in medicine, with the unique addition of practices devoted to learning disorders, genetics, and adolescent medicine.

With the continued movement toward subspecialization and the retirement of older general physicians, the long tradition of generalist care had declined and the ranks of its practitioners had thinned. These shifts, in turn, stimulated the concept of a group to renew generalist care, a direction that began to accumulate public support in the sixties and, at the MGH, had long had trustee backing. In their argument for a doctors' office building in 1954, the trustees had envisioned more than the housing of specialists; "It would," they noted, "enable the ambulatory patient to see the general practitioner and the specialists in one place." The attitudes of younger physicians also changed during the sixties. A survey by Leaf and Daniel Federman revealed nearly unanimous interest in future practice in a group rather than in a solo office. These elements and the better financing of ambulatory care through Medicare and Medicaid made the organization and financing of such a practice feasible.

In 1970 another committee on Ambulatory Patient Care, chaired by John Mills, was formed to engage these reawakening interests; this led the following year to the organization of a group practice within the Medical Services under the direction of Jerome Grossman. The new group practice, Internal Medicine Associates (IMA), began within the Medical Service with eight staff participants. In 1972 the initiative was strongly backed by Federman, acting chief of the Medical Services, and Benjamin Castleman, acting general director. Moreover, like his predecessors Means and Bauer, Leaf considered the group practice enterprise essential to the hospital and the Medical Service.

In this program both clinic and private practice were reorganized in novel ways, which altered traditional professional-hospital-administrative relationships. First, the medical clinics were decentralized from both hospital and department by establishing a board of managers (composed of a practitioner, nurse, and business manager) whose members held joint administrative, fiscal, and professional responsibility for ambulatory medical patients as well as for teaching and research. Second, the IMA became responsible for all patients seeking aid whether through individual private or institutional referrals. The practice had four goals: (1) to develop a primary care practice in internal medicine; (2) to integrate clinic and private patients in one practice with a single high standard of care; (3) to expand educational programs in primary care; and (4) to conduct research and evaluation of primary care practice. Professional fees became part of clinic charges, and the staff became salaried by the hospital, with salaries based on the quantity of clinical work. However, the medical staff had responsibility for practice management as they previously had in their offices. Continuity improved as the unpaid and part-time staff was reduced, providing a stable professional organization. The group practice accomplished patient-centered care and efficiencies only possible with full-time staff, a reform that had been advocated by Cabot in the early decades of this century.

This organizational model of group practice was eventually extended to pediatrics, psychiatry, dermatology, certain medical subspecialties (endocrine, diabetes, oncology, hematology), and the MGH health centers. By 1980 a sizable percentage of staff worked in group practices—39 percent of Medicine, 57 percent of Pediatrics, 50 percent of Psychiatry, and 33 percent of Urology. This reorganization also introduced a new class of professionals into the MGH, the business managers for ambulatory group practices. With their MBAs or MPHs, young administrators out of the business and public health schools of MIT and Harvard were responsible, together with the full-time professional staff, for the efficient, effective, and humane conduct of practice. The novel MGH arrangement for group practices drew the attention of other institutions and promised to deal with the continuing issues of comprehensive care and education.

Following the formation of group practices and prompted by the need to replace the Warren Building offices with a new facility, Charles Sanders appointed Jerome Grossman director of Ambulatory Care Planning and of the Ambulatory Care Division—the new name for the MGH Clinics—which now included group practices, the departmental clinics, and the emergency ward and health centers. In September 1974 plans for the Ambulatory Care Center were begun, and two years later a governance committee was formed to oversee its planning and operation. The center was unique in the hospital's divisions in being financed by rentals from practitioners and charges from services to patients—made possible because the ACC would have its own radiologic and laboratory services. In an even greater departure from tradition the committee recommended, and Sanders decided, to charge all staff for office rent, thus eliminating an old "perk" that went back to the 1930s when the new geographic full-time staff had hospital offices rent-free in exchange for part of their salaries.

The ACC was to be no mere doctors' office building, for its principles included common group goals: a single standard of care for all patients; cost-effective care that may also reduce hospitalization; a single center for coordination of ambulatory services; and instruction of students, residents, and health professionals in patient-centered ambulatory services—ideals that echoed the GEC statements of 1952.

After an arduous, difficult, and time-consuming approval process for the certificate of need, ACC construction plans received final approval from state officials in May 1978. Construction began in 1979 with the removal of the Moseley Building and Walcott House. The new structure contains a complex of practices in some 900 offices—examination rooms, an ambulatory surgical center, an expanded rehabilitation unit, a pharmacy, a cafeteria, and sufficient conference rooms for students, residents, and staff of the several services.

The development of the Logan International Airport Medical Station and the Pulmonary II Clinic merits special attention. Following a 1961 jet crash into Winthrop Bay off Logan Airport, the executive director of the Massachusetts Port Authority approached the hospital about organizing medical services at the airport. A survey suggested by Clark was conducted by the Harvard School of Public Health. The ensuing report proposed a clinic at the airport to meet the need for emergency care as well as for employees' health maintenance along the pattern used in large industries. In 1963 the Logan International Airport Medical Station of the MGH opened under the joint sponsorship of the hospital and the Authority, with Kenneth Bird as medical director. The station was an on-the-job medical practice providing emergency and walk-in services, annual examinations, and preventive vaccinations for travelers. It was staffed by one full-time physician and four nurses.

In 1966, under a contract with the Commonwealth's Division of Tuberculosis, the MGH established the Pulmonary II Clinic as part of the Pulmonary Clinic, the first general-hospital-based program for the care of tuberculosis patients. This was the first step in a statewide program to expand ambulatory treatment of tuberculosis and close existing sanitoriums; in 1980 there were 44 clinics in general hospitals throughout the state, and state sanitorium beds were reduced to ten. Drs. Homayoun Kazemi and K. Bird and Barbara Noonan, nurse practitioner, made up the clinic's initial staff.

Community-based Practices: The MGH Health Centers.

While the clinics at the MGH were taking steps to modernize, the movement for health centers away from urban hospitals staged a revival, stimulated by grants from the Office of Economic Opportunity in the "war on poverty." Bringing health services to the poor meant centers to replace the individual services of solo practitioners who had disappeared from inner city neighborhoods and implied the relocation of the group and technical services of hospital OPDs that were deemed inaccessible.

The MGH's history of involvement with neighborhood health centers had its roots in the 1965 Sackett Plan of the Boston Health Department which assigned the MGH "areas of responsibility" including the West End–Beacon Hill, the North End, Charlestown, East Boston, Chelsea, and Revere. The hospital responded by setting up two centers, the Bunker Hill Health Center (BHHC) in Charlestown and the Chelsea Health Center (CHC) while affiliating with the community-organized North End and Revere health centers through staff appointments to hospital services at the MGH.

The MGH started developing health centers in the late sixties when several of its departments (Pediatrics, Social Service, Nursing, and Medicine) and the MGH Clinics Administration joined community groups in planning such practices. Under the leadership of John Connelly, then chief of the Pediatrics Clinic, Nathan Talbot, chief of the Children's Medical Service, Mr. Murphy, Ms. Farrisey, and Dr. Knowles, what began as a pediatric survey of the health of Charlestown children grew into the BHHC. The development of the center proceeded despite alternatives that pulled temptingly in other directions. Leaf pushed for the community-based initiative while being pressed to affiliate the medical staff with the newly established Harvard Community Health Plan, a private prepaid practice plan sponsored by the Harvard Medical School, that served a young population of working adults. The needs and opportunities presented by Charlestown, an older community of low-income families, seemed greater.

The BHHC now occupies one of the old (1940) City of Boston Health Centers in Charlestown, a district with a population of 16,000. The early staff of the center included Roger Sweet, Robert Leet, Ann Godley, John Connelly, Leo Burgin, Edward Dyer, Henry Sicamore, and Kathan Kennedy. Currently under the direction of Catherine Beyer, the center has a physician staff of 18 pediatricians, internists, and obstetricians, along with nurse practitioners, physician assistants, a staff in community mental health, social work, nutrition, and dentistry, and specialty consultants.

Guided by a community advisory board, which was aided in its planning by Eleanor Clark, chief of MGH Social Service, the Chelsea Health Center—a community-based practice for a city of 32,000—was launched in the basement of the Horace Street Baptist Church in 1972. Andrew Guthrie acted as its first director. The CHC subsequently moved to the Remick House (the nurses' residence of the Chelsea Memorial Hospital) and has since reorganized as a complex of facilities of the now disbanded hospital, an arrangement negotiated by Lawrence Martin. The CHC facilities consist of an emergency ward and a 10-bed hospital unit from the old hospital, along with health center offices. The staff, now directed by Roger Sweet, numbers 23 physicians and 21 nurses, plus dental, nutrition, and mental health staff.

Both the BHHC and CHC are sites of clinical clerkships for undergraduate medical students and of rotations for dental students, student nurses, dietitians, and social workers. The CHC is also a training rotation for medical residents while the BHHC provides for psychiatric residents. In medical education, the centers have been sites away from the hospital "to see what practice is like" and for learning the basics of clinical method, providing second-year students supervised experience with patients outside hospital wards and clinics.

The health centers have realized an ideal of comprehensive health care, providing home visiting services that had been started but not sustained by the Family Health Program (1954–1961), developing hospice services for terminal cancer patients (Andrew Billings, 1978), addressing new services to the old but growing problems of child and elder abuse (Andrew Guthrie, 1978, and Terrence O'Malley, 1980) and, most distinctively, providing mental health services from the outset. At a time when federal and state mental health programs were building separate facilities, the MGH neighborhood health centers took a different tack and developed mental health services as part of their comprehensive programs by contracting with regional centers (Allan Jacobson, 1969).

Education, Training, and Research in Practice. The MGH

Clinics—and now its health centers and group practices—have always been distinguished among the Harvard teaching hospitals by maintaining a tradition of ambulatory clerkships for students in medicine and its subspecialties. In recent years there have been between 280 and 290 students in the clinics, figures close to those 270 reported by Cabot in 1919 for the entire hospital. The assigned resident participation has varied from 100 percent in Surgery, a completely resident-staffed clinic; to 30 percent in Medicine, a mixed resident and staff group practice; to none in those clinics such as gastrointestinal manned only by clinical fellows and staff physicians.

As an experiment in medical education in 1954, the Family Health Program introduced students to the comprehensive care of families. The FHP was aided by a five-year grant from the Rockefeller Foundation and organized as an interdepartmental enterprise that included preventive medicine. With 15 students each year, the program enrolled 170 "medically indigent" families who had traditionally used the MGH clinics and assigned each third-year student to care for one family under the supervision of a staff preceptor who, in turn, was also responsible for three or four other families. Patients were seen in the clinic, the hospital, and at home. The FHP managed to last until 1961 when neither the Medical School nor any clinical department wanted to make it an integral service or a required educational experience. Nonetheless, many of the ideas embodied in the FHP survived its demise.

After that experiment traditional outpatient clerkships and weekly follow-up practice for residents did not change—at least not until 1973. At that time, with stimulus from one of its first residents, Allan Goroll, a new medical residency track was introduced in which medical training was based on 50 percent experience in the newly formed IMA and 50 percent in the hospital, a major departure from the standard medical residency that was almost exclusively hospital-centered. While in ambulatory practice, the residents belonged to one of the IMA practice teams. For the first time in MGH history, ambulatory training was integrated with a staff practice. This primary care program, which became a model for other institutions, emphasized the learning of skills and techniques important for general medicine and developed a tradition of rounds on ambulatory patients as a major teaching exercise in which all the department's special units participated. By 1978 five medical residents a year—one-quarter of all medical residents—were on this special track. The program also influenced medical students who could now see the school and hospital acting out the values of patient-centered care in the person of residents and staff actually pursuing generalist careers that had only been espoused in the past.

The lack of research in the clinics, compared with hospital laboratory investigations, has been cited to explain the disinterest of academic clinicians in outpatient practices. Nevertheless, the clinics did stimulate research, particularly many clinical follow-up studies that developed from repeated contacts with patients and gave the medical subspecialists their early descriptive base and data on the outcomes of treatment. Meanwhile, study of the clinic developed as an important research theme. From 1959 to 1963 Irving K. Zola did his now classic study on "Cultural Factors in Seeking Medical Aid." During the same period Erich Lindemann, chief of Psychiatry, and his colleagues looked into the effects of relocation on West End residents, including their patterns of medical use. In addition, Lindemann's studies of the emotional crises surrounding illness and injury not only influenced the development of mental health programs in the health centers but also gave new direction to the care of both acute and chronic medical outpatients.

To facilitate the process of patient care, Kenneth Bird established telecommunication as a means to link distant to central site of care in consultation and education. Grossman's experiment with computer-based history-taking, with a view to standardization, was quite feasible but, like the automated medical record, not easily adapted to the traditional behaviors of medical practitioners. Videotaping of the medical interview, first used for the instruction of medical students by Stoeckle in 1967, has now become established in all programs in ambulatory practice. From nursing researchers at Boston University came the first analysis of the role and functions of clinic nurses which stimulated the development of work for nurse practitioners.

Reflections, Past and Future. Although one stimulus for practice reorganization was the declining OPD census of the fifties, a steady rise occurred from the 1952 low point of 118,063 visits to 567,453 in 1980. By then the Ambulatory Care Division had been defined as the MGH Group Practices and Clinics (360,774 visits), the Emergency Ward (82,548 visits), and the medical station at Logan Airport (13,663 visits). Visits to the ACD, combined with estimated visits (350,000) to MGH private practices, to the clinics of the MEEI (125,000), and to the affiliated health centers of the North End (30,000) and Revere (1,200), brought the total of ambulatory visits to practices at or affiliated with the MGH to over a million per year.

So numerous are these encounters with the public seeking medical aid that the MGH might, in fact, be viewed as an ambulatory care center with its own hospital. In retrospect it is clear that those ideas about practice originating in the 1950s and intermittently acted upon since then were completed by 1982, keeping the promise to improve treatment and learning outside the hospital in the tradition of the MGH charter. The newly organized ACC together with the health centers that reach out into local communities make the MGH distinctive, literally a hospital without walls, realizing those aspirations of the fifties that defined the modern hospital not as a tertiary referral center alone but rather a center for the health of the community. Whether the hospital can maintain this vision, with its promise of providing care outside, is problematic; yet that comprehensive goal is even more essential now than before, for the major problems of health and health care continue to be outside the hospital.

> With the assistance of *Daniel Ellis, Allan Sandler, George Baker, Kenneth Bird, Jerome Grossman, Walter Bauer, Edward Churchill, Alexander Leaf, Ruth Farrisey, David Crockett, Ruth Meehan, Gordon Scannell, John Mills,* and *Henry Murphy*

Dr. Leaf added the following comment:

Dr. Stoeckle has provided an extensive documentation of the development of the ambulatory medicine unit which he has headed since he was appointed to that position by Bauer in 1952. His history needs only one supplementary remark, namely the enormously important role he himself played in the developments which he documents. Through Bauer's tenure and through the period of Knowles' administration, Stoeckle held his peace while developing teaching programs in the ambulatory setting and awaiting the opportunity for more progressive leadership of the hospital to permit him to revise the entire medical ambulatory clinics system. This came only after Knowles had left the MGH and Castleman was the acting director. At that time, with the help of Jerome Grossman, Stoeckle, Dineen, and a few others managed to professionalize the ambulatory clinics, reducing the number of physicians from something over 170 members of the active medical staff, who looked upon their half day in the clinics as time in the stone quarries, to a handful of dedicated physicians who earned their living and developed their careers in the ambulatory medical practices of our outpatient clinics. This group, which organized as the Internal Medicine Associates, professionalized the whole practice of ambulatory medicine and served as the focus around which our primary care medical residency program could develop, and there was a marked increase in teaching of medical students in the ambulatory setting.

When the hospital became involved in the Bunker Hill Health Center, the adult medical group there became part of the outreach program of our ambulatory care unit; the Chelsea center provided a further extension of the outreach program. All these developments owe a great deal to the commitment and dedication and hard work that John Stoeckle put into them.

Emergency Ward

EARLE W. WILKINS, JR.

Nowhere within the MGH has the style of the practice of medicine changed more dramatically than in the Emergency Ward. It is no longer just a clinic for the management of accidents and other emergencies. In the three decades since the conclusion of World War II, it has become a center for the practice of family medicine, for consultation and decision about patients—often the elderly with complex pathology—and a portal of entry for nearly half of all admissions to the hospital. These phenomena were part of a national change which followed the disappearance of the endangered species of general practitioners and the increased sophistication in the diagnosis and treatment of the acutely ill patient. The movement ultimately generated a new specialty, the field of emergency medicine.

It is not totally clear when the name "Emergency ward" first appeared at MGH. Prior to 1900 the accident room was located on the first floor of Bulfinch East, now Ward 4. Washburn's history noted "difficulty in getting service for the EW from busy senior house officers in the mornings" and that in 1903 the EW was moved to the "glass rooms, sterilizing room and recovery rooms of the 1867 Operating Building." The ambulance approached via a drive along the rear of Bulfinch. The accident room was located at a considerable distance from the new Out Patient Building constructed in 1904; nevertheless, there the accident room remained until 1916 when it was moved to the basement of the new Moseley Building. It seems probable that the name Emergency Ward was firmly established in this facility. The quarters included four examining and operating rooms, sterilizing and instrument rooms, a recovery room, and two small wards, female and male. These constituted the emergency wards for overnight use, a concept first called for by OPD physicians and surgeons in 1898. The move to the White Building came just after Ether Day in 1939.

Whenever and wherever the sources of the names Emergency Ward and Overnight Ward, they remain such today despite obvious disparities between present nomenclature and usage. Their very busyness, however, makes them an appropriate topic for separate historic discussion for the first time.

A measure of the change of practice in the Emergency Ward in the past quarter century is provided by a consideration of the patient census. In this period there has been a three-fold increase in patients registered in the EW logs—from 28,209 to 82,757; and there has been a 100 percent increase in hospital admissions via the EW—from 7,001 to 13,674. In the past five years these admissions have accounted for 45 percent of all MGH admissions. Since 1970 this has been reflected particularly in admissions to the private services where there was a 33 percent increase, while admissions to ward services were actually dropping 5 percent.

Although the Emergency Ward has remained on the first floor of the White Building with ready access to the OPD, there have been some major physical changes. During the 1950s the burgeoning patient load and the demand for diagnostic x-rays created a crisis in patient care; finally, in 1964 a radiologic unit, designed by Jack R. Dreyfuss, was constructed in the open courtyard in the White Building, between the administrative offices adjacent to the White elevators and the Overnight Ward, providing four x-ray rooms, two supplied with fluoroscopic equipment. EW and Overnight Ward x-ray studies could be made without transfer by the inefficient elevators to the main radiology suite on White 2; in addition, all in-hospital patient x-rays at nights and on weekends were now carried out on White 1.

A major overhaul of the physical plant, again necessitated by the crush of patient load, was accomplished between May 1972 and October 1973. The renovation added 5,029 square feet to the original space of 6,414 square feet by (1) filling in the open courtyard north of the EW booking lobby, (2) utilizing space originally occupied by White admitting and cashier facilities (which had moved to the new Gray Building admitting area), and (3) assuming the space occupied by the insurance and discharge offices in the back corridor near the White elevators. This not only increased EW space by 78 percent but also made possible a dramatic improvement in traffic patterns, separate facilities for pediatrics patients, the separation of minor medicine transient patients from those with major illness requiring stretcher space, the opening of a complete dental suite, the development of a four-bed cardiac monitoring unit, and improved minor surgery and orthopedic facilities. Air conditioning permitted a more comfortable working atmosphere in this hotbed of continuing 24-hour pressure activity. This remarkable feat of renovation was accomplished without interrupting the function of the EW during the alteration. There have been several lesser changes in the physical plant since 1973. Meanwhile, over the years the bed capacity of the Overnight Ward dropped from 27 to 18.

The Emergency Ward continues to be a teaching facility with the resident staffs from all services participating in patient care. There has been an increase from one surgical and one medical resident assigned in the immediate postwar period to six surgical residents, 10 medical residents, two pediatric residents, and one resident each from neurology and orthopedics, all having full-time duties in 1979. In 1960 Earle W. Wilkins, Jr., was assigned the chairmanship of the supervising staff Emergency Ward Committee; in 1969 he was made chief of Emergency Services. In 1976 Peter Gross became his assistant, and later associate chief. The Children's Service was the first to provide daytime continuing staff coverage, beginning with the opening of the "new" EW in late 1973. At that time their EW facility became the center of all pediatrics walk-in, or acute care, activities.

There has been a comparable increase in the nursing staff, to an average total assignment of 19 registered nurses, 5 licensed practical nurses, and 5 nursing assistants. In 1975 adult nurse practitioners became regular participants in the provision of ambulatory patient care. There have, from time to time, been special nursing assignments, such as a liaison nurse, a psychiatric nurse, and an alcoholic therapy nurse. Since 1968 there have been just two head nurses or clinical team leaders, Geri Wittrock and Ginny Tritschler, who have provided formidable leadership as well as exemplary role models amid the drama of the department.

Administrative personnel has provided the third element in the troika of staffing. Their numbers have jumped to an average overall assignment of 5 administrators, 23 admitting assistants, and 10 clerks, adding to the huge force required to operate the emergency center. Michael P. Hooley has been senior administrator for most of the 23 years he has worked for the EW.

Perhaps the most noteworthy of all the contributors to the vitality of the operation was Henry J. Murphy, associate director of the MGH. He was not only administratively responsible for its function from the early fifties until 1974; he also thoughtfully and vigorously championed consideration of the patient as the principal obligation of the entire working staff. He was the main architect of the triage system, initiated in the late 1950s, in which patients were seen not according to the time of their arrival but in order of urgency and per subspecialty units available in the EW. At first this procedure was conducted by the senior resident, medical or surgical, who was in charge of the EW, in the interest of equality of resident experience and teaching. The authority with which the senior resident conducted his business was absolute. Ultimately, the passage of the patient triage function to specially trained nurses in the mid-seventies did more than anything else to change the system. It is a requirement that a third-year resident always be in attendance in the EW.

The Emergency Ward never functioned better nor its triage more smoothly than when General Director John Knowles took his day in charge. This was always on the occasion of the Medical Service annual picnic and party when senior staff went to the "pit"—as the EW was affectionately and accurately termed—to free the residents. Knowles had helped found resident triage when he was a resident, and he knew how to take command forcefully, generously, and compassionately.

Long a major contributor to the EW administration, Ferdinand (Bob) Strauss was its "godfather." His entire MGH career was spent trying to improve the EW until ill health prematurely limited his work capacity. He had succeeded Henry Murphy in 1963 and was in turn followed by Isabella Tighe (1974–1976) and then by Jerome Grossman, whose experience catapulted him into the directorship of the New England Medical Center in 1979.

Although during these decades of the evolution of the specialty of emergency medicine (it achieved conjoint board status in 1979) the MGH did not have a residency program in emergency medicine, it nonetheless assumed early primary leadership in the teaching of persons choosing this field as their specialty. In 1966 Stephen E. Goldfinger and Daniel D. Federman from the Department of Medicine prepared and delivered a pioneering course for three staff members of the Lynn, Mass., Hospital who were changing their medical practice styles to permit them as a group to provide continuous staff coverage for their emergency department. As a consequence, the Department of Continuing Education of the Harvard Medical School has sponsored a workshop in emergency medicine at the MGH, given thrice each year for 10 graduate physicians, in which the practical aspects of the specialty are taught in a two-week course of didactic lectures, laboratory practice, and patient observation. Many of the current national leaders in the field have participated—a total of 269 participants between September 1969 and March 1980.

In 1978 the MGH published its *Textbook of Emergency Medicine* (Williams & Wilkins Co.), compiled largely from lectures and demonstrations developed in the emergency medicine workshop course and edited by Wilkins, James J. Dineen, and Ashby Moncure. Beginning in 1971 the MGH Emergency Medicine sponsored again by the HMS Department of Continuing Education. In this program, for a single scholar each year, a full year's curriculum is especially designed to round out the residency exposure and education in whatever aspects of emergency medicine had not been adequately covered in the individual's prior residency training in general medicine.

In this eventful era of exploding health care provision in the hospital emergency departments of this country, the Emergency Ward at the MGH was never for even one minute closed. Its reputation for prompt attention has often been taxed by the burden of demand. Other hospital facilities providing patient care regularly shut down nights and weekends; some temporarily suspend function because of overload of patients or unavailability of staff. Never the EW: For 24 hours a day, each day of the 365, it is there with doors open ready to look after any and all problems coming its way.

Fortune had kept us from another disaster of the magnitude of the Cocoanut Grove fire in 1942, but lesser disasters make an impact on the EW at all too regular intervals: the North Station train accident (1962), two Logan Airport plane crashes (1974), the Charlestown amusement park accident (1974), the Charles Station subway crash (1977), the Somerville trichloroethylene spill (1980). Readiness for these and uncounted mini-disasters has maintained the reputation of the MGH Emergency Ward as the busiest and the finest in New England.

The continuing challenge to the EW has, perhaps, never been more dramatically illustrated than in the Everett Knowles case. On May 23, 1962, 12-year-old "Red" Knowles arrived at the EW with his right arm severed at the shoulder when caught between the side of a train and a stone abutment. Under the imaginative and innovative leadership of vascular surgeon Robert S. Shaw and chief surgical resident Ronald A. Malt, the arm was reattached by a multiservice team (including David C. Mitchell, John D. Constable, William H. Harris, L. Henry Edmunds, and John M. Head) in the first successful limb replantation effort in the United States.

16. Dermatology Service

THOMAS B. FITZPATRICK AND IRVIN H. BLANK

In 1948 Chester North Frazier was summoned from the University of Texas in Galveston to become chief of the Dermatology Service and the Edward Wigglesworth Professor of Dermatology. He came with a 10-year grant from the Rockefeller Foundation and the specific charge to establish a first-class department.

Frazier had a somewhat unique approach to teaching and to topical therapy of skin diseases. He felt that dermatology could be taught best to medical students and residents if emphasis was placed on well-worked-up inpatients; he seldom involved outpatients in teaching. He also believed that there was little proof of the efficacy of many of the topical therapeutic agents and reduced the MGH formulary of dermatologic agents from over 100 to 25.

When Frazier arrived at the MGH he found a research staff consisting of a single biochemist, Irvin Blank, who had been at the hospital since 1937. Blank was the principal basic research scientist from 1948 to 1959 as well as the key person in planning the research facilities on the fifth floor of the Warren Building. His own research, in collaboration with Robert Scheuplein—later of the Food and Drug Administration—was concerned mostly with percutaneous absorption.

Walter Lever, a diligent teacher, clinician, and investigator during those years, concentrated on proteins and lipids in collaboration with Edmund Klein. Meanwhile, contact with Benjamin Castleman, chief of Pathology, quickened Lever's interest in the pathology of skin disorders. He later became one of the outstanding dermatopathologists in the United States, and his textbook on that subject has been a standard reference through five editions. In 1959 Lever left for Tufts Medical School where he became professor and chief of Dermatology.

In June 1958—in the wake of Frazier's departure—Thomas Fitzpatrick, professor at the University of Oregon Medical School, was selected to be the Wigglesworth Professor of Dermatology and chairman of the Department of Dermatology at the Harvard Medical School and, simultaneously, chief of the Dermatology Service at the MGH. Fitzpatrick had spent one year (1958–1959) as a Commonwealth Advanced Fellow at Oxford, doing biochemistry research in melanin biology. When Fitzpatrick arrived in August 1959, Blank came to the new chief's assistance. So, too, did Maurice Tolman, an astute clinician and teacher, who had during 1958 and 1959 been managing patient care and clinical teaching in dermatology and who continued to inspire generations of residents until his retirement in 1977. Together, Blank and Tolman helped Fitzpatrick with the early development of the present Dermatology Service at the MGH— the former helping to build and stabilize the research facilities, the latter focusing on patient care and teaching.

In 1959 the Rockefeller Foundation again agreed to provide funds for five years in a second attempt to build a department. Furthermore, it was a fortuitous time for the enlargement of research facilities because the NIH had awarded a dermatology training grant which provided stipends for trainees and staff from 1960 onwards. The grant enabled the department to find and train a large number of investigators between 1959 and 1980. During that period the Dermatology Service served the field of dermatology in the United States, Canada, and Japan by training more academic dermatologists than any other training program in the United States; there are now ten professors and department heads, and 44 full-time dermatologists.

Fitzpatrick's interests were largely centered on the biology of melanin. His contributions included (1) the first demonstration in humans of the pigment-forming enzyme, tyrosinase; (2) the isolation of the basic metabolic unit, the melanosome, in which pigment is synthesized in the cytoplasm of melanocytes; and (3) the discovery of differences in concentrations of tyrosinase in normal melanocytes vis à vis malignant melanocytes in melanoma. This striking difference provides a mechanism for concentration of toxic metabolites in melanoma cells and offers a unique opportunity for chemotherapy of melanoma.

This broad interest in melanin biology led Fitzpatrick to begin a study of melanoma in humans. To aid in this research and to replace Lever as the dermatopathologist at the MGH, Fitzpatrick invited Wallace H. Clark, associate professor of pathology at Tulane, to come to the MGH in 1961. Clark established for the first time at the hospital a dermatopathology unit jointly sponsored by the Dermatology Service and the Department of Pathology.

Clark, with Fitzpatrick, Martin C. Mihm, Jr., and the late John Raker, a surgeon, established the Pigmented Lesion Clinic as a subgroup in the Tumor Clinic to study the pathology and natural history of malignant melanoma. From this study came Clark's and Mihm's contributions to the pathology of melanoma which have reoriented the thinking about melanoma of the skin; the Clark-Mihm classification of melanoma is now accepted throughout the world. In addition, the definition of early clinical characteristics of primary melanoma by Fitzpatrick, Clark, and Mihm enabled, for the first time, an early diagnosis; these criteria are now widely used, and some believe the marked increase in the survival rate, from 40 percent primary survival rate in 1946 to 75 percent in 1980, is related to the early detection of the lesions using these criteria. In the years since Clark left for Temple University and later the University of Pennsylvania to head its dermatopathology unit, Mihm who, as professor of pathology, has appointments in both dermatology and pathology, has served as a focus for a host of trainees in dermatopathology.

When Fitzpatrick came to the MGH in 1959, there were two first-year residents already involved in research who were later to play an important role in the department and in dermatology in America. These two—Howard P. Baden and Irwin M. Freedberg—were fresh from the Harvard Medical School and medical residencies in the Peter Bent Brigham Hospital and Beth Israel Hospital, respectively. They collaborated on the biosynthesis of keratin and on the study of keratinization disorders. They had also had a year's stint in biochemistry at Brandeis University. As a now tenured member of the department, Baden is a distinguished physician-scientist; he is actively involved in the curriculum organization and serves as a member of the Board of Advisors to the students. Freedberg returned to the Beth Israel Hospital after finishing his training in dermatology to become chief of the Dermatology Service and to build that unit to its present excellence. He sparked a new era of dermatology in the Peter Bent Brigham Hospital and Beth Israel by combined teaching and patient care rounds. This combined program was further strengthened when Harley A. Haynes left the MGH to head up a clinical unit at the Peter Bent Brigham Hospital in 1974, and in 1978 when Arthur Rhodes, who was trained in the Harvard program, became chief of Dermatology at the Children's Hospital. Freedberg went to Johns Hopkins as chief of Dermatology in 1977, and an able clinician, Kenneth Arndt, became chief of Dermatology at the Beth Israel Hospital.

In 1959 Fitzpatrick brought with him from Oregon a biochemist, Madhu A. Pathak, to continue their collaboration in the study of vitiligo, a disease known for several thousand years in Egypt and India, and still prevalent throughout the world. A traditional treatment in North Africa and Asia had been the use of psoralens, a naturally occurring group of plant photosensitizers, in combination with exposure to the sun. Fitzpatrick and Pathak undertook a study of the interaction between the drug and ultraviolet radiation and its use as a therapy for vitiligo. Acting on evidence that topical psoralens plus sunlight gave some improvement to psoriasis sufferers, Fitzpatrick and Pathak, joined by John A. Parrish and Lewis Tanenbaum, began using oral psoralens and long-wave ultraviolet light (UVA) as a therapy for intractable cases of psoriasis. They learned that the UVA-wavelength (290–320 nm) in sunlight, administered two hours after psoralen ingestion, was the effective wavelength of the light spectrum to activate the psoralens systemically. Fitzpatrick called the process photochemotherapy, and it later evolved into the first medical application of a photobiologic principle.

The amount of UVA light needed to be effective requires too long an exposure to natural sunlight. Therefore, a high-intensity light source was developed by engineers at the nearby G.T.E. Sylvania Lighting Products group in Danvers in collaboration with the MGH research team, particularly Parrish. Special bulbs were built into a light box within which the patient could stand. The PUVA (Psoralen–Ultra Violet A) was reported in 1974 by the four investigators and is now used worldwide for the most difficult cases of psoriasis and for a T-cell lymphoma of the skin, mycosis fungoides. A new phototherapy center was established at the MGH in 1975 with eight UVA irradiators and a new large laboratory facility. Parrish, associate professor of dermatology, now fully trained in basic photobiology, heads this research unit, the Wellman Laboratories. New laboratories will be located in the Wellman Building, built with a $15 million gift to the MGH by Guillan Wellman, a patient of Fitzpatrick and Parrish, and Arthur O. Wellman.

The Dermatology Service has not lagged in outpatient care which has been carried on under the sequential leadership of Harley Haynes, Richard Johnson, and, since 1972, Ernesto Gonzalez. The inpatient service has long suffered from space problems, with only ten beds and, therefore, a long waiting period. Inasmuch as the MGH has the only dermatology inpatient facility in New England (except for a small unit at Dartmouth), there is pressure for beds to accommodate the large number of referrals. Arthur Sober, a dermatologist-internist, ably heads the inpatient service, including consultation.

This span of two decades has witnessed the growth of the Dermatology Service into a unit with nine full-time physician-investigators devoted to the highest standard of patient care, to the pursuit of new knowledge in the biology of melanin and of keratin, skin optics, and photobiology, and to the successful application of this basic knowledge to the diagnosis and treatment of certain diseases of the skin: a new method (photochemotherapy) for control of severe psoriasis and certain skin malignancies, early diagnosis of primary malignant melanoma of the skin, and the development of effective methods for the prevention of sunburn by the topical application of chemical solutions that shield the skin from damaging ultraviolet radiation.

A new era was begun for the Dermatology Service in 1981 as quarters in the Ambulatory Care Center became available. This provides a much-needed facility for the large outpatient population seen every year—over 35,000 patients, the largest in New England. The new facility includes a Day Care Center with beds, personnel, and equipment for treating dermatologic diseases on an outpatient basis.

Dermatology at the MGH has in the past two decades taken its place alongside internal medicine as a serious specialty with a critical mass of dermatologist-scientists, good clinical facilities, and excellent laboratory space and equipment. Most important has been the increasing number of high quality young physicians who elect dermatology as a career. This fact more than any other assures the future of this burgeoning specialty.

17. Neurology Service

RAYMOND D. ADAMS

Neurology as a medical specialty has had a long and illustrious history at the MGH. James Jackson Putnam was one of the first professors of neurology in an American or European hospital. He and E. Wyllys Taylor, James B. Ayer, and Charles S. Kubik succeeded in forming and maintaining first an excellent clinical outpatient clinic and later a neurology ward and a consultation service that became internationally renowned. Many diseases received their first or most definitive clinical or pathologic descriptions through the astute observations of these neurologists. Moreover, they established a residency training program. Ayer recognized the importance of laboratory methodologies in facilitating clinical diagnosis and in the quantification of neurologic phenomena. Kubik was invited to develop a laboratory of neuropathology; Robert Schwab created the first laboratory of electroencephalography in a U.S. hospital; Edwin Cole, a cortical (psychological) testing laboratory, and Ayer himself, the first spinal fluid laboratory in the country.

These were the facilities available at the MGH and the Harvard Medical School when Raymond D. Adams was invited to return from Boston City Hospital as chief of Neurology in 1951. It was immediately evident to him that a primary objective must be the maintenance of an outstanding clinical service to which the most difficult neurologic problems would be referred and young physicians indoctrinated in the principles of medical neurology. But more was coming to be expected in a university hospital by 1951: New diseases must be singled out; causes, mechanisms, and potential therapies must be investigated. To do this effectively required a staff of clinical scientists and new laboratories for all the science fields that offered promise of aiding neurology. Neurologists must specialize and concentrate on certain diseases, and they must acquire aptitude and skill in the fields of science (neuroscience) relevant to the diseases in which they were interested. In fact, Adams' selection as chief was undoubtedly influenced by the fact that he had received training in psychology, physiology, and cellular neuropathology.

Finding neurologist-scientists to buttress the staff at that time was difficult, if not impossible, for the traditional training of neurologists was in internal medicine followed by one or two years of a neurologic residence (one year at the MGH from 1934 to 1946). Fortunately, in the early fifties the National Institute of Neurology decided to appropriate funds to support training programs in order to overcome a deficiency of clinical neurologists in the United States and of teachers of neurology with academic qualifications in American medical schools. The MGH was the recipient of one of the first grants, and this enabled the expansion of the residency staff. The new residency training was to include two years of internal medicine and three years of neurology and neuropathology. The grant thus gave MGH the opportunity to prepare five, and later seven, neurologists per year. Unique to the program was the provision that each potential neurologist should devote himself to the study of diseases of the human nervous system in living patients as well as to the study of neuropathologic bases.

158

An equally important development was the expansion of the research staff and provision of facilities. When Adams returned to the MGH in 1951, Maurice Victor, who had become interested in nutrition and alcoholic neurologic diseases, accompanied him. Within a few years Victor earned international recognition for his contributions to knowledge of nutritional disorders of the nervous system. The factor of abstinence was proven to be the mechanism of delirium tremens; Korsakoff's psychosis was shown to be the mental component of Wernicke's disease and thiamine deficiency was confirmed as its cause; the pathologic substratum of alcoholic cerebellar degeneration was demonstrated for the first time, and an atlas of the human cerebellum (the normative control for these studies) was written with Yakovlev, Mancall, and Angevine; the neuropathology of nutritional optic neuropathy was discovered; a new disease, *central pontine myelinolysis,* was found; and an authoritative monograph on Wernicke-Korsakoff disease was issued from the nutritional laboratories. Adams' studies with Roy Swank on the effects of pyridoxine and pantothenic acid deficiency on the animal nervous system were completed. Near the end of the decade, as these studies were being concluded, Victor, Eliott Mancall, Pierre Dreyfus, and Jay Angevine accepted prestigious appointments in academic medicine elsewhere.

In 1951, when immunology was beginning to show promise of clarifying a number of neurologic diseases, particularly multiple sclerosis, Byron Waksman joined the MGH Neurology Service to establish a neuroimmunology laboratory. For a decade thereafter, working in association with Adams and others, experimental allergic and infectious demyelination were brought under laboratory scrutiny. The first experimental model of an allergic polyneuritis was created; the purely toxic nature of diphtheritic neuritis was determined; the basic processes of delayed cellular immunity were explored; blood-nerve barriers were investigated; the viral nature of multifocal leukoencephalitis was predicated; and, most importantly, a generation of young neuroimmunologists was prepared for further research. Barry Arnason, one of the recruits, succeeded Waksman when the latter was invited to Yale Medical School as professor of microbiology. Arnason carried on his studies of lymphocytic typing and reactions in the autoimmune diseases until 1977 when he went to the University of Chicago as chairman of the Neurology Department.

Consonant with the theme of promoting clinical neurologic science, C. Miller Fisher joined the service in 1954 at the time of the opening of a new floor of laboratories in the Warren Building. Fisher, a Canadian with unusual war experiences, had early revealed a talent for original clinical and pathologic observations. Prepared for a career in medicine and science at the University of Toronto, he realized that the study of cerebrovascular diseases required most of all accurate bedside observations and clinicopathologic correlations. Working in his inimitable style at night on the wards and in the emergency rooms of the MGH, he probably did more than anyone of his generation in bringing cerebrovascular diseases under scrutiny, and many of the advances in this field can be traced to his original observations. To mention a few, he was one of the first to appreciate the high incidence of embolism as a cause of strokes—nearly one-third in a series that he and Adams collected in 1949. Hemorrhagic infarction was traced most clearly to the migrating and vanishing embolus, a new concept. The importance of carotid atherosclerosis and its relationship to amaurosis was demonstrated. The pathology of atherosclerosis of the cerebral arteries was made the subject of a special study. Anticoagulation and carotid artery surgery were explored as therapeutic methods. Cerebellar hemorrhage was defined as a clinical entity for the first time, subject to accurate diagnosis and successful surgical intervention. Buerger-Winiwarter disease was shown to be most often a misinterpretation of atherosclerotic arterial occlusion and its peculiarities in brain pathology related to the stasis in the meningeal anastomotic systems between the cerebral arteries. Fisher himself had earlier helped to define the role of the latter in a study with Henry Vander Eken and Adams. Dissecting false aneurysms of cervicocranial arteries were delineated in collaboration with R. Ojemann. The current language of cerebrovascular disease reflects Fisher's conceptualization of many such diseases: the stroke in evolution, the completed stroke, TIA (transient ischemic attack), the subclavian steal syndrome, and amaurosis fugax.

Fisher's influence on clinical medicine at the MGH has been equally important. He has been able to excite young physicians about the necessity of the bedside study of disease, of intensive training in neuropathology, and of precise quantification and description of the phenomenologic aspects of disease. His examples and his standards have been reflected in the quality of clinical neurology practiced by MGH residents and staff over the past 25 years.

The neuromuscular diseases were also brought into the focus of clinical study during the 1950 to 1970 period. Stimulated to some extent by Adams' interest in myopathology, a succession of research fellows came to the MGH for study in this field; they included Sir John Walton, Carl Pearson, and Byron Kakulas. Hayes, Victor, and Adams showed that the oculopharyngeal paralysis of late life was a unique form of senescent myopathy and not a nuclear atrophy as E. Wyllys Taylor had postulated in 1915. To carry out the biochemical studies of muscle diseases, a working arrangement was established with John Gergely and his staff at the Boston Biomedical Research Institute. They became members of the Neurology Service staff. Asbury, who came as a resident in neurology, went to work on peripheral nerve diseases. Following Banker, Victor, and Adams who made the original studies of uremic polyneuropathy, Asbury collaborated in the most complete neuropathologic study on acute idiopathic polyneuritis (Landry-Guillain-Barré syndrome) and on hypertrophic mononeuritis multiplex. With Raff he made the first complete pathologic study of the vascular lesion of subacute mononeuropathy multiplex as a cause of the so-called diabetic myelopathy. Many other studies of nerve came under the purview of Asbury before he left the MGH to become a professor at the University of California and thence to the University of Pennsylvania as chairman of Neurology.

Investigations of metabolic disorders of the nervous system were also encouraged. Hyperammonemia was a topic of considerable interest, and a natural collaboration developed with William McDermott, the surgeon, who at that time was preoccupied with the effects of liver disease on the nervous system. A singular opportunity was offered to observe the neurologic manifestations of Eck fistula in man, which was shown to be based on a state of hyperammonemia. McDermott reported the first human case of the syndrome with Adams in 1955. The neuropathologic effects of Eck fistula were studied in animals, and later Cole, Victor, and Adams described the chronic clinical effects of acquired hepatic diseases on the nervous system of man. Hypoxic encephalopathy was another metabolic disease that came under observation when James Lance, now the first professor of neurology in Australia, studied at the MGH. He and Adams described the syndrome of *intention myoclonus,* contrasting it to the asterixis of metabolic disease earlier described by Adams and Foley.

In 1952–1953 children's neurology was a neglected field. Bronson Crothers, Randolph Byers, and Adams were the only neurologists in the New England area who had experience with the neurologic diseases of infants and children. They decided to establish a division of children's neurology at the MGH; this was made possible through the cooperation of Allan Butler, then chief of the Children's Medical Service. Philip Dodge, a resident in neurology, was chosen as the person to help in this development. In 1956, with David Crockett's help, a large grant was obtained from the Joseph P. Kennedy, Jr., Foundation to support research in this field, and part of the grant was used to add three floors of laboratories and work areas on top of the Burnham Building. There followed an active period of training of pediatric neurologists, assisted by one of the first training grants from the NIH for this purpose. Research activities were directed to the study of toxic and metabolic encephalopathies, the epilepsies, and developmental and chromosomal disorders of the nervous system. Many talented young neurologists were graduates of this division of the service.

Aware of the difficulties of studying in a general hospital the diseases of the child's nervous system that resulted in mental retardation, we undertook the establishment of a new research center for the study of mental retardation on the grounds of the Fernald State School in Waltham in 1959. Once again with the backing of David Crockett, funds were obtained from federal and state government sources for the creation of one of the first of 12 such centers in the United States. This research center was named the Eunice Kennedy Shriver Center in honor of the gracious lady who had staunchly supported our research and training program in children's neurology for many years.

The new Shriver Center Building was dedicated in October 1970. During the decade that has since passed, the center has flourished. In 1980 its staff numbered 200, including 36 senior scientists. The center's objectives are the diagnosis, treatment, and prevention of neurologic diseases causing mental retardation and other disabilities. The building in Waltham consists of four floors of laboratories for biochemical, genetic, neuropathologic, and psychologic studies of the neurologic diseases of children. The center is an integral part of MGH neurology, with Adams serving as its director. Through an agreement between the trustees of the MGH and the state Division of Mental Health, the Shriver Center has brought the Neurology Service into contact with one of the largest unexplored groups of neurologic diseases in society. Students and residents are becoming interested and involved in this field and are specializing in it.

For several years the need for a firm association between MGH neurology and the McLean Hospital was recognized. Pierre Dreyfus acted as consultant, and when he left the staff, Larry Embree assumed this responsibility. Embree's subsequent departure for the University of Louisiana dramatized the importance of improving our service to McLean patients. Brian Woods was invited by Shervert Frazier, psychiatrist-in-chief at McLean, to form a neurology service and to survey all admissions for diseases of the nervous system other than schizophrenia and manic-depressive disease. Five consultants go to McLean each week to assist Woods in this task. Once more the idea of training residents as neuropsychiatrists emerged. All MGH neurology residents rotate through McLean for two months in their second year of training, and McLean residents come to the MGH service in their first year. Collaborative research, long encouraged by the late Professor Folch-Pi, continued between Alfred Pope and the staff of the MGH Neurology Service. Joint scientific meetings are held with the staff of the Shriver Center and the Mailman Research Institute directed by Professors Seymour Kety, Pope, and Bird.

A significant development upon the death of Robert Schwab was the expansion of the laboratories in clinical neurophysiology. With the completion of the Gray Building, part of the 11th floor became available for this purpose, and the most modern laboratories for the investigation of the function of the diseased nervous system by electrophysiologic methods became possible. Shahani, an Oxford-trained neurophysiologist, was brought to the MGH by Robert Young who had succeeded Schwab. Later Keith Chiappa joined the staff and assumed responsibility for the introduction of evoked potential methods utilizing computers. A large number of neurophysiology fellows receive training in these laboratories.

In all this period the neuropathology laboratories—which were directed by E. P. Richardson after the retirement of C. S. Kubik and are now named the Kubik Laboratories in honor of their founder—have continued to provide the link between the Neurology Service and the Department of Pathology. Our insistence that every neurologic resident spend a year studying the morphologic aspects of disease has kept the relationship to pathology closer than that of any other clinical service. Many neuropathology residents and fellows have gone on to professorships of neuropathology in other universities, not to mention countless others who are professors of neurology and whose activities in research have been strongly influenced by the year spent in the neuropathology laboratory.

Coincident with the development of children's neurology, an expansion of the service's activities in neurochemistry became necessary. A part of one floor of the Joseph P. Kennedy, Jr., laboratories in the Burnham Building was assigned to Mary Effron who, because of her contacts with Professor Dent in England, was able to exploit new methodologies for detection of disorders of amino acids. Her death at a time when her laboratory had become a national center, extremely productive in finding new diseases and treatments, was felt keenly. Two of her assistants, Vivian Shih and Harvey Levy, have continued this work. Hugo Moser became interested in metabolic diseases and was helpful in setting up the neurochemistry division of the Shriver Center. When Moser left to go to Johns Hopkins, Edwin Kolodny took over. He and Ira Lott, both of whom had worked at the NIH Institute of Neurology in Bethesda, supervised and participated in an active program of biochemical research, aided by an able staff of full-time biochemists. The facilities—which include a lysosomal laboratory, an electron microscopy laboratory, and the Golgi laboratory, aided by mass spectrometry and gas-liquid chromatography—are unexcelled.

Genetics research has also been encouraged. Milunsky is in charge of the amniocentesis program and the alpha-fetoprotein studies; and Atkins of the Pathology Department, until recently, has done all of the chromosomal work. Morphologic studies of the genetic and other pathologic bases of mental retardation were pursued by Yakovlev until he retired and, since then, by Verne Caviness. Roger Williams has recently joined his staff. They have two floors of laboratories, including a modern electron microscopy unit.

Laboratories of behavioral science were installed with the opening of the Kennedy Laboratories at the MGH. Murray Sidman, Barbara Ray, Paul Touchette, MacKay and Stoddard developed methodologies for the study of brain function in nonverbal humans. This imaginative work attracted the attention of scholars in the field of mental retardation. Much of it was transferred to the Shriver Center when it opened, and it continues to flourish. A cluster of young neurologists interested in behavioral science have been indoctrinated in this field and continue to do research in it.

When viewed in retrospect over the past 25 years, the MGH Neurology Service has changed from a fine clinical service to one in which research has been promoted in all the neurosciences; where young physicians are trained successively in clinical neurology and the neurosciences for careers as neurologist-scientists; where categories of nervous diseases not previously recognized as part of neurology have been encompassed; and where postgraduate students come regularly for instruction.

At the time of Adams' retirement as chief of service in 1978, there were eight floors of well-equipped laboratories made possible through the generous support of the MGH, the NIH, and the Commonwealth of Massachusetts. Twenty-one residents were in the training program each year. More than 30 clinical neurologists from all over the world were carrying an ever-increasing load of clinical cases, and more than 30 senior neuroscientists were collaborating with the clinical staff.

With the arrival of Joseph Martin from McGill University to serve as chief and with new facilities provided by the MGH and Harvard, another dimension was added to the teaching and research program. Martin's eminence in the field of neurotransmitters is expected to shape the careers of another generation of young neurologist-scientists and maintain the standards of the Neurology Service in a way of which the MGH will be proud.

One of the important events early in Martin's tenure was the funding by the NIH, in July of 1980, of The Huntington's Disease Center Without Walls, a Massachusetts consortium. The program project grant was a five-year, multi-institution award to permit the development of a cooperative approach to clinical and basic research studies of Huntington's disease, an autosomal dominant genetic disorder. The projects include studies involving the sociologic implications of the disease, analysis of memory deficits in patients, molecular genetics, and studies in neuropathology, neurochemistry, and neuropharmacology. Martin directs the program, and the MGH heads the consortium.

With the assistance of *Gerald F. Winkler.*

C. Miller Fisher adds this observation:

What of Raymond Adams himself, clearly the central and moving figure in all of the prodigious accomplishment just described? Calm, indefatigable, knowledgeable far beyond human expectation, and completely devoted to teaching and demonstration, he seemed never to be too busy to discuss with colleagues, fellows, students, or staff, any neurological point be it clinical, pathological, or experimental. A gifted speaker, even his extemporaneous presentations flowed in perfectly arranged sentences, clear, concise, and authoritative, often to the amazement of his audience. His thoughtful, gentle bedside manner was a model for his generation. He was the ablest neurologist of his time. The many important discoveries already referred to were largely his or were instigated or guided by him. He found time to author or co-author some seven neurological works in which his clear thinking and well-marshalled views are set in pleasant prose that delights as it informs the reader. Any one of these works would itself be a source of great pride. And last, but not least, through his scholarly example and leadership, students and colleagues were led on or lifted up to academic achievement they had not dreamed of. Truly, Adams ranks with the giants of neurology.

18. Psychiatry Service
Stanley Cobb

Stanley Cobb was one of Harvard's great men of medicine. Born and bred in the Harvard atmosphere, during his life he held three important Harvard posts: From 1926 until his retirement in 1954 he was the Bullard Professor of Neuropathology; from 1925 to 1934 he was chief of the Neurology Service at Boston City Hospital where, as Penfield has said, he founded "the strongest school of contemporary neurology in the United States"; in 1934 he became chief of the newly created Psychiatry Service, in a sense created for him, at the MGH. It was in this third post that he achieved his greatest distinction, for he brought to psychiatry the background of experimental and anatomic neurology and a wide clinical experience in both neurology and psychiatry. Physically crippled by arthritis for the last 30 years of his life, he maintained his intellectual vigor until his death in his 81st year, in February 1968.

Born in Brookline in December 1887, Cobb spent his boyhood in Milton where he attended Milton Academy. He graduated from Harvard College in 1910 and from the Harvard Medical School in 1914. After a surgical internship under Harvey Cushing at the Peter Bent Brigham Hospital, he went to Johns Hopkins for postgraduate study with Howell and Adolph Meyer. During the First World War he served in the Army Medical Corps.

His service to the Harvard Medical School started in 1919 when he was appointed instructor in physiology and neurology and assistant neurologist at the MGH. In 1920 he was promoted to assistant professor of neuropathology and in 1923 to associate professor. At this time he was given charge of the course in neuropathology and of the laboratory at the Medical School quadrangle. In preparation for these responsibilities he was sent by the Rockefeller Foundation to Europe for study from 1923 to 1925—to London, Paris, Berlin, and Oxford. While he was in Europe, his appointment to the Neurology Service at the Boston City Hospital was arranged. Upon his return in 1925 he thus divided his services between clinical neurology and neuropathology. The following year he was promoted to the Bullard Professorship.

The direction of Cobb's academic activities was forecast in a remarkable way in the terms of the bequest of the Bullard Professorship, written in 1906: "This professorship shall embrace study, research, investigation and teaching in relation to all diseases of the nervous system, whether functional or organic in origin; and it shall include not only those affections ordinarily classed under Neurology but all diseases and disturbances classed under Psychiatry and any others that may exist. The method and detail of work under this Professorship are not in any way restricted. It should include any form of research and investigation which may lead to the knowledge of the nervous and mental disease. It comprises the comparative study of these diseases in animals and all other living forms."

The years from 1925 to 1934 at the Boston City Hospital were productive ones, an expanding phase of Cobb's life. In the hospital he studied patients with neurologic diseases. With Lennox he wrote the classic monograph on epilepsy and introduced Dilantin therapy. Cobb's Neurology Service also treated patients with psychiatric disorders, for there was no Psychiatry Service at the hospital at that time. In the laboratories of neuropathology, he not only encouraged the study of microscopic neuroanatomy and pathology but carried out himself, with his brother-in-law Henry Forbes and others, the classic experiments in the cerebral circulation that still stand as the fundamental work.

Cobb's transfer to the MGH in 1934 to build the Psychiatric Service was a natural sequence in his life's pattern. Of this transfer Cobb himself said that it came about because "Howard Means, chief of Medicine, had the vision to see what could be accomplished by treatment of the mentally ill in a general hospital." The new service was generously supported by the Rockefeller Foundation, for whom Alan Gregg reported in 1948: "The first grant to Harvard Medical School and the MGH in 1933 was for the purpose of setting up a new kind of Psychiatric Service. Until that time, institutional psychiatry had been practiced and taught almost entirely in hospitals remote from medical schools and scarcely related to the practice of medicine as a whole. . . . The example set by the Harvard–Massachusetts General Psychiatric Service has been and may continue to be a valuable stimulant in the growth of psychiatric teaching and the hospital study and care of emotional disorders."

Cobb flourished at the MGH. Support came not only from the Rockefeller Foundation and the Hall Mercer trustees but also from Means, Dr. Faxon, the director of the hospital, and many of the staff. Through his insight and his ability to deal with people, Cobb became the most influential figure in the hospital. He attracted topflight men and women from all over the world. His associates and assistants constitute a list of distinguished scientists, clinicians, professors, and heads of departments too long to enumerate here.

His contributions to scientific and clinical aspects of neurology and psychiatry were prodigious, many magnificent and classic. Some, as already indicated, were in experimental neurophysiology. Others were in the fields of comparative neuroanatomy and neuropathology. Many of these were described in his book *The Borderlands of Psychiatry,* published in 1944. This monograph, which he considered one of his best writings, is a timeless treatise on comparative neuroanatomy and neurophysiology.

Cobb approached the patient with emotional and psychiatric troubles from his background of neurology, his experience with Adolph Meyer, and his continuing experience with psychoanalysis. He was a monist: "No biological process takes place without change of structure. Whenever the brain functions, there is organic change. The brain is the organ of the mind. Therefore, all function is organic, and mind and body are one." His volume *The Foundations of Neuropsychiatry,* which went through six editions before his death, summarized his thoughts about man and his brain. So simple and fundamental, it is still to be surpassed in its wisdom.

Cobb's bearing was commanding. He had the look of a crested bird. Always handsome, his face grew handsomer with age. He was a brilliant and devoted teacher. His vistas were wide, and he was not a specialist by exclusion; he took the "all-else" into his specialty. Added to this was an uncommon lucidity. Perhaps because of his lifelong affliction of stuttering, he chose his words with discrimination, and his use of language was powerful and inspiring.

In matters academic at the Medical School, Cobb was a force to be reckoned with. Though not a member of the World War II Curriculum Committee, he made himself heard. Despite much opposition, he got the faculty to accept a month of psychiatry as a requisite of the fourth year. Though not a member of the Committee on Examinations, he succeeded in getting that committee to reduce the number of examinations in the second year. He almost succeeded in getting the clinical faculty to see the importance of the Behavior Examination.

As a psychiatrist, he was not an analyst, but he appreciated what psychoanalysis had contributed to our knowledge. He encouraged the growth and development of analytic psychiatry on his service at the MGH and in Boston generally in the direct and indirect support he gave the Psychoanalytic Institute. Without his breadth of wisdom and support, the institute might not have been founded and certainly would not have flourished as it has. His first contact with analytic psychiatry came when he was in Europe; he studied for three months with Leonard Seif in Munich. Then, in Boston, after the arrival of Hanns Sachs in 1934, Cobb himself undertook an analysis with Sachs. From the early 1930s on, he encouraged all his close associates and assistants to undergo analysis. Though many, like Cobb, did not wish to practice analytic psychiatry, he considered an analysis a part of their education.

Cobb's social and political activities were characteristic of his wide interests. He wasn't just a do-gooder; he was a working liberal. He was the first to appoint a black physician to the house staff of the MGH—in 1938. With the rise of Hitler to power, few did as much, and nobody more, to support and recognize the refugees from Nazi Germany. At a time when anti-Semitism was still present, he fought it at every turn—in the hospital, in the university, and in the American Medical Association.

Born in a conservative Republican family, he supported the liberal social policies of the New Deal. He loved to tell a story about his mother. A rock-ribbed Republican, she detested Franklin Roosevelt. In 1945 Cobb went on a secret mission to Washington to visit the training camp of the OSS. His mother put her own interpretation on his mission: "Stanley has gone to Washington, and he cannot say why. Stanley is a psychiatrist. Roosevelt is crazy. Therefore, he has gone to see Roosevelt."

All through his life, from early boyhood to his last days, Cobb had a consuming interest in birds and wildlife. He made several noteworthy contributions to his avocation. In a classic article in *Auk,* in October 1945, he described the change in ecology of the birds of Milton Hill from 1904 to 1944, the effect of urban civilization, and the wholesale redistribution of the bird population as a result of the encroaching civilization. Upon his retirement he and Mrs. Cobb spent much of their time at Little Compton, Rhode Island, and at Cotuit on Cape Cod. At Cotuit he wrote another classic, *The Death of a Salt Pond,* in 1962; he had watched the devastating effects of insecticides.

Two last items. First, Cobb's thoughts about religion, in his own words: "I believe in all humility that the directiveness which I see in the evolutionary drive toward making whole organisms and whole societies is God. . . . It is enough immortality for me if I may become even a very small part of advancing wisdom, hoping that I have done my part to make the world a better place."

Second, his reaction to a new trouble, for he was a tireless observer and investigator to the end. In mid-December of 1967, ten weeks before his death, he suffered a mild stroke. This happened just as he was to have gone to New

York to receive the medal of the American Psychiatric Association. The medal and citation were sent to him instead, and in acknowledgement he wrote, on January 2, 1968:

You must have wondered what happened to me. . . . A cerebral stroke knocked me out of contact enough so I couldn't do anything for a week or so. But now, the earliest effective time, I would like to write to you what happened and say that it is just as well I did not go to New York because if this episode had occurred there it would have been pretty troublesome all around. What did happen was I realized one morning that something had seriously gone wrong with my brain and only 24 hours later did I realize that I had a slight weakness of the left arm and leg. Then I figured it would get well quickly. . . . The weakness only lasted three or four days and then I began to get used to using crutches. The surprising thing to me was that the motor weakness was really quite unimportant and that I was left with a fine selection of partial agnosias that are much more incapacitating than the motor element ever was. These have been very interesting to me and . . . I thought I should write (imitating Gunther) a book on "Inside Neurology." This is a fascinating subject. But the ludicrous part of it is that you can never learn it in time to teach it to anybody because by that time no one will believe what you say. This is one of the paradoxes of postgraduate study. I can lie quietly and think about these important subjects, but as soon as I try to express them I realize that I am afflicted by mild global aphasia, so well-described by Harold Wolff, and that this happens with all cerebral injuries, from the very slight to the quite severe degree. Mine is very slight, but as I dictate this letter I realize that something suddenly went when this CVA occurred. I can lie and think about it and it brings up some very important subjects, but my cerebrum just is not equal to handling them with the keenness and finesse that I formerly enjoyed. The main point is, of course, when does a man die? The usual medical opinion is so far from the truth that one knows the general diagnosis of death makes no sense. And, of course, this brings up a raft of legal questions. But, this is about where I am now and although friends will keep on telling me "you look fine" and "your mind is as good as ever" and that sort of thing, I just know it's foolishness. I am not going to write anything more except what is already in press. . . . My mentality is about at the level of the average reader of the *Reader's Digest*. I have lost the ability to choose *le mot juste* which used to be a hobby.

And, in a postscript:

I used to think I knew a lot about cerebral strokes. Well, I know a lot more now.

Cobb died six weeks later.

> Adapted from a Memorial Minute, *Harvard University Gazette*, Vol. LXIV, No. 38, June 7, 1969

Erich Lindemann

JOHN C. NEMIAH

It is important to take a brief look at Erich Lindemann's professional interests and the direction of his work in order to understand better the history of the service during the period he was in command. Born in Germany in 1900, he studied psychology, medicine, and neurology at the universities of Marburg, Giessen, and Heidelberg before he came to the United States in 1927 to work as a clinician and laboratory investigator in the Department of Psychology and Psychiatry at the University of Iowa. He joined Stanley Cobb's staff at the MGH in the late thirties and immediately focused his investigative interests on psychosomatic medicine. Unlike many analysts, however, whose concern centered on the internal psychologic conflicts of the individual patient, Lindemann was acutely aware that the sick person was part of a human social network and that a significant factor in his psychologic disturbance was the result of stressful changes in his physical and human environment. This was evident in his early investigation of the response of patients to major surgery, but his ideas were crystallized as a result of his participation in the Cocoanut Grove fire studies in 1942 to 1943.

In this endeavor Lindemann's attention was directed not at the mutilated victims of the fire themselves but at the relatives of those who had lost family members in the flames. His observations of the correlative psychologic and physiologic manifestations of their response to sudden tragic loss led to the publication of his classic paper "The Nature and Management of Acute Grief."

Lindemann's clinical experience during these studies was decisive for the direction of his future work and ideas. For a time he continued to study patients within the general hospital setting in a collaborative clinical investigation with Chester Jones on ulcerative colitis. Here his recognition of the importance of the nature and changes in human relationships as a factor in the production of physical illness was readily evident, and the interactional aspect of psychiatric and psychosomatic phenomena guided his observations.

But Lindemann's emphasis on the stress resulting from changes in human relationships had effects on his scientific thinking and activities that went far beyond the arena of the general hospital. Psychologic stress, he recognized, was a universal phenomenon and if severe enough constituted a crisis situation for the individual involved. For many, the crisis could be weathered without serious lasting damage, but in a significant number of people it formed the starting point of a downward spiral that could lead to chronic debilitating emotional and physical illness. It was evident that therapeutic intervention during the crisis period might prevent the development of serious consequences. Crisis intervention and prevention, therefore, became the key concepts as opposed to concern with the treatment of well-established disease processes that represented the late stages of a long process of deterioration. Prevention, however, entailed early case-finding as well as working with and training individuals (general practitioners, clergymen, teachers, police, social workers in community agencies) to whom people under stress initially turned for help. For this reason Lindemann directed his efforts away from the clinical activities of the hospital, and, with the help of a generous award from the Grant Foundation, he created the Wellesley Human Relations Service, the prototype of the modern community mental health center. Indeed, Lindemann may with justice be considered one of the prime movers and originators of the mental health movement that changed the face of American psychiatry during the 1960s and 1970s.

By the time Lindemann was appointed chief of Psychiatry to succeed Stanley Cobb at the MGH he was already thoroughly entrenched in his work at the Wellesley Human Relations Service (the HRS), and it was perhaps that fact more than any other that determined the future course of the MGH Psychiatry Service for good and for ill. Established primarily as a clinical research and teaching unit, the service under Stanley Cobb had nonetheless developed a tradition of providing psychiatric care for the population who looked to the MGH for diagnosis and treatment. As Lindemann took over the reins, there was a strong potential for the development of the hospital-based service along these lines, as general hospital psychiatry and psychiatric residency training programs were strengthened throughout the country by the rapid influx of federal funds in the form of NIMH training and research grants. Although Lindemann's interests and research activities were already following a different direction, he recognized the need for strong leadership in the clinical area, and one of his earliest moves was the appointment of George Saslow as clinical director. According to Avery Weisman, "Saslow was—and is—an outstanding, enthusiastic, assertive, knowledgeable man, who had strong opinions that he did not bother to temper. In some respects he would have been an ideal complement for Lindemann, had the arrangement worked out. When Saslow found that Lindemann encouraged him to make decisions and then would fail to support him on grounds that he was usurping authority, he went to the Dean, protested, made demands, and lost his case. Patience and tact were not among Saslow's virtues. While he was highly critical of some phases of psychoanalysis, he had too much integrity to deal in prejudice. After his departure, Lindemann never filled the post of Clinical Director; instead, he chose three comparatively junior staff men as his lieutenants—John Nemiah (inpatient), Peter Sifneos (outpatient), and Gardner Quarton (teaching). I was appointed to be in charge of consultation/liaison work on a very part-time basis. Nemiah, Sifneos, and Quarton actually ran the department, selecting residents, teaching, and doing much more than any job description should have called for. That the department functioned with reasonable smoothness and productivity can be attributed to their inability to do a mediocre job."

Clinical Activities. After Saslow's departure the various clinical units continued to function under the guidance of the several unit chiefs who formed an informal but cooperative federation under the rather remote direction of Lindemann himself. Although this may have somewhat weakened the overall strength of psychiatry in the hospital as a whole, it provided considerable autonomy to the unit chiefs and gave them a degree of responsibility for the direction of their own units that enabled each to mature and grow professionally and academically.

The Child Psychiatry Unit, initially headed by Lucie Jessner and then by Gaston Blom, came under the direction of John Lamont, ably assisted by Norman Bernstein, when Blom moved to Denver in 1957. Lindemann added two important clinical units as a result of his concern for preventive and community psychiatry. An Alcoholism Clinic was created with the help of state funding under the leadership of Alfred Ludwig and later of Morris Chafetz when Ludwig moved to a similar position at the Peter Bent Brigham Hospital. Even more significant was the organizing of the Acute Psychiatric Service (APS). From the time of the founding of the Psychiatry Service at the MGH by Cobb, it had always provided psychiatric consultation for patients admitted to the Emergency Ward with emotional problems. Lindemann recognized an opportunity to intervene early in emotional disorders during the initial crisis phase of the development of the illness, with a view to preventing the often chronic sequelae through prompt and intensive treatment of the patient during the acute stage of illness. Plans for the APS were formulated during the late fifties, and when Fred Frankel (a former clinical fellow under Cobb) returned from South Africa in 1962, he was assigned to implement them. As a result, the contribution of the Psychiatric Service to the Emergency Ward was considerably increased and strengthened, and as its usefulness became evident to the community, its activities increased even further. When Frankel, in the early sixties, turned his attention to the development of a state community mental health center, Chafetz became the first formal head of the APS, an appropriate appointment since his activities with the Alcoholism Clinic were centered in the Emergency Ward setting. The eventual acquisition of funds to build the Tilton Building contiguous to the Emergency Ward for the care of patients with alcohol problems provided the opportunity to create space specifically designated for the increasing tasks of the APS, and the role of the Psychiatric Service as a provider of care for all kinds of psychiatric emergencies was consolidated in a unit that became a model for such care in the community mental health movement.

The latter movement was officially inaugurated on a national scale by a congressional act in the early sixties that mandated the creation of community mental health centers (CMHCs) throughout the country, each to provide complete psychiatric service for a population of an officially defined catchment area. Since the guiding principle of the CMHCs was the treatment of the patient within his own community, it was necessary to create inpatient beds within each catchment area to avoid sending the acutely ill patient often miles away to one of the existing state hospitals. Even before the formal passing of the congressional CMHC act, Harry Solomon, then Commissioner of Mental Health of the Commonwealth of Massachusetts, had been setting up mental health centers within the state. High on his priority list was what eventually became the Lindemann Community Mental Health Center, a facility for which he and Lindemann had begun planning in the late 1950s. When Frankel arrived from South Africa, a part of his time was spent in the Department of Mental Health (DMH), not only assisting the Commissioner in creating outreach psychiatric clinics in the North End but also helping to provide liaison and coordination between the MGH and the DMH in planning for the construction of the building to house the activities of the CMHC designated to fall under the direction of the MGH Department of Psychiatry. Shortly before Lindemann's retirement in 1965, Nemiah joined in the planning of this facility which ultimately became a reality—named in honor of Erich Lindemann—after Leon Eisenberg had become chief of Psychiatry.

Finally, mention must be made of clinical activities that were carried out in the community under the active interest and direction of Lindemann himself. As a counterpart to the suburban setting of the Wellesley HRS, he also created an urban mental health clinic at Whittier Street, designed to provide help to a portion of Boston's inner-city disadvantaged population. In this endeavor he had the invaluable help of Gerald Caplan who, with Lindemann, ultimately founded and headed the Laboratory for Community Psychiatry under the aegis of the Harvard School of Public Health—a facility that rapidly developed an international reputation for the teaching and research carried out by its staff.

Despite the excellence of these various community activities, however, there was little contact between them and the hospital-based facilities. Lindemann's energies were largely focused on the former, and the latter, as has been hinted earlier, functioned relatively autonomously, neither segment of the overall clinical activities being fully aware of the nature of the work of the other.

Teaching and Training.
Lindemann's arrival as chief of Psychiatry coincided with a major expansion of psychiatric teaching at the Harvard Medical School. At that time there were two academic departments of psychiatry at Harvard, one based at the MGH, the other at the Boston Psychopathic Hospital (later the Massachusetts Mental Health Center). In the organization of the new curriculum, responsibility for the first two years was assigned to the MGH, for the last two clinical years to the MMHC. Clinical psychiatric rotations had been available to medical students since the ending of World War II, and the major innovation in the revised curriculum was the addition of a series of lectures in the first and second years. Under Lindemann's general direction, Gardner Quarton was responsible for the first-year lectures, which were devoted to a survey of behavioral science, and Nemiah for the lectures in psychopathology given throughout the second year. In addition Nemiah was charged with the administration of the psychiatric participation in the second-year Introduction to the Clinic course, which was taught at all of the general hospitals where students were learning physical diagnosis under the aegis of the various departments of medicine and surgery. The MGH Department of Psychiatry also played a major role in providing month-long clinical clerkships to students in their fourth year. This general program continued in force until the first of the significant medical school revisions of the curriculum in the early seventies effectively dismantled the systematic teaching of psychiatry to medical students.

During Cobb's tenure the training program in psychiatry comprised three formal residents and a handful of advanced fellows in child psychiatry. The advent of more stringent criteria for training promulgated by the American Board of Psychiatry and Neurology and the provision of funding for training by the NIMH brought about a major expansion and regularization of training programs in psychiatry throughout the country. Psychiatry at the MGH was no exception, and the early years of Lindemann's chairmanship saw the development of a formal three-year training program in adult psychiatry and of a two-year advanced program in child psychiatry. The adult program, initially based only at the MGH, soon enlarged its scope to include clinical experience for residents at the McLean Hospital under a joint training program inaugurated by Lindemann and Alfred Stanton, the chief of Psychiatry at McLean, and worked out in respect to details by Nemiah, who was appointed coordinator of psychiatric training at the MGH, and Merton Kahne, director of training at McLean.

The joint program, though well-coordinated on paper, was perhaps less successfully implemented in practice owing to the ten miles of city traffic that separated the two institutions and to an equally inhibiting distance in ideologies and practice. It was effective, however, in providing MGH residents with experience with chronically hospitalized psychotic patients and in giving McLean residents an opportunity to learn the techniques and concepts of psychiatric consultation. In order that residents at the MGH might have further exposure to patients with chronic mental illness in a structure that was more closely under the direction of the MGH training staff, negotiations were started with Danvers

State Hospital in the late fifties, and under the guidance of Sifneos and Nemiah a formal arrangement was created for training at that facility. Several young graduates of the MGH training program focused their time and energies on the Danvers program, notably the late Donald Fern, who made major contributions to the teaching of residents and the care of patients at that institution.

Finally, brief mention should be made of the teaching provided for interns on the Medical Service, half of whom spent a month on the Psychiatric Inpatient Service. Supervised by Nemiah as head of the Inpatient Ward, a large number of young physicians were introduced not only to the phenomena of emotional disorders but also, perhaps more importantly, were given the opportunity to learn how to explore and observe the important psychologic stresses and conflicts that play a central part in all forms of human illness.

Research. Like the clinical services, the research activities of the department were carried out in isolation from one another, leading to a relative lack of communication among three major groups of individuals involved in clinical research, laboratory research, and the investigation of social and community processes.

In one sense, the whole of Lindemann's professional activities may be considered a form of research, for the Wellesley HRS was set up as an experimental project, and from the experiences gained there many basic principles of group process were discovered, later to be refined in the studies undertaken by the Laboratory of Community Psychiatry. The HRS, however, was in large part service-oriented, and it was not until it was decided, as part of Boston's urban renewal plan, to destroy the West End and relocate its population that an opportunity was provided for a detailed scientific study of a population undergoing the crisis of a major transition. Accordingly, fortified by another large award from the Grant Foundation, Lindemann gathered around him a team of social scientists, including Paul Hare and Marc Fried, to study the behavior of some 12,000 West End inhabitants before, during, and after the stress of losing their traditional homes and surroundings. Unfortunately, the findings from this study were never published in a detailed systematic monograph, but it became clear from the extensive investigations that the form of urban renewal to which the West End was subjected was a major psychologic trauma to many of the individuals who were forced to move. In this sense the project, a pioneering venture of its kind, provided significant guidelines for those responsible for later programs of urban renewal.

Shortly after Lindemann became chief, he added a major unit to the department in the form of the Stanley Cobb Laboratories. Housed on Warren 6 and named in honor of Lindemann's distinguished predecessor, the laboratories provided space for a number of important laboratory investigators. Perhaps foremost among them was George Talland, an experimental psychologist who came to the MGH from the University of Cambridge and whose death in the 1960s put to an end a scientific career that was in full flower. Talland's main area of study was the function of memory, and through his study of defects of this function in patients with Korsakoff's syndrome, he pioneered the development of the concepts of short-term and long-term memory, which brought him world renown as an investigator. Talland's interests were catholic within and without the pale of science proper, and he was one of the few laboratory investigators who had significant contact with the clinicians of the department—to their mutual pleasure and profit.

An early tenant of Warren 6 was Frank Ervin, who came at Lindemann's invitation to direct the Stanley Cobb Laboratories and to undertake a pioneering investigation into the function of the limbic system (especially the amygdala) and its relation to violence and disturbances of mood. After completing his residency training in the MGH program, Jack Mendelson joined the laboratory unit to begin, in conjunction with Nancy Mello, a life's work of studies on the behavioral and physiologic aspects of alcohol consumption. Similarly, Michael McGuire moved from residency training to Warren 6 where he developed a program of investigation of the process of psychiatric interviewing through the use of computer technology.

Most of the clinical research carried out during Lindemann's tenure was done without funding and accomplished through the systematic recording and analysis of data derived from observations made during the clinical activities for which individual members of the clinical arm were responsible. Weisman, beginning with an interest in the problem of suicide, soon shifted his focus to the experiential phenomena of dying, and in this endeavor became one of the pioneers of the now widespread discipline of thanatology. Thomas Hackett, charged with a major responsibility for the consultation activities of the service, focused his attention on coronary artery disease and has become internationally known for his research in this area. As head of the Outpatient Clinic, Sifneos began his investigation of brief, anxiety-provoking psychotherapy which, at first frowned upon by the Establishment, has now become a staple in the therapeutic armamentarium of the modern psychiatrist. Nemiah pursued his interest in psychosomatic medicine, with a particular focus on the psychology of chronic illness and disability and the psychologic problems complicating the process of rehabilitation. Together with Sifneos, he contributed to the observations of the psychology of patients with psychosomatic diseases that have led to the formulation of the concept of alexithymia, a concept that is currently the focus of considerable interest in this country and Europe and has helped to stimulate renewed activity in clinical psychosomatic research. Finally, mention should be made of the work of Howard Blane, a clinical psychologist attached to the Alcoholism Unit, whose study of the behavior of individuals with major drinking problems clarified the nature of the difficulties in their treatment.

Perhaps a concluding word of assessment of Lindemann's eleven years as chief of Psychiatry may not be out of order—subjective as it must unavoidably be. Lindemann was a brilliant clinician, observer, and theoretician, who despite his unique talents as a clinical psychiatrist turned his attention to group, community, and social processes. Here his genius for seeing familiar facts in a new light led him to develop original formulations and theories that provided the basis of what later became the Community Mental Health Movement. He had a peculiar knack for stimulating those who worked with him to amplify his basic observations and ideas, and for those who shared his interests in community process he was an inspiring leader. It is perhaps to be regretted that he abandoned his clinical concerns when he turned to more sociologic investigations, for this meant that, although chief of a clinical service, he did not provide the attention and leadership to the clinical arm of his department that were necessary to provide the cohesion and direction to make it a truly strong and effective organization. Given what appears to be a fundamental incompatibility between the approaches of clinical and community psychiatry, perhaps this was inevitable, and certainly many of us, who were enabled to grow and to develop our own interests as members of the clinical hospital staff during his chairmanship, are grateful for the opportunities he afforded us.

Avery Weisman, the Psychiatry Service's senior staff member, offered this "sideline view" of Erich Lindemann:

One of the happier by-products of long-term staff membership is that I retain reasonable recollections, plus those modifications of judgment which we generously call "perspective". . . . Everyone has a store of Lindemann anecdotes, most of which, I think, have their punchline in showing Erich as the forgetful savant, bewildered by everyday responsibilities, trying to be a good guy, but failing ludicrously. . . .

Even after these many years, two questions are still alive: Why was Erich Lindemann chosen? Why did he accept? Those who really knew Erich came to see the man beneath the ruddy cheeks, piping voice, and Father Christmas image. He was capable of giving and taking away, of showing interest, and then forgetting all about it. Some of us even had an affection for this visionary, almost spiritual man, even as he griped us by falling prey to those whom we considered opportunists. He was a spellbinder on the podium because he had a knack for simplifying complex issues with a colorful phrase or a dramatic formulation which everyone could understand. This gift had its drawbacks. For those who looked for simple answers, particularly colleagues who didn't want to be bothered with the metaphysical ideas promulgated by other psychiatrists, Erich's talent, eloquence, and eagerness for acceptance were an irresistible combination. Perhaps this contributed to his selection.

Erich knew that he was not an administrator, that he was not by nature one to lead the troops, to battle it out, and to enjoy political frays. In later years he once told me that the offer had been too attractive; one did not turn down a Harvard professorship lightly. In my opinion, he never got over feeling like a foreigner, or a misfit. Consequently, he remained very sensitive, long-suffering, and quick to anger—at his friends. It was easy for him to alienate colleagues, and not easy for him to make friends. He tried to please everyone and, of course, failed.

Finally, without lingering long over the Lindemann era, my assessment is that Erich's remoteness and indifference towards the hospital side of the department permitted an autonomy which led several of us to develop along similar, but independent, professional tracks. I suppose it was discouraging to Erich through the years; I know that at the time of retirement, he became depressed, and wondered if he had accomplished anything at all. I am glad that with time his reputation has grown until now he has become more legend than man.

Psychiatry After Lindemann: "A View from the Bridge"

LEON EISENBERG

The interregnum between Professor Lindemann's retirement and my appointment, three years in duration, was a difficult and trying time for the department, as seems always to be the case during the "deliberate speed" of the Harvard search process. An acting chief, no matter how distinguished and competent (and John Nemiah was both), lacks the authority to make long-term commitments. Staff members, overdue for promotion, have to await the new appointee because the imperative is to preserve the new chief's options. The longer the hiatus grows, the more intensely staff members come to feel that neither the hospital nor the medical school gives a tinker's dam about psychiatry. Academic worship for Matthew's Law (13:57: A prophet is not without honor, save in his own country and in his own house) makes it highly improbable that the new chief will be chosen from the existing staff. When the acting chief is clearly an individual with the scholarly and personal qualities appropriate for the succession, as was true for John Nemiah, his many supporters become further offended by the Search Committee's failure to take their preferences into account.

To add to the discomfiture of the staff, some MGH physicians and surgeons undertook to circulate a petition urging the Search Committee to appoint a chief of Psychiatry with a biologic orientation, one who would be more responsive to the problems of hospital consultation than (in their view) the previous incumbent had been. In part, their concerns were understandable; Lindemann had devoted his energies to research in social psychiatry, for which he became an internationally known scholar, but his presence within the hospital was neither as visible nor as vigorous as that of his predecessor, Stanley Cobb.

However, there was more to the petition than a proper concern for clinical service. Psychiatry has always had to struggle for its legitimacy in a general hospital. Psychoanalytic psychiatry, the dominant school in Boston in the mid-sixties, was particularly unacceptable to many of the internists and surgeons who found its concepts confusing, its practices heretical, and its practitioners too unlike other physicians. A number found themselves far more in sympathy with the handful of Boston psychiatrists who professed their allegiance to biomedicine and who proclaimed electroshock therapy a universal panacea (though they were less forthcoming about its income-generating potential).

The Search Committee undertook its task at a time in the history of American psychiatry when the post-World-War-II ascendence of psychoanalysis was under serious challenge for the first time. For 20 years it had dominated the academic scene. Now there were new developments: a concern for precision in diagnosis and classification; the excitement generated by effective psychopharmacology with its development of quantitative measures for controlled clinical trials; a revival of interest in brain biochemistry; and a new thrust to the study of the genetics of mental disorder. To most members of the Search Committee, these developments, with their roots in basic science, had great appeal in contrast to the arcane concepts of psychoanalysis. On the other hand, to break with what remained the dominant trend in academic psychiatry was not to be lightly undertaken (in 1967 the department heads at Boston University and Tufts as well as at all the Harvard hospitals were card-carrying analysts).

Candidates came and went before the Search Committee. Some were clearly outstanding but refused to consider a move. Others were only too available but far less appealing. The debate about the schools of psychiatry was bitter and wearing. After all, a committee searching for a chief of Medicine doesn't have to decide among an allopath, a homeopath, a naturopath or what have you; that nonsense was settled with the birth of scientific medicine in the last half of the nineteenth century. What Adolph Meyer once called the doctrine of exclusive salvationism is pretty much on its way out of psychiatry as I write this chapter, but it was still very much alive 15 years ago. And it bedeviled my colleagues.

I had participated in a conference on medical education jointly chaired by Gerald Zacharias of MIT and Oliver Cope, the MGH surgeon, in Swampscott in the fall of 1966. The participants included a number of leading MGH physicians who were later to become friends and colleagues. Not long after, I was invited to spend a week at the MGH, to meet individually with members of the Search Committee and to give several lectures, all in the guise of serving as a "consultant" to the Search Committee. It seemed a pleasant way to go about being a candidate; if I palled on closer view, we could all pretend that I had never been a suitor and thus never rejected. Since I was perfectly happy with my position at Hopkins (second only to the MGH according to the *Ladies Home Journal*), I had no particular anxieties about being considered and really hadn't given much thought to whether I would serve if nominated.

Two things stand out in my recollection of that week. The first was meeting John Knowles and going on his clinical rounds for residents and medical students. I was thoroughly charmed. He was bright, enthusiastic, warm, and full of confidence about the greatness of the MGH and the bright promise of its future. I began to be excited at the prospect of an offer. What I saw and John's portrait of the hospital resonated with the image I had formed as a medical student when I first encountered Ben Castleman's CPCs (clinicopathologic conferences) in the *New England Journal* and the lectures I heard then and later from some of its distinguished physicians. The ward rounds were an eye-opener. I saw my first (and last) case of acute brucellosis and watched John arrive at the diagnosis through a careful occupational history. The second major event was my meeting with Bob Ebert, so recently the physician-in-chief at the MGH and now the dean of the Medical School. It was in my conversation with Bob that I first broached my dream of inviting Seymour Kety to head the department's laboratories if I were to be asked to take the chair.

The visit ended with a dinner and discussion with the full Search Committee during which I gave voice to my views on the future of psychiatry, one that would see psychiatry reintegrated with the rest of medicine—using, but not dominated by, the concepts of psychoanalysis and developing the foundation for more effective clinical care through a commitment to basic and clinical research. I was thanked for my comments, gracefully told that it had been a long day for me, and invited to retire to my hotel so that the committee could continue its deliberations *in camera*. I had just about fallen asleep when my phone rang. John Knowles and Bob Ebert were in the lobby of the Ritz Carlton and invited me down to have a drink. I was not fully awake when I was told that I was the "unanimous" choice of the committee. (That turned out to be a bit of poetic exaggeration; the committee had voted 12 to 1. The one holdout—a psychiatrist—gave in when the other members of the jury pointed out that they had been locked in long enough.)

Back in Baltimore, I phoned Seymour Kety in Paris, where he was on sabbatical, to ask him to join me at Harvard where both of us were wanted. I do not believe that it is in any way to minimize my own worth (I've never suffered from excessive modesty) to acknowledge that what made the prospect attractive to the Search Committee was that it was a package: a clinical scholar-administrator and an internationally known investigator. Seymour responded as enthusiastically as I had done, and we settled on a date for both of us to journey to Boston to settle the details: such small matters as space, budget, staff, and personal salary, none of which, in the best New England traditions of good taste, had been bruited about when we had accepted our posts.

Seymour had long been a hero of mine. When I was a medical student, he was a newly appointed instructor in pharmacology at the University of Pennsylvania. His lectures were a model of clarity, logic, and precision. He was, I had decided, what I wanted to be when I grew up. If I never quite made it, I comfort myself with Browning's moral admonition that a man's reach should exceed his grasp. Seymour's research career had begun with a fellowship under Joseph Aub at the MGH before he had been invited to return to Pennsylvania. There he developed the first quantitative method for measuring cerebral blood flow by using inspired nitrous oxide, measuring the carotid-jugular arteriovenous difference, and employing Fick's principle. Seymour was so popular with the medical students that when he moved on to Penn's Graduate School of Medicine the students invited him back to give them a short course on their own time after hours. He moved on to Washington as the first scientific director of the National Institute for Neurological Diseases where he put together a first-rate intramural program. Having recruited an outstanding staff, he defied all bureaucratic laws by stepping down from that directorship to a lesser position in the civil service pecking order because he wanted to do his own research as a laboratory chief at the NIMH. There, he and his colleagues pioneered research in biogenic amine metabolism in schizophrenia and created what still remains the leading national resource for the training of postdoctoral fellows. He had also, incidentally, served on the MGH Scientific Advisory Committee from 1956 to 1960.

Seymour and I had briefly been colleagues when he had become the Phipps Professor of Psychiatry at Hopkins. The appointment was a daring one because Seymour had had no clinical training; unfortunately, it did not work out for him at a personal level because he found it uncomfortable and unrewarding to be responsible for a large clinical service. Despite the brevity of his tenure at Hopkins, he was so charismatic as a leader that the clinicians on the hospital staff petitioned him to stay. He returned to the NIMH where he began a research program that he continued at the MGH: He and his colleagues conceptualized an ingenious model for discriminating between the genetic and the cultural hypotheses for the transmission of schizophrenia. By studying the psychiatric status of the families of children adopted in infancy who became schizophrenic as adults, he was able to contrast rates of psychosis in biologic as against adoptive relatives and to demonstrate that the preponderance was found in the biologic relatives. At the MGH he invited Ross Baldessarini and later Steve Matthysse to join him in a research program that has become a world center for the study of neurotransmitters, psychotropic drug actions, and the genetics of psychosis.

In the months before I arrived at the MGH to take up my responsibilities, I was faced with a crisis in the resident staff. For many years the NIMH had provided stipends for psychiatric residents as a federal response to the shortage of psychiatrists that had become evident during and in the years immediately after the Second World War. For 20 years psychiatric trainees had been the privileged recipients of federal stipends when residents in other medical and surgical specialties were still living on their patrimony. But times had changed; hospital stipends had come to exceed the NIMH allotment. John Knowles at once recognized the propriety of having the MGH assume the responsibility for a uniform level of payment for all resident staff; NIMH support, so long as it lasted, was to serve as an offset against the hospital pledge. That decision, parenthetically, became increasingly important to the department when the Congress substantially reduced its support for psychiatric training over the succeeding decade.

But that was only the half of it. The department of psychiatry at the MGH had lost repute as an academic training center because of the long interregnum and the failure of the hospital to provide adequate space and support for research. Although we continued to get some superb residents, our applicant pool was disappointing and even embarrassing in comparison with the other clinical specialties. Indeed, in the first several years I had the unpleasant necessity of terminating several residents with prejudice. Happily, it was not long before the enthusiasm of the new program began to attract the quality of applicants we wanted. But we did succeed in competing, and a number of our graduates have already become leaders in American psychiatry.

Within the first year of my tenure, John Nemiah was offered and accepted the professorship at the Beth Israel; with him departed several of the key people in the outpatient clinic. With some urgency I had to find a promising young person to take on this crucial role. I was singularly fortunate when a colleague called my attention to a young man, trained at the Massachusetts Mental Health Center, who was on the staff at Yale. When I met Aaron Lazare, I knew I had found a winner and my only task was to recruit him. From the day of his arrival, he transformed a good but somewhat pedestrian outpatient program into what has become a premier clinical service, teaching program, and research center. In the Acute Psychiatric Service of the MGH, young physicians under close supervision learn to recognize and manage a greater number and variety of acutely disturbed patients than are seen anywhere in the metropolitan Boston area. Aaron's research on the nature of patient requests, on the negotiation of a contract between the patient and the physician, and on the effective treatment of acute and chronic psychiatric problems is not only outstanding but feeds back into more effective service and training in an integrated fashion. His recent text, summarizing a decade of systematic research and clinical experience, is certain to become a landmark in outpatient psychiatry.

Liaison psychiatry and psychosomatic medicine had been the strong points of MGH psychiatry from the time the department was established by Stanley Cobb. For reasons I cannot fully understand, the service had languished under Lindemann, perhaps because his own interests lay elsewhere. But personal foibles played a part as well. He objected to hypnosis; Freud had abandoned it for the method of free association and that was that. When Lindemann found that Tom Hackett used hypnotic treatment for selected patients, Tom was in the doghouse and never received any recognition for his contribution. When I arrived, Tom was on the periphery of the staff, understandably perplexed by the way he had been treated but quietly going about his own excellent clinical work. It did not require much judgment on my part to recognize his clinical skills and organizational talent. Once he was given a modicum of support, Tom went off like a house afire. Within a very short interval he had made liaison psychiatry what it should always have been: one of the gems in the diadem of a department of psychiatry in a general hospital. It became an increasingly major component of the residency training program to the very great advantage of resident education and to the benefit of clinical care throughout the hospital. Tom was the one with the perspicacity to recruit Ned Cassem; together they developed one of the very best research programs on the psychologic aspects of coronary care.

I was fortunate enough to inherit another outstanding scholar in the interface between medicine and psychiatry in the person of Avery Weisman, a long-time member of the staff who, like Tom Hackett, seemed to be in exile. Avery's scholarly research on death and dying and on the psychologic aspects of patients with terminal cancer soon became central to the department. Both Tom and Avery were MGH born and bred; it was simply a matter of letting them do what they knew how to do and getting out of the way. Both provided sage counsel to a new chief who needed a good deal of advice in order to avoid the follies of improvident decisions.

The remaining clinical area to require revitalization was the inpatient unit; it suffered from too low a census, too long an average length of stay, and a tendency to select admissions on "teaching" criteria rather than on the clinical needs of patients. I had been impressed by a young resident I knew at Hopkins, Bernie Levy, who had taken two postdoctoral years at the NIMH on an inpatient program designed as a therapeutic milieu. Bernie agreed to undertake the redesign of our ward along similar lines and did so with brio. In short time the change was dramatic: full census, rapid turnover, responsiveness to the needs of other hospital services. However, we had not fully appreciated the complexity of the attempt to incorporate first-year residents into the social system of an inpatient unit whose driving force was group process. The residents, still struggling to consolidate their own medical identities, were unable to cope with the egalitarian staff structure. Despite the clinical excellence of the patient care, resident antagonism mounted to a crescendo, so painful to all that no constructive resolution seemed possible. When he was offered an attractive post elsewhere, Bernie decided to accept it; ultimately, it had been my failure to recognize and deal with the problem earlier that led to the impasse. In the end, all worked out well. The inpatient program remains the better for the fresh ideas and leadership he provided. Bernie heads a major private psychiatric hospital in Boston and continues to be a much admired teacher by HMS medical students. If my account of my stewardship lists mainly accomplishments, let me acknowledge that this episode is one I still recall with discomfort; I was asleep at the switch until too late.

One of the valuable heritages Lindemann had left to the department, although it was one that seemed to me at first to be a splendid opportunity artfully disguised as an insoluble problem, was the state planning that eventuated in building a community mental health center one block away from the MGH. It was designed to have academic ties as close to the MGH as the Massachusetts Mental Health Center had enjoyed with the Harvard Medical School. The building was already under construction before I arrived. My task was to recruit a superintendent, mutually acceptable to the state Department of Mental Health and to MGH/Harvard. Seymour headed a joint Search Committee on which I served as a member, and the two of us canvassed the nation for academic psychiatrists. Although there were a number of first-rate candidates, the one who was clearly the most outstanding was Gerald Klerman, then director of the Community Mental Health Center at Yale. It took several years of negotiation, but Gerry finally did join us. With his high level of energy, his willingness to mix it up with the state government when necessary, and his scintillating array of innovative ideas, the Mental Health Center, later to be named in honor of Lindemann, became a very considerable asset to the psychiatric training program. It provided a venue in which psychiatric residents could learn to treat patients in the community, an option that was not available so long as all their support derived from hospital-based stipends. Moreover, LMCH provided an opportunity for direct clinical experience with a population of chronic psychiatric patients who could not be managed within the small acute inpatient unit at the MGH. Gerry's research in psychopharmacology, in the interaction between drugs and psychotherapy, in the study of depression, and in the epidemiology of psychiatric disorder in the community became benchmarks in American psychiatric research. His lectures and seminars produced such intellectual excitement that they became a major point of recruitment to the residency program. For sheer intellectual brilliance, depth of scholarship, and breadth of vision, he is without equal in clinical psychiatry. His national recognition led to his choice as the director of the Alcohol, Drug Abuse and Mental Health Administration in Washington, a position for which he took leave of absence from the MGH.

So much, then, for an account of the major departmental activities for the period from 1967 to 1974. As a service chief, I was also privileged to sit on the MGH General Executive Committee during a period crucial to the development of the hospital. Perhaps my outstanding impression after seven years of service was the remarkable quality of the MGH as an institution and the dedication it evoked from its staff and its trustees. Although each chief of service might be guilty from time to time of a parochial view that what was good for his specialty was necessarily good for the hospital, most of us most of the time were able to subordinate special interest loyalties to the greater good of the institution. In my experience, this is rare; many institutions suffer an unbalanced centrifugal pull from specialty demands. Moreover, the quality as well as the quantity of trustee input to hospital policy was remarkable; it was not merely that the hospital had a distinguished group of trustees (many do, on paper) but that they contributed long hours to hospital affairs. I cannot recall an instance in which the trustees transgressed on what were properly decisions to be made by the medical staff (although I can remember the frequency with which we told the trustees what *they* ought to do). I did not always agree with their decisions but I did recognize the sincerity of their civic concerns.

Afterthoughts. Why, then, did I resign as department chairman at the MGH? The hospital had been every bit as exciting, clinically as well as scientifically, as I had expected it to be. Most of my colleagues were a joy and a delight; if I acknowledge that a few were considerably less so, such would be true of any place short of heaven. My problem, by no means unique, is one that plagues the heads of clinical departments at teaching hospitals—namely, the extent to which administrative demands displace opportunities for personal scholarship.

In the period since the Second World War, the size, scope, and budgets of clinical departments have expanded almost exponentially. The time and skill required to manage them are correspondingly greater; yet few chiefs have had other than on-the-job training for what has become a decisive aspect of the job description; few are able to enjoy what they do most of the time. Being a good manager *is* important; the skill of the chairperson makes or breaks department morale. But what is required for durability in the role is more than ability to do the job well; one has to be able to derive enough personal satisfaction from remote outcomes to provide sustenance during the long and lonely days and nights when difficult and unpleasant decisions must be made.

I still remember vividly a colleague who described to me with evident glee several of his administrative triumphs. They were triumphs indeed, for they enabled his department to maintain its national reputation for excellence. When I won an administrative battle, I was less depressed having won than I would have been having lost, but I continued to regret the time consumed by an activity I didn't enjoy while I was doing it. It isn't a matter of the relative importance of administration versus scholarship. By that criterion, few of us could make a case for getting back into the laboratory or the clinic. It is the rare investigator who has as much impact on a department as the average chief. What is at stake is that, for many of us, "professing" is closer to our dreams of glory than "administering" and a lot more fun.

I had suggested several times to my colleagues on the GEC that they consider limited terms of tenure for department heads but the proposal was never accepted. If, however, one surveys the national scene, it is becoming evident that even without formal strictures the half-life of department heads is well below what it was a generation ago. That, I suggest, is not because there were giants in those days but because the nature of the job has become so much more demanding that a periodic renewal is necessary for survival.

I don't regret my seven years as chief for a moment. They provided a superb postgraduate education in the problems of contemporary medicine in the company of outstanding teachers and under the aegis of two of the greatest hospital directors of our time. I am much the richer for the experience. What I gave to others, particularly the young men and women in the department, is a long-term investment that continues to yield dividends of satisfaction as I watch their careers mature. But there is a time for endings, when affairs are at high tide and new challenges beckon.

Editors' Note

When, in 1974, Thomas Hackett was appointed to the post of chief of Psychiatry at the MGH, a tradition of overlooking MGH-trained talent finally ended. Hackett brought to his job not only an engaging personality which was both forceful and compassionate but also an unexcelled and unusual combination of talents. His research record stretched back many years and, despite his relative youth, he was already a "master clinician"—in Dr. Weisman's words—when he first came to the hospital in 1956.

As chief, Hackett soon showed a unique ability to enjoy and actually thrive on administrative duties, tasks that others often found onerous and unrewarding. His vision and persuasive manner rapidly brought a degree of respect to the Psychiatry Service that it had not known before.

Ned Cassem succeeded Hackett as head of the Consultation Service which grew in size and regard until other teaching hospitals also recognized its merit and sought to emulate its contribution to resident training. Hackett's personal popularity and familiarity with the MGH scene eliminated much of the misunderstanding that marred previous tenures. And he expanded the range of services and specialties within his department in keeping with changing times for the economy as well as patient care.

Avery Weisman offers some final reflections "from the sidelines" on the broad subject of MGH psychiatry and psychoanalysis:

Much has been talked about, and even more surmised about the place of psychoanalysis in the Boston area, and at the MGH in particular. For many years MGH was known as "anti-analytic," meaning that psychoanalytic concepts or even psychoanalysts were said to be scoffed at here and regarded as a contaminating influence. Consequently, prospective residents interested in psychoanalysis were dissuaded from applying to the MGH in the belief that they would receive better training elsewhere. When it came time to appoint a new chairman, both to replace Cobb and Lindemann, the Search Committee explicitly said that it wanted to get away from someone who was "heavily psychoanalytic" and turn MGH psychiatry back to medicine, where it belonged. Thus two views prevailed: the notion that MGH opposed psychoanalysis and the belief that MGH psychiatry was "too analytic."

As one who has worked under every chief of Psychiatry in the history of this department, I can attest that neither accusation was ever correct. MGH was never "anti-analytic," whatever that means, nor was there any split between psychiatry and medicine because of psychoanalysis.

In the early years after Hitler came to power, psychoanalysts who had been among Freud's followers became refugees. Many landed in East Coast cities, along with other physicians, scientists, artists, and business people. But it was through the help of Stanley Cobb that several outstanding psychoanalysts were able to settle in Boston and begin putting their lives together again. He invited a few to participate in the department's teaching program, although most preferred to resume practice and to establish themselves in a new institute. Shortly after World War II, however, the link with psychoanalysis became stronger with the popularity of analytic training among psychiatric residents. Men and women continued to work in hospitals, teaching and consulting with the newer generations of students, but maintaining themselves by office practice of psychotherapy. I must emphasize that in those days there was no other opportunity for post-graduate training than in psychoanalysis. Today, newer fields have opened up, but the contribution of psychoanalysis to the teaching and practice of psychiatry continues. Although the medical community may feel that psychoanalysis can be rooted out of departments of psychiatry, we must recall that long before the influx of refugees psychoanalysis had imprinted itself throughout the artistic and literary world. Consequently, it is part of our common culture and cannot be denied. Most of us realize that psychoanalysis has disappointed our naive, early expectations, but we went into analytic training because it held out a promise. It is no longer a question of being analytic or not, but rather how well one learns the importance of psychotherapy.

But I cannot explain the antagonism expressed for psychoanalysis by medical colleagues who are otherwise fair and objective. Why the establishment feels threatened by the mild, inconspicuous efforts of some staff members with analytic training is a mystery that I do not care to solve. Those chiefs of service who opted not to get analytic training themselves have not, at the same time, been unsympathetic or threatened. Cobb, Eisenberg, and Hackett, along with John Nemiah, encouraged residents to get training in anything that might broaden their psychiatric weaponry and perspective.

Part III. Children's Service

19. Allan Macy Butler

Allan Macy Butler, chief of the MGH Children's Service from 1941 to 1960, was born in Yonkers, New York, the son of a stockbroker. Even at an early age, we can discern some of his creative organizational talents: In carpentry class it was Allan who held the fruits of the labor; his brothers held the tools. In 1912 he entered Princeton and, upon graduating, was slated to become a bond salesman on Wall Street. His desk in that institution happened to be next to that of James Forrestal. On a Saturday morning following New Year's Day in 1917, Allan said to him, "Jim, I have decided that I am not going to have an eighth of a point on the stock exchange as a major interest in my life, so I am resigning today." Forrestal indicated that he didn't want this as a major interest either, but said he was going to stay on the job until he made a million. He stayed, made his million, became the first secretary of defense, had a mental breakdown, and took his own life just before the end of World War II. Butler never made a million, but he did receive the Howland Award of the American Pediatric Society in 1969.

Less than a week after resigning, he joined a British Infantry Reserve Training Corps at Oxford and eventually was commissioned second lieutenant in the Field Artillery, a discipline in which he had no training or experience. While serving as supply officer, Sixth Field Artillery, Butler displayed some of the independence of thought and action for which he is so well known. Although on two occasions he was cited for court-martial, the first time for not obeying a regimental order to hold a 6:00 A.M. reveille (his reason was that the men had difficulty getting their cold swollen feet with wet socks into their wet shoes) and the second time for some minor infraction, he was later cited as having "shown the greatest efficiency and zeal in the performance of his duties. Under the most trying conditions of weather, roads and traffic, he has by constant effort kept his vehicles and animals in such excellence of condition and appearance as invariably to elicit the commendation of his superiors."

In 1919, following the end of World War I, Butler got a job as efficiency expert on the docks of the Cunard Steamship Company in New York. His shift from industry to medicine came a year later when his branch of the company was dissolved, and he found himself out of a job. To gain some perspective while thinking over what he would do next, he took a job as a coal miner in Pennsylvania where, as a result of nearly being blown up, he gained a strong sense of the need for public safety measures. This led to a decision to study physics and chemistry. Shortly afterwards, while he was eating lunch with his newly acquired bride, Mabel, on the lawn at the Columbia University Summer School, a Princeton classmate by the name of Stewart Mudd came along and asked what he was doing. On learning that he was studying chemistry, Dr. Mudd asked Butler why he was not pursuing this within the framework of medicine. The end result was that Butler matriculated in the Harvard Medical School in 1922, at the age of 28 years.

His course at the HMS was somewhat unusual. For instance, when he found that a course in physical chemistry conflicted with courses in pediatrics and psychiatry, he skipped the latter two. Likewise, when he disagreed with Professor Hale of pharmacology about the use of the English system of dosages, he felt that the best way to argue his point was to give dosages only in the metric system, so he was given a failing mark. When he came up for graduation, it turned out that he had not attended courses in two major subjects, had a failure in another, and yet, *mirabile dictu,* was graduated in 1926 an AOA student. Since it was difficult for married men to get positions as interns, Butler went to the Rockefeller Institute as a fellow with Van Slyke for two years, after which he returned to Harvard as a tutor in biochemical sciences with L. J. Henderson. In the ensuing years he became associated with James Gamble at the Children's Hospital, began to work on the wards, and became an instructor in pediatrics at the HMS. Subsequently, he maneuvered the authorities of Massachusetts, Michigan, and California to grant him a license to practice medicine in their respective states; one wonders whether he had the distinction of being the only physician in the United States licensed to practice in three states who had never either an internship or residency.

During the thirties and forties his long and strong interest in chemistry and metabolism yielded a series of significant contributions in respect to the clinical measurement of sodium concentration, the early recognition of renal tubular acidosis, the use of potassium ion in the repair of dehydration, the chemical pathology of ascorbic acid deficiency, the treatment of rickets by means of citrates, the phenomenon of renal hypertension, and, during World War II, the development of life-raft rations for sailors and airmen wrecked at sea. His talents and drives were not limited, however, to the pursuit of these highly acceptable and proper forms of academic endeavor, for he was among the first to recognize the need for better means of delivering and financing health care services. His interest in this subject was catalyzed by a series of discussions starting in 1928 and culminating in 1932 in the publication of the "Report of the Committee on the Cost of Medical Care." In recognition of his lively interest in this subject, he was made a member of the Legislative Committee of the Massachusetts Medical Society. Later, in his capacity as associate editor of the *New England Journal of Medicine,* Butler wrote a series of editorials which, as you might guess, were not exactly supportive of American Medical Association policies. Indeed, the AMA not only complained to the Massachusetts Medical Society about these editorials but also went so far as to demand that the editor of the *Journal* be fired. Rather than be the cause of such an unhappy eventuality, Butler decided to drop out as associate editor. However, this did not by any means mark the end of his literary expositions on the subject, for it happened that the Committee on Physicians for the Improvement of Medical Care came into being at about this time, and Butler wrote all the editorials and articles about this committee for the *Journal.*

In the years since, his contributions in these regards continued to be of major national significance. He was one of the group that argued for the National Health Program against strong opposition at the National Health Conference held in 1938, and he has been a familiar figure on Capitol Hill, where he has appeared before most of the congressional committees considering medical legislation, including Medicare. Concerning the latter, he received a personal message from President John F. Kennedy in a letter from Theodore Sorenson, then special consultant to the president, dated September 14, 1961: "The president has asked me to thank you for your testimony before the House Committee on Ways and Means in support of his bill for health insurance for the aged. The president believes health insurance for the aged through Social Security is an important and essential part of the program. He looks forward with your help to the enactment of the legislation next year."

Adapted from remarks by *Nathan B. Talbot*, at the presentation to Allan M. Butler of the American Pediatric Society's Howland Award. *Pediat. Res.* 3:471–474, 1969

20. Service History

NATHAN B. TALBOT

By the time Butler reached retirement age as chief of the Children's Medical Service in 1960, he had succeeded in establishing it as one of the two main divisions of Harvard's Department of Pediatrics. Moreover, as a result of his many other accomplishments, the service that he headed for 19 years had become recognized nationally as a high quality, although small, teaching service. Most of Butler's achievements have already been recorded in Faxon's history, and many of his other activities are covered in the foregoing chapter. In view of these, the current section concerns itself primarily with the evolution of the service since 1960.

Upon Butler's retirement, leadership of the Children's Medical Service passed to Nathan B. Talbot who had served as Butler's full-time associate throughout the latter's administration. The service's physical resources consisted of 85 beds located on three floors of the recently constructed Burnham Memorial wards for children, a small office suite, and two research laboratories housing the service's Endocrine-Metabolic Research Unit. In addition to Talbot there was only one full-time senior staff member, John Crawford, who, while playing a major role in all departmental patient care and teaching activities, headed the Endocrine-Metabolic Unit, a responsibility that he has carried with distinction ever since. The service benefited substantially from close partnerships with two pediatrically skilled clinicians who were primarily members of other services: Philip Dodge, a pediatric neurologist, who functioned simultaneously as a member of the Children's Medical Service, and W. Hardy Hendren, a pediatric surgeon. Hendren had been cultivated by Edward Churchill, chief of the Surgical Services, to fill the hospital's need for a highly qualified pediatric surgeon "who would work closely with the medical pediatricians in developing excellent resources for the care of all types of child patients on the pediatric service of the MGH." At the time he was appointed in 1960, he had completed training as chief resident of the Surgical Services at both the MGH and the Children's Hospital Medical Center.

In view of subsequent developments, it is interesting to reflect on the fact that Hendren was quite concerned that he might not be able to earn a living as a pediatric surgeon in a general, as opposed to a specialized children's, hospital. Fortunately, it turned out that with the strong support tendered him by W. Gerald Austen, Churchill's successor as chief of the General Surgical Services, Hendren's outstanding skills as a diagnostician, operating surgeon, and consultant soon became widely recognized. His untiring willingness to come in at any time of day or night to attend to the needs of a critically sick child gave patients and referring clinicians a high sense of confidence in him as a caring physician. Furthermore, his imagination, courage, and skill enabled him to devise and implement successfully new and improved ways for correcting hitherto incurable maladies. The value of having a person with these capabilities as a senior partner in developing the Children's Service can be understood readily when it is realized that roughly half of pediatric admissions are apt to be primarily or secondarily for surgical reasons. (See Page 259 for more extended discussion of pediatric surgery.)

Those familiar with the never-ending, multitudinous responsibilities of even a moderate-sized university teaching and tertiary referral clinical service will understand the gratitude felt towards another cohort of senior staff members—namely, our pediatric generalist practitioners. Among the many who contributed are Leo Burgin, Leroy Eldredge, Lawrence Essember, Nathan Fearer, Robert N. Ganz, Andrew Guthrie, M. Edward Keenan, Thomas Peebles, John C. Robinson, Ralph A. Ross, Robert T. Sceery, Rudolf Toch, and Eleanor Zaudy. These highly capable, ever-willing, and largely unpaid physicians carried a major portion of the service's overall patient care and clinical teaching responsibilities. They literally enabled it to function in the early sixties pending the development of a full-time staff of adequate size.

In laying out plans for the future of the service, we were intrigued with the expectation expressed by Dean George P. Berry of the Harvard Medical School that we would demonstrate that one could render exemplary child care, offer high quality pediatric teaching and training, and conduct significant research on problems related to child health in the setting of a large general hospital. Underlying this thought was the realization that most children the world over are cared for in general hospitals rather than in specialized children's medical centers and that much might be gained in our understanding of the origins of disease and their effects on the health of people in their later years. The long-range significance of developmental deviations could be studied by cultivating a wide variety of collaborative arrangements between child- and adult-oriented experts in diverse aspects of medicine, surgery, and allied disciplines.

This thesis was attractive per se, but it also served the useful purpose of suggesting how we might get around a seemingly nearly insurmountable obstacle—that of having no spare space to house additional staff or much hope for such space in the immediate future. As will become clear shortly, this was without question a blessing in disguise: It forced us to bypass any thought of developing a mini-Children's Hospital within the framework of the MGH. Instead, the collaborative approach suggested above was pursued.

As a first step in this direction, the position and responsibilities held by the then Children's Medical Service within the MGH underwent redefinition. Since Hendren was working closely with the service as a pediatric surgeon, it was clear that the term *Medical* within the title was misleading and could only continue to promote the public image of the service as one of limited capabilities. Moreover, by tradition, members of the adult medical and surgical services could admit and care directly for young patients in the Children's Service if they so desired. As a consequence, many of the children so admitted did not receive specialized pediatric attention. Accordingly, we recommended that the service be made officially responsible for the overall welfare of all child patients, that its age span be widened to cover the entire human developmental period from birth through adolescence, and that its name be changed to The Children's Service, Burnham Division for Children, MGH. This recommendation was approved by the General Executive Committee and trustees in 1961. Six years later the chief of the Children's Service was made a regular member of the General Executive Committee, enabling the pediatric point of view to be represented regularly in the hospital's top professional administrative group.

A second major factor in our planning related to the major changes in the nature of childhood diseases and disabilities which were occurring as a result of advances in medical science. Many of the erstwhile life-threatening and disabling problems, which at one time necessitated hospitalization, could now be handled on an outpatient basis. Meanwhile, new ways were emerging almost daily for identifying, correcting, and/or preventing hitherto unmanageable disorders. Moreover, there were indications that disease and disability should no longer be viewed as just biophysical phenomena; rather, it should be borne in mind that they are often the result of a closely interwoven mix of physical, biologic, social, and behavioral pathogens. While this reality was considered to be deserving increasingly of systematically objective attention, we concluded that our first developmental goal should be to equip our service to deal competently with all major biophysical aspects of children's diseases. Drawing on the experience gained by bringing Hendren and Dodge into the service, physicians were added in the fields of genetics, cardiology, infectious disease, pulmonary pathophysiology, gastroenterology, and hematology-oncology. Fortunately, the chiefs of these MGH units supplied financial support and space for these individuals. Gradually the Children's Service added representation or developed cooperative arrangements with all appropriate medical and social areas. The following Children's Service staff members headed activities in each field: Ronald Benz (ambulatory care–emergency ward), John P. Connelly and Andrew Guthrie (Bunker Hill Health Center), Allen Goldblatt (cardiology), Philip Porter (community hospital), Joseph Warshaw (developmental biology), John Robinson and Thomas Peebles (education), Allan Walker (gastroenterology), John Littlefield and Richard Erbe (genetics: see also p. 195), John Truman (hematology-oncology), Richard Talamo (immunology), David Lang and Daniel Keim (infectious disease), Daniel Shannon and David Todres (intensive care), Daniel Shannon (pulmonary), John Herrin (renology), John D. Crawford (trauma-burns).

Other MGH services and departments spontaneously added to their staffs individuals fully trained in the pediatric aspects of their specialty: David Todres and John Ryan (anesthesia), Ann Sheetz (nursing), Michael Ehrlich (orthopedics), Ann Dvorak (pathology), Spencer Borden (radiology), and Barbara Zenn (social service).

Another major category of advances demands attention, namely, the gains in patient care facilities at the MGH. These included improvements in the Children's Service's ambulatory care unit, the establishment of a new Emergency Ward unit specifically designed for infants and children, and the creation of a fully staffed and equipped Intensive Care Unit on one of the Burnham floors. With the strong support of the MGH administration, our ambulatory "clinic" was completely transformed into an attractive facility where so-called public and private patients alike could be seen in a personalized manner. To ensure adequate oversight and developmental leadership, a fully qualified pediatrician was named head of this unit. He functioned with the support of additional full-time physicians plus other part-time members of our staff as needed to cover generalist and specialty service needs. House officers and students work alongside this staff in much the same manner as they do on the inpatient services. These changes effectively erased the erstwhile picture of hospital clinics with patients sitting for hours on benches waiting to be seen by whoever happens to be available—usually a different physician each time. They also have confirmed the impression that with adequate ambulatory resources many of the problems that once were thought to deserve inpatient admission can, in fact, be handled as well or better on an outpatient basis. In this connection, Hendren was among the first to perform selected categories of child surgery on a daytime transient as opposed to an overnight or longer inpatient basis. The Anesthesia Department enhanced this service by creating a room where children could be induced with parent-at-hand—a move that substantially reduced the anxiety so often associated with hospitalization and surgery.

We were also enabled to develop for the first time an Emergency Ward unit specifically designed for child patients within the framework of the MGH's Emergency Ward. As with the ambulatory services, it was felt to be highly desirable to make available senior staff oversight of our EW activities on a full-time basis as necessary. This responsibility was assigned to the ambulatory service team which shared it on a rotating basis. The net result has been that physicians in training were enabled to learn how to make quickly oftimes critical decisions concerning diagnosis and treatment with minimized chances of making avoidable errors.

With the increases in expertise enumerated above, increasing numbers of critically sick infants and children were referred to the MGH for care. This soon led to an uncomfortable awareness that we lacked a fully developed and specifically staffed intensive care unit. With the collaborative support of the surgical, anesthesia, and nursing services and Henry Murphy of the MGH administrative staff, it became possible to restructure completely one of our Burnham Building floors into an exemplary intensive care facility equipped to care for infants and children from birth to approximately 18 years of age. Upon its completion on July 1, 1971, a full-time pediatric intensive care team was inaugurated with staff assigned thereto by the surgical, anesthesia, and nursing services as well as the Children's Service as indicated. The resources of this facility were made readily available to community physicians and hospitals throughout Massachusetts and neighboring states through MGH-pediatrician-staffed land and coast guard helicopter airlift ambulance services on a 24-hour-a-day basis. These otherwise generally unavailable resources were sought at a rapidly increasing rate as it became evident that the unit was capable of saving the lives of many children whose chances of recovery without this type of care were very limited. In addition, the opportunity to work with the unit staff became much sought after by students, house officers, and practicing physicians. The unit also provided opportunities to make significant advances in the management of a number of life-threatening conditions, among them the sudden infant death syndrome. Shannon and his colleagues deserve much credit for all these accomplishments.

The third category of gain was undertaken in an effort to create opportunities to care for children in close relation to their home community life experiences. One opportunity to do so was arranged by the development of a working relationship with the Pediatric Service of the Cambridge Hospital, which agreed to allow the MGH Children's Service to appoint a member of its staff chief of their Child Service. Philip Porter has filled this post for many years in a thoroughly successful manner. The teaching and training provided by him and his staff with respect to community hospital pediatrics have become highly sought after by our house officers and Harvard medical students. Additionally, an opportunity arose for us to play a primary role in the formation of the Bunker Hill Health

Center to care for children and their families in Charlestown, Massachusetts. At the beginning, this center perforce dealt chiefly with children. Subsequently, as originally envisaged, it became a comprehensive, multidisciplinary community care center in which all the MGH clinical services were actively involved.

Andrew Guthrie, who succeeded John P. Connelly as executive director of the Bunker Hill Health Center in Charlestown, also contributed to the welfare of older children and adolescents as chairman of a joint effort of the Children's Service and Bridge over Troubled Waters. Recognizing the high risk being experienced by many youngsters living on the streets of Greater Boston, they initiated a medical van service running on a regular schedule so that these children would know that they could obtain medical and human support without risk of losing privacy. The van, staffed by a large number of volunteer physicians, nurses, social workers, and others, helped to get many young people out of serious trouble before it was too late.

The final category of effort was concerned with the fulfillment of the teaching and training responsibilities of this division of Harvard's Department of Pediatrics. As the spectrum of departmental disciplines broadened, the variety of patients increased markedly, thus enriching our teaching-training. As a result, the number of Harvard clinical clerks *choosing* to obtain their principal clinical pediatric experience at the MGH increased from 54 in 1960 to approximately 100 per annum in recent years. These gains were due on the one hand to the generous and deeply interested teaching efforts of our resident and senior staff and on the other to the sensitive, personalized attention given by John Robinson in his role as director of this part of our teaching program. Much credit is due also to Thomas Peebles for the entrepreneurial skills that he has demonstrated in managing the postgraduate continuing medical education courses in pediatrics given by our department annually. Perhaps the best indicator of his successes is the fact that the number attending these courses each year has grown from modest beginnings to the point where the Shriners Burns Institute auditorium has been filled to overflowing on several occasions. Moreover, the fact that students are coming from far and wide attests to the reality that this offering has become broadly recognized as one of the best available.

All these developments have yielded major functional, physical, and financial gains. For example, bed occupancy, which was fluctuating around the 60 percent level in 1960, gradually increased to a point near saturation. The assignment of a whole floor of the MGH Research Building to house our newly formed genetics and immunology units increased the service's original allotment of office and laboratory space from 2,700 to 7,500 square feet. This was further augmented by the assignment by the Shriners Burns Institute of quarters into which Dr. Crawford could expand his metabolic endocrine unit. It has also been heartening to observe that the number of well-qualified applicants for residency and research traineeship positions have increased manyfold over the past two decades. Accordingly, we have been experiencing to an ever-enlarging extent the mixed blessing of having many of our senior staff sought for positions of leadership in grade A medical schools, teaching hospitals, and research institutes across the country. In association with all this, our budget has grown proportionately as a result of major increases in departmental allotments from the MGH and Harvard Medical School and the winning of very substantial grants-in-aid from U.S. government and various private agencies.

While it is beyond the scope of this review to set forth in detail the research accomplishments of the staff of the Children's Service, it can be said that they have been notably productive of top-quality publications, most of which are recorded in the annual MGH research booklets.

In closing, we would like to emphasize our appreciation for the thoughtful and very solid support provided by John H. Knowles and Charles Sanders as general directors as well as the trustees, whose combined backing was essential to making the advances recorded here. We would also like to underscore the highly notable extent to which essentially all the other major MGH services and departments contributed to the development of the Children's Service over these years.

Talbot retired as chief of service in June 1977 and was succeeded by Donald N. Medearis, Jr., who noted the outstanding base that had been developed for the Children's Service since 1960. "Our obligation," he wrote, "is to utilize it to build and continue our development."

Genetics Unit

JOHN W. LITTLEFIELD AND RICHARD W. ERBE

Medical genetics as we know it today emerged about 20 years ago. It combined immunogenetics, population genetics, biochemical genetics (which began in the late 1940s with studies on hemoglobins and on urinary aminoacids), cytogenetics (which provided a simple and rapid method to analyze the chromosome complement of an individual), and clinical genetics (which had been a relatively tranquil and descriptive subspecialty). I [JWL] believe the MGH first recognized genetics as a new, valid, and useful subspecialty about 1963. Victor McKusick, then and now one of the great pioneers in clinical genetics, visited the hospital to provide advice. He was most enthusiastic and even recommended a new separate department of genetics at the MGH. Because most severe inherited conditions are encountered in childhood, and also to fortify research in the department of pediatrics, the hospital made the wise decision to locate the new subspecialty in the Children's Service.

The relation of my research and publications to genetics plus my eagerness to return to active clinical involvement led to my inclusion in the new unit. I got the required "union card" by attending McKusick's human genetics course in Bar Harbor in the summer of 1964; and in 1966, after a sabbatical in Naples, I returned to the MGH to get the Pediatric Genetics Unit underway. At first I had to learn clinical genetics as well as a lot of pediatrics in order to provide consultations and make known the new enterprise. Within a few years, however, Richard Erbe, Lewis Holmes, and Lee Jacoby joined the unit and strengthened markedly its clinical and research activities. We developed affiliations with Leonard Atkins in the Chromosome Laboratory and Vivian Shih and Harvey Levy in Neurology. The number of inpatient consultations increased from 100 in 1968 to 400 in 1973, and an active ambulatory clinic was established. A prenatal diagnostic laboratory was established in 1970, and in 1973 about 300 cases were studied. To amplify the variety of patients available, we arranged affiliation with the Fernald School. Thus a number of different opportunities in clinical and research genetics were available for medical students, house staff, and faculty.

Furthermore, in conjunction with the pediatric genetics group at the Children's Hospital Medical Center under Park Gerald and with Henry Cohn, a Harvard Center for Human Genetics was created. Funding for fellowship training was obtained. We worked vigorously for the establishment of a full-fledged department of human genetics at the Medical School.

The initial years saw considerable growth of the MGH unit. Our laboratories moved from two rooms in the Huntington Laboratories to several makeshift rooms in the "Temporary Building." These we vacated just before an enormous flood, moving back to the present quarters which occupy a floor carefully renovated for us in the Research Building. From 1967 to 1973 the total budget of the unit increased over tenfold. The number of individuals involved increased from four to 28, and the publications generated went from 11 in 1968 to 50 in 1973. That same year I departed for Johns Hopkins, and leadership of the Genetics Unit passed to Richard W. Erbe, who comments on subsequent events as follows:

Littlefield left the Genetics Unit very well equipped and housed. I became chief in February 1974 and spent the initial period working to replace the research grant support that went with him. I was permitted to succeed him as program director of both the Developmental Medicine Training Grant and the Genetics Training Grant so that training support remained available. Like Littlefield, my clinical training had been in internal medicine, with postdoctoral training in biochemistry and molecular biology. The transition period went quite smoothly, and two main research groups emerged, each pursuing laboratory research and conducting laboratory research training largely for Ph.D. and M.D. postdoctoral fellows. One group, headed by Lee B. Jacoby, has focused on the urea cycle enzymes and pathways. The other, which I head, has concentrated on the pathways of folic acid and methionine metabolism. In their respective areas each group has helped to understand the normal metabolic pathways using various types of cultured human cells, to characterize the alterations of these reactions by inherited defects, and to make possible the prenatal diagnosis of new inborn errors of metabolism. The scientific group expanded with the addition in 1980 of a third major research group headed by James F. Gusella; he had just completed his graduate studies at MIT and brought to our program the approaches in the new area of recombinant DNA research. His group is also a key component of the Huntington Disease Center Without Walls.

By 1977 the demand for prenatal genetic diagnosis had expanded to exceed the capacity of the MGH-affiliated laboratory at the Shriver Center. Thus we decided to establish the Prenatal Diagnostic Laboratory as part of the Genetics Unit and selected as director Wayne A. Miller, an obstetrician-gynecologist who had recently completed his genetics training at MGH. Whereas clinical genetic services had been offered since the early years of the unit, the Prenatal Diagnostic Laboratory was the first instance in which laboratory services were also provided. At the same time we brought together the key persons involved in prenatal diagnosis from throughout the New England states to form the New England Prenatal Diagnostic Group which is now responsible for coordinating prenatal genetic diagnosis throughout the region. This group was the prototype for the establishment a year later of the New England Regional Genetics Group, by Allan C. Crocker and myself, to provide for regional coordination and planning in all aspects of genetic service. Thus the MGH Genetics Unit has helped to provide leadership in bringing the benefits of genetics to persons throughout New England.

Moreover, during this period the field of medical genetics came of age, with steady expansion of demand for clinical and laboratory services, greatly improved financial support, and the formation of a subspecialty board for formal certification of practitioners in genetics. In 1980 the long-standing hope for a Department of Genetics at Harvard Medical

School culminated in the vote by the faculty that such a department be established. Philip Leder was selected to guide the formation of this new department as its first chairman. One of his first acts was to join with the MGH in selecting Howard M. Goodman to be part of the department at HMS and to head the Department of Molecular Biology at MGH. These additions reflect the explosion of new knowledge capabilities in human genetics and signal a promising future for genetics at MGH and HMS.

Part IV. Surgical Services

21. Edward D. Churchill

J. GORDON SCANNELL

Edward D. Churchill was for 30 years John Homans Professor of Surgery and chief, first of the West and later of both, General Surgical Services at the Massachusetts General Hospital. As the Warrens, Bigelows, and Richardsons had done before him, he left an indelible mark on the growth and development of the Surgical Services and, indeed, of the hospital as a whole. His influence is sufficiently profound that a summing up of the Churchill years, 1931 to 1962, is appropriate, rather than a limited consideration of the final period. There is a wealth of biographic material; in fact, a first draft of memoirs is among his unpublished papers currently gathered in the Countway Library. The memoirs, dictated to Saul Bennison, carry him through his early years as professor and chief. They help form the basis of this essay.

Churchill was born in Chenoa, Illinois, of transplanted English and New England stock. He came to the Harvard Medical School with a master's degree in biology from Northwestern in 1917. One might say that he remained a surgical biologist through his entire career. He graduated cum laude from the Medical School in 1920 and spent the next four years as a member of the house staff of this hospital. With the introduction of a full-time system by Edward P. Richardson, Churchill became the first West Surgical resident. The following year, 1925, he spent as a Dalton Scholar with Cecil Drinker. In 1926 he was awarded a Moseley Travelling Fellowship, which provided an opportunity to work with Krogh in Copenhagen and to visit the major surgical clinics in Britain and Germany.

Churchill returned to the MGH in the summer of 1927 to join the full-time surgical staff which Richardson had gathered about him—young men of promise including Munroe McIver, James C. White, Robert Linton and, later, Oliver Cope. Richardson's successful efforts to establish a full-time professorial service in the context of a clinical tradition are interesting in the light of a letter written in 1909 by his father, Maurice H. Richardson—a clinical giant and former Moseley Professor and chief of Surgical Services—to Harvey Cushing, then at Johns Hopkins: "I feel that my men, although they make splendid practitioners of surgery, failed to get from me any inspiration towards so-called research work . . . seems that the coming generation needs a broader field in which to work; that the men should be more than purely clinical observers. . . . I feel, too, that we get to be very narrow in Boston. I advised Doctor Homans to go to Baltimore. . . . I hope later to have my son, Edward, get the inspiration from your example." As it happened, it was Cushing who came to Boston in 1913 to establish a full-time professorial service at the Peter Bent Brigham Hospital. Preoccupied by World War I and the subsequent period of readjustment, the MGH did not follow suit until the twenties with the appointment of Edward P. Richardson as John Homans Professor of Surgery and chief of the Third Surgical Service—a temporary arrangement, for this unit was subsequently merged back into the West Surgical Service. Churchill was Richardson's first resident in the modern sense.

On his return to the full-time staff in 1927, Churchill addressed himself principally to the problems of cardiopulmonary physiology and shock. His clinical activities were directed toward the development of thoracic surgery, which was then enjoying satisfactory, but not spectacular, development under Wyman Whittemore. It was at this time that Churchill carried out in collaboration with his medical colleague, P. D. White, the first pericardiectomy for constrictive pericarditis to be done in this country. This pioneering and spectacularly successful effort in the field of cardiac surgery—a demonstration of bringing the physiologic laboratory to the operating room—together with his accomplishments in thoracic surgery (in productive collaboration with Frederick T. Lord and Donald S. King) very early projected him into a position of national leadership. Although many years their junior, he became a close friend and valued colleague of Graham, Alexander, Eloesser, Eggers, and other leaders of this rapidly expanding field.

In the fall of 1928, with Richardson's approval and encouragement, Churchill accepted the challenge of heading a full-time unit at the Boston City Hospital. The hope of creating a surgical counterpart of the Thorndike Laboratory did not succeed. In the following year he turned down an offer to assume directorship of the surgical laboratories at Columbia-Presbyterian and a similar overture from the New York Hospital in favor of an invitation to return to the MGH to reestablish his laboratory and clinical activities on a permanent basis. The premature disability of Richardson in the summer of 1930 profoundly changed the course of events.

The official appointment of Edward Churchill as chief of the West Surgical Service on April 21, 1931, marked the beginning of 30 years of leadership that were to see the integration of a research-oriented full-time staff into a clinically oriented matrix of unusual depth. These years also saw the development of a basic concept of residency training which was to challenge the precepts of Halsted and, in so doing, win nationwide acceptance. Finally, the last ten years of Churchill's regime saw the reconstitution of a surgical staff after four years of disruption by war and the reorientation of that staff in an environment modified by an extensively responsible residency system.

The circumstances of his appointment illustrate the relationship that survives to this day between the hospital and the Harvard Medical School. Fundamentally it is a relationship of great inherent strength; but it can have its awkward moments, and this was one of them. For six months Churchill's appointment as chief of the West Surgical Service was held up by the failure of the Medical School to appoint him John Homans Professor, by recent tradition a concurrent appointment. It must be remembered that at this time there was an open difference of opinion between Harvey Cushing and the then dean, David Edsall; to establish a full-time university department outside the Quadrangle ran counter, perhaps, to Cushing's grand scheme of things. After six months the academic smoke cleared, and the designation of Churchill as Homans Professor then facilitated his appointment as chief of the West Surgical Service.

It is interesting to recreate the situation that Churchill inherited in 1931, particularly with respect to the surgical staff and the groundwork so solidly laid by his predecessor. As Churchill assumed his duties, the General Surgical Services were represented on the one hand by clinical masters such as Daniel Fiske Jones, Richard H. Miller, George W. W. Brewster, Lincoln Davis, Robert Greenough,

Beth Vincent, and Charles Scudder. Most of these men were at one time, or were to be, chiefs of the East Surgical Service. Each had his special forte, and each had his talented clinical assistant waiting in the wings, his star in the ascendant: Arthur Allen, Leland McKittrick, Joe Meigs, Channing Simmons, Ernest Daland, and so on down the list. It was a strong group, all clearly products of a master-apprentice system and, as time was to prove, extraordinarily able clinical innovators.

On the other side of the scale were the full-time surgeons recruited by Richardson. To assign priority is dangerous, especially on hearsay evidence at this late date. James White was the senior among them; already his course in neurosurgery had been charted among the reefs and shoals of the autonomic system. In this endeavor he would work closely with Reginald Smithwick, at this time a clinical assistant of Hugh Williams but shortly to display a clinical virtuosity of extraordinary degree. Next to White was Munroe McIver who in 1930 had departed the Harvard scene to head up the Mary Imogene Bassett at Cooperstown, New York. Recently recruited, but active in the laboratory, was Robert Linton, an individual of uncommon force and positive imagination. The relationship between Linton and Richardson had been a close one—indeed, in the light of Churchill's unpublished papers, perhaps closer than that which had existed between Churchill and Richardson. Linton was to remain on the full-time staff throughout the thirties and then develop an impressive clinical practice on a local, national, and international scale but always centered on the MGH. In many ways his experimental approach varied greatly from that of Churchill, but there always existed an atmosphere of mutual respect. To complete the picture in 1931 was Oliver Cope, then a resident, his clinical and academic promise clearly evident and already enlisted in the Richardson cause. Later, Churchill was to enlist John Stewart and Fiorindo Simeone among his full-time staff, and Ralph Adams in a clinical capacity.

To describe the surgical *dramatis personae* in such an oversimplified fashion runs the risk of diminishing the individuals involved. This, of course, is not the intent, but a brief overview illustrates the tremendous challenge that Richardson had faced and now abruptly transferred to a brilliant "young" man of 36. One cannot overlook the factor of age: To become professor and chief of Service in one's mid-thirties was a real break with MGH tradition, though on the Harvard scene Cushing had acceded to the Moseley Chair at the age of 35.

In 1931 General Surgery included the Department of Anesthesia. This department had suffered the sudden loss of its clinical chief, Freeman Allen. He had no official successor until the appointment in 1933 of Howard Bradshaw, one of Churchill's men, a sound surgical investigator particularly interested in pulmonary physiology. Bradshaw left the MGH in 1936 and was succeeded by Henry K. Beecher, later to become Dorr Professor of Anesthesia. Beecher's subsequent brilliant, at times tempestuous, but tremendously productive career is well known (see Chapter 32). One can cite Beecher as a clear example of Churchill's ability to encourage independence of development not only of the man but also of the department and discipline he came so ably to represent. This relationship between Churchill as chief and the men who were eventually identified as his full-time lieutenants is indeed a complex one.

In 1931 Orthopedics and Urology were already separate specialty services encompassed within the Department of Surgery, and throughout the Churchill years they remained so. Neurosurgery and Gynecology were the only two traditional specialties to split off from the General Surgical Services during his administration. Indeed, Gynecology was not to become a separate service until 1942 with the absorption of the Vincent Memorial Hospital and the appointment of Joe V. Meigs as professor of Gynecology. It is worth noting, however, that while Gynecology became administratively separate, its staff—both permanent and resident—were part of the General Surgical Services. Unwillingness to fragment General Surgery into its component specialties was the Churchill way. For example, before the American Association for Thoracic Surgery in 1941 he warned that other special societies had often become preoccupied with technical proficiency and operative experience which could lead to "an encouragement of myopic regional technical surgery."

During the early Churchill years clinical growth and innovation were encouraged by a "special assignment" system which distributed challenging clinical problems to members of both the part-time and the full-time staff in reasonable proportions. There were also special clinics, notably the vascular clinic and rounds, led by Allen and McKittrick and later Linton and Smithwick.

The first ten years of Churchill's tenure were marked by the establishment of surgical laboratories with a separate-but-equal status with those in the Quadrangle. The full-time staff were all on the West Surgical Service; the East Service was under the forceful leadership of Arthur Allen with his associates—first Claude Welch, then Gordon Donaldson. As the first decade drew to a close, however, it was apparent that instead of the services drawing apart, the East and West, in defiance of Kipling's dictum, did in fact meet on common ground. It would seem that this concert of effort, rather than divisive rivalry, was no accident. Churchill had, in fact, strong views about the importance of encouraging independence of thought and action among junior staff, for he well knew the repressive features that an uncontrolled master-apprenticeship system could contain. He spoke often of "gifted amateurs," a phrase borrowed from Kipling, but at the same time he recognized the professionalism and talents of the Allens, the McKittricks, the Welches, the Taylors, and the Sweets, and he worked effectively in accord with them.

Although certain names stand out among the permanent Churchill contingent—Cope, Stewart, Lyons, Simeone—there were a host of men who came to work with Churchill and his staff as clinical fellows and then went on to academic and clinical posts of national visibility. Among those who stayed on was Edward Benedict, once a surgical house officer, then a pioneer and the "first and last" (EDC's words) endoscopist at the MGH.

Oliver Cope (in 1982 still active and perhaps the most youthful-appearing elder statesman on record) exemplifies Churchill's ability to manage an environment in which individual development could flourish, though in this, as in other fields, skillful integration with the medical service was essential. A surgical resident from 1930 to 1932, Cope was a Moseley Travelling Fellow in 1933 and returned to the staff and the Surgical Laboratories, fourth floor rear of the Bulfinch, in 1934. He worked closely with the Thyroid Clinic, a long-time interest of E. P. Richardson, an activity that was to lead to the parathyroid research and all that stands for in the annals of the MGH surgical world. The achievement was a brilliant synthesis of exacting technical accomplishment and sound biologic understanding of endocrine disease. And it was a superb example of cooperative effort on the part of a strong medical service with its Means, Aub, Albright, and Bauer. Nor, in the clinical excitement, should the participation of the Department of Pathology be passed over. (See page 220 for more on Cope.)

The mention of Cope, who was clearly involved in resident training, leads naturally to a second of Churchill's major accomplishments in the first decade. By 1939 Churchill was ready to propose a new concept of surgical residency training and education which was to introduce a new dimension into university and teaching hospitals. On the surface the change seems straightforward—a matter of geometry, a rectangular structure instead of a pyramid. In a letter to the Office of the Surgeon General in 1948, Churchill explained his rationale: "Our whole program in graduate education is to keep the framework flexible and adapted to the needs and interests of the individual. If technical training dominates these years of a young surgeon's life he will emerge as a pure technician. It is very essential that he be taught to understand the nature of the tools that he is using, and develop a critical judgment in regard to new procedures and new tools, not merely attain proficiency in existing techniques." Reflecting on the revisions he had stimulated, Churchill remarked in 1961, that "the greatest change in this program came between the years 1940 and 1960, and if I were to sum it up . . . I would say, the transition from the classical and ancient master-apprentice training to a more contemporary age-peer group educational effort."

Basic to Churchill's plan was the assumption that one can select a given number of men in their final year of medical school and plan to carry this number through the requisite five years of training in the parent institution or program. It was his belief that such a system not only allowed a more practical and productive use of the teaching facilities of a large hospital but also maintained a far better level of morale and industry than did a pyramidal competitive system. Churchill's proposal went into effect in 1940; the basic concept survived the dislocation attendant upon World War II and remains the basis of the MGH Surgical Residency to this day.

Returning to the clinical accomplishments of the Surgical Services in the pre-war years, many areas can be cited. These were years of explosive expansion of thoracic surgery, particularly with respect to the surgical management of bronchopulmonary suppuration, bronchiectasis, lung abscess, and cancer of the lung. In these areas Churchill was an acknowledged leader, and he attracted a succession of clinical fellows which included Jack Gibbon, Howard Bradshaw, Gus Lindskog, Ronald Belsey, Max Chamberlain, and Ralph Adams.

One of the by-products that always provokes interest is the story of Jack Gibbon and his earliest work with extracorporeal circulation. A young woman was dying of a pulmonary embolus, the victim of progressive right heart failure. Gibbon was part of a final desperate effort to remove the embolus, but the situation was clearly beyond salvage. Recognizing that she might have lived had temporary circulatory support been available, Gibbon worked for a year in the MGH surgical laboratories on the problems of extracorporeal circulation. His wife, Mary Hopkinson, worked closely with him. It seems odd, perhaps, that Churchill with his pioneering and ongoing interest in pericardial disease did not pursue the grail of extracorporeal circulation; indeed the relationship of Churchill to the whole cardiac effort was one of the enigmatic and complex features of this most unusual man.

That Churchill played a leading role in the history of thoracic surgery is evident. His exposure during his Moseley year to Brauer Sauerbruch intensified an interest already apparent in his early work with Drinker and later with Cope, Beecher, and others in the area of pulmonary physiology and its relevance to surgery. He had a basic knowledge and understanding of tuberculosis and pioneered its surgical treatment. He was fortunate, also, in his association with clinicians of the stature of Frederick T. Lord, Donald King, and Helen Pittman who formed the nucleus of the Thoracic Clinic. The position of Richard Sweet in the thoracic surgical assignment is interesting. By the late 1930s his clinical indenture to Daniel Jones ended. Sweet's clinical judgment and masterful technical accomplishments plus a high degree of self-discipline were increasingly channeled into the thoracic field. A long period of collaborative work on the esophagus began at this time, and he became an acknowledged master of esophageal surgery. As the war clouds gathered and Churchill went off to his great adventure, it was Sweet who took on the thoracic assignment with a series of thoracic surgical residents and established himself as a master in this field.

Perhaps one of the most important features of the first Churchill decade was the balance he maintained between his acknowledged leadership in thoracic surgery and his strict insistence on the generalism of surgery. Forward motion on all fronts with basic cooperation of full- and part-time staff was the key—though this should not imply an idyllic, unruffled surgical utopia. Examples are many: The thyroid, parathyroid, and endocrine front was spearheaded by Cope with strong support of the Medical Services; surgical metabolic problems and the liver were the territory of John Stewart; later, surgical infections became the special area of Champ Lyons; the field of vascular surgery and shock became the province of Fiorindo Simeone. All of these areas advanced *pari passu* with the active peripheral vascular clinic—Arthur Allen, Leland McKittrick with his special expertise in the diabetic complications of vascular surgery, Smithwick with his knowledge of the autonomic system, and Linton with his special interest in veins and the lymphatics. Gynecology was infused by the personal dynamism of Joe Meigs and the clinical support of Marshall Bartlett and Langdon Parsons. And all this time the plans for surgical residency matured. It was an exciting era.

Then came the second decade of Churchill's tenure, World War II and its aftermath. Base Hospital No. 6, activated in 1940, drained off a major portion of the surgical staff. (The history of the hospital is amply reported in Faxon's volume.) Churchill was held in reserve, so to speak, not to leave until early in 1943. Before his departure, on November 28, 1942, a civilian disaster of titanic proportions, the Cocoanut Grove fire, put all the emergency planning of the MGH to an acid test. There can be little doubt that this single event—the hospital's Night to Remember—had an enormous influence on the direction that research and development in this hospital would take in the ensuing decades, not only as a burn center but also as a trauma center.

Churchill left in January 1943 to assume a key position as consultant to the Mediterranean theater. Arthur Allen remained as chief of the East Service, Leland McKittrick as acting chief of the West, Oliver Cope in charge of resident and student affairs. With a large proportion of the staff overseas, the elaborate plans of the extended surgical residency had to be drastically modified. A few "unfit" by Army or Navy standards—4Fs—were left as senior residents (your author among them), and the ranks were filled by "nine-month wonders." From a resident's point of view it was a time of tremendous delegation of authority that was to persist and grow in the aftermath of the war, particularly as individuals who had borne responsibilities imposed by the war returned to complete their residency training. Because of the greatly increased intake of resident trainees during the war, beyond the educational and training limits envisioned by prewar planning, an extensive degree of individual career management was inevitable; born of necessity, it persisted during the years of an uneasy peace. Finally the Korean conflict converted a resident program into a complex structure of career planning. Since flexibility was basic to Churchill's concept of a residency, the pattern of development continues today.

In 1948 Arthur Allen, chief of the East, reached retirement age. It was a crucial year for the Surgical Services. By vote of an ad hoc committee of the trustees, the following resolution was passed:

The Trustees reaffirm their belief that the care of the patient is and must remain the primary function of the Massachusetts General Hospital, but that teaching and research are and must always be essential functions of the Staff in promoting the welfare and care of the patient.

The contributions of the part-time unsalaried staff to all three of these functions is of great importance. This group contains many men of great skill and experience. Their interest in and service to the Hospital must be maintained and the development of able men in all grades must be assured through continuing for them participation in Hospital policy.

The Trustees believe that the foregoing can best be achieved under the guidance of Doctor Edward D. Churchill and have accordingly created the position of Chief of the General Surgical Services and have appointed Doctor Churchill as that Chief.

The vote speaks for itself and yet omits a tremendously important personal equation: the natural expectation that Leland McKittrick, heir to the tradition of the East Service and acting chief of the West during the war, would succeed Allen. McKittrick remained as a clinical tower of strength, of incalculable influence on the training of residents, but clearly his center of gravity shifted uptown to the Deaconess Hospital.

The late forties and early fifties saw the memorable presence of Grantley Taylor whose surgical wit was as sharp and therapeutic as his courageously skillful dissections. He worked with Ernest Daland, and the Tumor Clinic flourished. Marshall Bartlett and Claude Welch, both returned from the 6th General, came into their clinical own. After Smithwick left for Boston University in 1946, Linton became the unchallenged—though not undisputed—leader of the Vascular Clinic. There were no specialty services, but increasingly thoracic surgery was identified with Richard Sweet, particularly with Churchill's time so heavily pre-empted by Washington. Even cardiac surgery began to send forth its branches. During the war Sweet had divided a few ductuses. A technical challenge seemed to delight him, and he had, in fact, dealt with a vascular ring at about the same time that Gross first described this at the Children's Hospital. Coarctation of the aorta had fallen to Linton's lot, as had sporadic attempts to deal with tetralogy of Fallot. Sweet collaborated with Edward Bland, successor to Paul Dudley White, to apply the principles of shunt surgery to mitral stenosis, which resulted in the so-called Bland-Sweet operation, an anastomosis between a pulmonary vein and the azygos. This ingenious method of decompressing an engorged lung—incidentally, an operation of great technical challenge—was soon to give way to the direct approach to the valve. In 1948 the Cardiac Catheter Laboratory was organized as a joint venture of cardiologists, surgeons, and radiologists; major credit must go to Gordon Myers for his critical energy and drive. The evolution of cardiac surgery in the late Churchill years is a story in itself and leads us away from our central theme, except that it emphasizes once again Churchill's insistence on the general nature of surgery. The author of this essay was actively engaged in the evolution of cardiac surgery at the MGH in the fifties, the last of the Churchill years. Except for surgery of the pericardium, Churchill did not involve himself in the explosive development of this field. Much of this was undoubtedly caused by the distractions of many other pressing priorities, among them the Hoover Commission and the reorganization of the Department of Defense.

In the late fall of 1953 Churchill had a cerebral vascular episode from which he recovered well, but thereafter he set limits on his direct clinical participation. He remained extremely active, however, in the administration of the department and in the development of younger surgeons.

Following the war and into the early fifties, only Oliver Cope remained of the original full-time staff in a full-time capacity. A new generation was in the resident stage—Raker, McDermott, Waddell, Nardi, Shaw, Russell, Grillo, Burke; later Ronald Malt, Charlie Huggins, John Constable. All were to metamorphose in the later fifties; all were to be involved in the time of succession. Once again a pattern emerged: a residency suited to the individual needs and talents with the necessary allowances for the exigencies of the armed services. The pattern permitted time away in the basic sciences.

A model comes quickly to mind in the person of Francis Moore, West Surgical resident during the war as one of the "unfit." In 1941—with the kind of intellectual imagination and energy that always characterized him—Moore spent a year with Aub and Cohn learning how to work with radioactive bromine, phosphorus, and sodium. In 1942 he returned to the resident staff, served a somewhat abbreviated term as chief resident on the West, and in November 1943, at the invitation of Oliver Cope, moved into the academic side of surgery at the MGH while joining Leland McKittrick in the conduct of a busy clinical practice. In his surgical laboratory he set up the groundwork of body compositional study by isotope dilution. In 1946 he was asked by Churchill to remain with the department as tutor. In many ways Moore epitomized the MGH Surgical Services during the later forties. In 1948, with the tragic and premature death of Elliot Cutler, Moore succeeded to the Moseley Chair as chief of surgery at the Peter Bent Brigham. Clearly, most of this spectacular achievement was Moore himself; how much was Churchill, how much Cope, is something that those of us who watched the passing scene can speculate on with pleasure and without resolution.

In this welter of names and personalities, one name and one person should not be left out: Edward Hamlin, West Surgical resident, 1939, another of the "unfit" who devoted much of his surgical life to a generation of third-year students. Radiating a sort of comfortable wisdom, he lent continuity to the teaching effort of the department without apparent desire to mount the academic ladder. In a sense Hamlin bridged the gap between Richard Miller, who had so wisely and generously given way to Churchill's appointment in 1931, and the development of the academic staff. Hamlin's clinical interests were varied; with Marshall Bartlett he strengthened the ties of the MGH to the Faulkner; he was an active clinical member of the Thyroid Laboratory; and in the days before the emphasis on academic position, he was quite willing to forego the formalities of academic advancement.

Following his temporary disability in late 1953, Churchill involved himself less with clinical matters and more with the internal administration of the Surgical Services and the problems facing the hospital at a time of major social change. An example is the evolution of the Surgical Associates. The groundwork and leadership for this enterprise came from Marshall Bartlett. Churchill—while approving in principle and obviously an important factor in the development—nevertheless avoided direct commitment of the department.

The latter fifties were for Churchill a time of mature reflection. He expended an enormous amount of effort in the publication of *To Work in the Vineyard of Surgery,* about which he wrote, "Indeed, the Warren Reminiscences have afforded an opportunity to look upon the Vineyard in which we have both worked from two vantage points separated by half a century." He chose an unusual mode of presentation: On the one hand is a superb account of J. Collins Warren, both his personal development and his key role in the development of the HMS and the MGH; the material on Warren is accompanied by a voluminous series of footnotes in which Churchill's reflections on surgery become evident—an *apologia pro vita sua.* Close reading of the notes discloses some of the rigorous intellectual discipline of which he was capable.

Most of 1958, the year the *Vineyard* was published, found Churchill on a Rockefeller grant visiting the medical centers of India and participating in the organization of surgical teaching at King George's Medical College in Lucknow. He returned in late 1958 to a most unusual department dinner held in The Great Hall of the Harvard Lampoon. It was a relaxed informal gathering, a prelude to a difficult period in the department which, for want of a better term, we can call the time of succession.

By force of circumstances, Churchill's clinical practice following the war was not a large one. It was my privilege to assist Churchill in the care of his individual patients and to see one side of this complex man that was often obscured by his "intellectual" eminence. His sensitivity to the human needs of his patients was exquisite. He borrowed from Kipling to illuminate this facet of a surgeon's life: "And, meanwhile, their days were filled, as yours are filled, with the piteous procession of men and women begging them, as men and women beg of you daily, for leave to live a little longer, upon whatever terms."

In 1962 Churchill retired from the hospital and the Medical School. At his homes in Belmont and in Vermont he filled the role of Cincinnatus in a most appropriate fashion. The field that he plowed were his thoughts on the treatment of the wounded in battle. His summers were spent in Strafford, Vermont, where for 40 years, whenever time permitted, he had blended into the rural life of the community. One late summer afternoon in 1972 he went for a walk among the hills and did not return.

Bert Dunphy, at that time professor of surgery at the University of California but formerly a key figure with Cutler at the Brigham and then at Boston City Hospital, has summarized Churchill perceptively: "His writings will continue to have a major impact on American surgery if only we can find a way to encourage the future generation to learn from the past."

The closing lines of Churchill's Presidential Address to the American Surgical Association in 1947 suggest the measure of the man: "In times of change there is need for wisdom both in the external social order and within the profession. Spokesmen who loudly proclaim measures based on self interest will not be tolerated. A hold-fast in Science is essential, but this represents only a part of the strength of Surgery. By maintaining the ancient bond with humanity itself through Charity—the desire to relieve suffering for its own sake—Surgery need not fear change if civilization itself survives."

22. Eminent Surgeons

Arthur W. Allen

CLAUDE E. WELCH

Arthur Wilbur Allen was born in Kentucky in 1887, attended public schools in his hometown of Somerset, and later graduated from Georgetown University. The years in Kentucky were enormously important in that there he acquired those habits of living and thinking that directed and colored his future performance and growth. Christian morals were inculcated; he developed a magnificent physique and a love of the outdoors and of people. He lived in an environment of gracious, courteous relations to others, one that emphasized independence of spirit and dignity of the individual. He also acquired a nickname, Jimmie, from his father's name; and, more importantly, he found a wife, a boyhood sweetheart, Vida Barthenia Weddle, whom he married in 1913. So that when he left Kentucky he took much of it that was good and attractive with him.

Dr. Allen graduated from the Johns Hopkins Medical School in 1913, having been a bookseller and a carrier of trays to pay some part of the tuition. During his last school vacation he toured Eastern cities, looking over their hospitals. He decided rightly or wrongly that the patients in Boston hospitals were treated by the staff with more human interest than in some other areas, and therefore he decided to apply here for graduate education in surgery. Happily for him and for the hospital, he secured an internship at the MGH.

At the time Dr. Allen began his surgical career, surgery was still dominated by the mechanistic viewpoint: Surgery was learned largely by the apprentice system; the operation was all important; the state of the patient was accepted as an uncontrollable but frequently unfortunate factor. The experience of surgeons in World War I demonstrated the fallacy of this view and also showed the importance of a broad, planned graduate education, the value of an experimental approach to problems; the role of a teacher of surgery changed from that of a prima donna playing to an anonymous supporting cast to that of a man eagerly and humbly searching for truth while acting as captain of a team, every member of which played an important and honorable part in its performance. Arthur Allen entered surgery at a time when he could have stayed with the old or moved with the new. He became one of the pioneers in the development of a new concept of surgery and its teaching. However, he brought to the new that which was good in the old, namely a devotion to his patients, each of whom was to him a human being with peculiar reactions that he stored in his memory. This added an element, sometimes uncanny, to his diagnostic and prognostic skills and, naturally, made him adored by his patients.

Dr. Allen's scientific interests and contributions were many, ranging from all aspects of trauma to all organs and lesions in the abdomen, to peripheral vascular disease, to preoperative preparation, to postoperative care and complications. He shed clear and logical light on every problem he discussed. His last work, a book entitled *Operative Surgery in the Abdomen,* published after his death, maintained his customary standards of excellence.

Dr. Allen was a lecturer in surgery at the Harvard Medical School from 1936 to 1948, but his most important and effective teaching occurred at the graduate level while serving on the staff of the MGH. He rose through the hospital's grades and served as chief of the East Surgical Service from 1936 to 1948. I worked with him from 1937 to 1942—after serving as chief resident on the East Surgical Service in 1937—and have a rich stock of memories from those years. There was no period in my life in which I learned more or which molded my life more firmly. It represented work every day and every night except for a two-week vacation during the summer, but it was exciting and thrilling and made very easy by the fact that one knew that the chief subjected himself to the same stern discipline.

And, indeed, Dr. Allen was the chief. He was not only the chief of the East Surgical Service for over a decade, but wherever he was found his dominance was easy to comprehend. His extremely quick response, his intimate knowledge of all the surgical literature, and his rapid intuitive analysis of a person's character and ability were hard to match. In many respects he was the personification of the Old Testament Jehovah. His underlings viewed him with awe, respect, admiration, and—to a certain extent—fear. To his equals he was also a jealous god: Anyone who attempted to take away one of his patients incurred his everlasting wrath.

Dr. Allen was first and foremost concerned with patient care. He often said that the surgeon who did not wake up at 2 A.M. and worry for an hour about his patients did not deserve to be a surgeon. He thought about them day and night. Once when he returned from one of his operations in an outlying hospital with the local surgeon, he sat down to recount the whole story of the difficult procedure to me. As he progressed in the tale, it became apparent that he had made a technical error in the operation. He immediately dashed out of his seat, went back to the operating room, had the patient anesthetized again, and repaired the error. Thereafter the patient made an uneventful convalescence.

Every morning after I had finished rounds, he arrived at 8:30 for the first operation. His opening sentence always was "What is the BN?" BN, of course, stood for bad news, and it was possible to recount bad news in great detail at that time. In fact, in those days the major abdominal operations were followed by serious complications in nearly 30 percent of the cases and a postoperative mortality of approximately 10 percent. Many of the problems were due to anesthesia but, of course, antibiotics, fluids, and electrolytes and blood have made a tremendous difference.

There were operations essentially every morning. However, perhaps once in six weeks there would be a momentary hiatus. On those days Dr. Allen would have more time to spend with patients. As a general rule rounds were so hurried that one patient once complained that all the people on the floor would catch pneumonia from the speed with which Dr. Allen and his entourage swept through the room, stirring the air currents. But on those rare days when he had additional time, he would spend an hour and a half or two hours on rounds talking with the patients.

He reveled in the niceties of operative procedures. Every step was considered very carefully in advance, and then all was supposed to go in exact routine just as a symphony orchestra would replay its favorite composition. Dr. Allen's exacting approach led to some of the finest technical accomplishments ever seen in the MGH—and in those days technical accomplishments were absolutely essential to avoid the ills inflicted by our lack of knowledge in many other areas.

He was a firm believer that the papers he wrote should be based upon actual experience in clinical fields. If operating happened to be a little slack, he gathered his material together and prepared another paper. His most important writings dealt with the subject of gastric surgery or peripheral vascular surgery. In addition he wrote long review articles on developments in abdominal surgery for the *New England Journal of Medicine;* he kept his ear so close to the ground as far as surgery was concerned that he could compose these articles over the weekend.

Dr. Allen served as a trustee of the MGH from 1953 to 1958. He also served on the General Executive Committee of the hospital when it was a small select group that conducted its business rapidly and effectively. He would probably have very little sympathy with the large committee that now exists. As a matter of fact, he was very jealous of any diminution in his authority. There was the usual competition between him and the other members of the staff in an era when it seemed more important to gain ascendancy in one's own hospital than to promote a unified spirit.

Later in his life Dr. Allen became greatly involved with important professional organizations. As president and as chairman of the Board of Regents of the American College of Surgeons, he performed very important services. In the mid-forties he became president of the Massachusetts Medical Society; he put all his energies into this assignment and impressed on his assistants the necessity of involvement in extrahospital affairs. As president of the Boston Medical Library for five years, he almost singlehandedly raised the great sum of money which led to the amalgamation of the Boston Medical Library with the Countway Library of the Harvard Medical School.

For the last 17 years of his life he remained under the shadow of a fatal disease. A very private operation was performed by Leland McKittrick, and for month after month he required radiation therapy, that being the only treatment then available for lymphoma. He did remarkably well, but in the periods of his incapacity his patients were operated upon by his assistants; then he returned to take up his usual difficult schedule when he felt better. He never spared himself. He frequently asked me to tell him when he was becoming incompetent so he would know when to stop operating. I never had to warn him because he was always superb in the operating room.

An extremely warm person, Dr. Allen made deep friendships and loved conviviality. He always dressed exquisitely in a double-breasted suit. (His wife, Vida, always disliked the portrait that now hangs in the operating suite because it portrays him with a white shirt and an open single-breasted coat, a result of the artist's desire to emphasize Allen's face rather than his clothing.) He was also a very generous person. When I returned from World War II in very straitened circumstances—since the monthly salary of some $250 was barely enough to support a family—he put a check for $1,000 on my desk. I am sure that he approved of the actions of the young surgeons during that war and wished that he might have contributed more than the work he was able to provide by staying in Boston.

Dr. Allen left a number of assistants: Henry Faxon, Richard Wallace, Gordon Donaldson, Grant Rodkey, Glenn Behringer, Philip Giddings, James Shannon, and myself. All of them have been imbued with one or more qualities of his many faceted character and have tried in some way to emulate what he did so well.

He died at the Phillips House on March 18, 1958.

> With material extracted from an obituary written by the late *Frederick A. Coller*

Leland S. McKittrick

Leland Sterling McKittrick was born in 1893 in Thorp, Wisconsin, as the first of six children of a physician with a large and busy rural practice. His father died at age 44, leaving Leland, at age 20, the patriarch of the family and sharing the responsibilities with his mother. These can be regarded as simple facts or can be interpreted as having significant bearing on his career and on his moral and ethical standards. His admiration for his father undoubtedly led to the emergence of one of his own particular characteristics—dedicated, intensive, and thoughtful concern for the welfare of his patients. In addition, one could reasonably presume that his assumption of early responsibility within the family led to the compassion and firmness that he directed toward the care of his patients and was exemplified by his frequently repeated comment that "skill and discipline as well as kindness are required to cure disease and alleviate suffering."

McKittrick's early education was at the University of Wisconsin from which he graduated in 1915; he then entered the Harvard Medical School. The onset of World War I led to an acceleration of the curriculum, and McKittrick was awarded his M.D. degree in February of 1918. He enlisted in the Medical Reserve Corps, which ultimately led to six months of medical internship at the University of Minnesota before he returned to the MGH as a house pupil in 1919.

Formal hospital training was short in that era, and surgeons were expected to develop their skills and experience during a long apprenticeship to a master surgeon. Thus, after 18 months of resident training, he became associated with Daniel Fiske Jones, one of the leading surgeons of that era and a man who had enormous impact on the development of McKittrick's professional skills. It was through Jones that he developed his initial associations both at the MGH where his first appointment was surgeon to outpatients and at the New England Deaconess Hospital where Jones was an active senior surgeon.

At the MGH McKittrick advanced steadily in the department of surgery, both in terms of appointment and, perhaps more important, in the enormous respect that he engendered among his colleagues and the young surgeons in training. All those who were at the hospital during his decades of service remember him as a person of great integrity, honesty, and judgment who furnished an outstanding example of a superb clinical surgeon. His aphorisms urging a hesitant young surgeon to "fish, cut bait or go ashore" or his expression of finality—"it is just as certain as God made little green apples"—served as powerful stimuli when associated with the analysis and management of problems of a disease. During World War II he and a few remaining senior surgeons held the hospital together in the absence of the large numbers of staff who had entered the armed services; these were years of intense work, endless hours of administration and supervision, and an immense sense of responsibility that patient care should not suffer because of attrition of the staff. After the war he served briefly as chief of the West Surgical Service before East and West were amalgamated into one department under Churchill. As Scannell remarked in the foregoing pages, that decision to merge the two services perhaps deprived McKittrick of the "natural expectation" that he would become chief of the East Service.

McKittrick's surgical career covered a wide scope. Introduced to Joslin and Root by Jones, he became interested in the diabetic patient. By close medical and surgical teamwork, and with the introduction of insulin, diabetic patients for the first time were brought through all types of surgery safely. He also became concerned with diabetic foot problems, identified the difference between those brought about by ischemia and those in which neuropathy was the cause of the lesion, and tailored the operative approach appropriately. Whereas formerly most patients with ulcers or infections required above-knee amputations, soon many of them needed only lesser amputations in the foot or lower leg. McKittrick introduced the transmetatarsal amputation to diabetic problems, a procedure that has saved thousands of legs. In one paper reporting a 19 percent mortality for major amputations, he forecast a drop to 5 percent once some agent to control infection became available. The drop is exactly what occurred in the 1940s. McKittrick developed his expertise in surgical problems of the diabetic patient largely at the Deaconess Hospital, where he was chief of staff from 1932 to 1953 of the Palmer Memorial Division. He and Howard R. Root coauthored a classic volume, *Diabetic Surgery*, which gained him an early reputation and brought him a great many patients through the Joslin Clinic at the Deaconess. McKittrick's MGH patients were more apt to be varied in scope. And, of course, residency training at the MGH attracted him immensely.

Another of McKittrick's interests was gastric surgery for ulcer disease. Distressed by the occasional death from postoperative duodenal leakage, he devised the two-stage gastrectomy to be used when the duodenum was highly inflamed and deformed. The procedure saved a number of lives until it became obsolete when vagotomy was discovered. McKittrick also made important contributions to colon surgery. Chester Jones enlisted his help in caring for ulcerative colitis patients. For some years McKittrick carried out this assignment at the MGH and influenced the change from ileostomy alone for the very ill patient to the more aggressive and effective ileostomy plus colectomy. He was also concerned with cancer of the colon and pushed for wider resections. Another innovation, which he refused to publish because, as he said, everyone knew of it, was the use of the end-to-side low rectal anastomosis. By using this technique anastomotic leaks are avoided, and the need for temporary colostomy is obviated. His operative techniques were superb and his complication rate incredibly low.

Francis D. Moore remembered one peculiarity of McKittrick's operating room behavior: "During an operation, about 10 or 10:30 in the morning, the head nurse would come into the operating room and say, 'Dr. McKittrick, will it be convenient for you to see Mrs. McGillicuddy at 3:30 P.M.?' He would then give either a positive or negative answer. On first acquaintance one wondered why he was asked almost daily about seeing one specific patient in the afternoon when it was common knowledge that he saw lots of patients almost every afternoon. Gradually it became clear that this was the coding system—used in a sort of conspiracy between his office nurse and the operating room head nurse—to signal whether or not he would play a squash game at that particular time."

McKittrick had a strong impact on students and on young surgeons in training. His approach was characteristic of his own intense desire for perfection in the analysis and management of clinical problems. Rarely did a young man or woman receive direct praise, but on the other hand justifiable censure was always delivered in a kindly and dispassionate way which proved to be extraordinarily effective in the shaping of the careers and attitudes of the young. These qualities and years of devotion to teaching were reflected in his appointment as clinical professor of surgery at the Harvard Medical School.

McKittrick's characteristics of articulate leadership in local and professional societies led to his election as president of the Boston Surgical Society, the New England Surgical Society, and ultimately the American Surgical Association, one of the highest honors in peer recognition that can come to a surgeon in the United States.

He had a home in New Hampshire and loved to go deer hunting there. He rowed on the Charles River in the spring and fall. He had a rule when he got home at night that no one was to mention a telephone call or a patient call for a half an hour unless there was an extreme emergency. From all these safeguards to maintain an even humanistic equilibrium, one might think of him as one of those surgeons who try to insulate themselves from patients and families. But that was not the case. McKittrick never shirked the extra trip; he never wanted to be shielded from bad news. He just knew in his soul that he had to arrange his life in a way that would permit a high level of work and accomplishment while still preserving his normal physical fitness and his sense of well-being, vigor, and humor.

McKittrick had determined that he would retire in his late sixties, not because he wished to but to protect his patients. However, upon reaching that age he still felt capable of continuing his high standard of surgery, so with typical pragmatic objectivity he set three criteria for himself: physical fitness—when he could no longer enjoy a good game of squash; dexterity—every week he tested his ability to thread needles; and most importantly, complications—acknowledging that with his experience he should have fewer complications than the younger staff, he routinely attended rounds to check the results. Failure to meet any one of these criteria would indicate retirement. After several productive years, still active at squash, threading needles skillfully, and with excellent operative results, he finally retired at age 78. Several years later, on December 30, 1978, a brilliant career ended.

Adapted from an obituary by *Frank C. Wheelock, Jr.,* and a Memorial Minute, *Harvard University Gazette,* December 14, 1979, with the assistance of *Francis D. Moore.*

Robert Ritchie Linton

R. CLEMENT DARLING

Robert R. Linton, one of America's pioneers in vascular surgery, died quietly after two years of declining health, at the age of 79 years, on July 21, 1979. In the words of a friend, "Bob knew when to die, and not a minute sooner."

Linton was born in 1900 in Grangemouth, Scotland. His father, a doctor who became an invalid after service in the Boer War, took Robert as a toddler with his older brother, James, to begin a new life in the Puget Sound area of Washington, leaving behind his wife who was unwilling to abandon her own family for the challenges of the Northwest. Growing up in Burton on Vashon Island, Bob soon acquired a love of sailing. He was to find relaxation and escape from the cares of a busy practice during his later professional years by sailing in Penobscot Bay.

Linton went to the University of Washington, was elected to Sigma Xi for his research, and was graduated summa cum laude in 1921. His medical education was at Harvard, where he was elected to Alpha Omega Alpha. In 1925 he began an internship in medicine at Johns Hopkins Hospital, where he met Emma Bueermann, daughter of a German-born Baptist minister. At this time Linton was an athletic young man with a full head of brown, curly hair. In 1926 he moved to Boston to begin his surgical residency at the MGH. Emma followed, and they were married in 1928. By this time Linton had developed total alopecia. Later he was to joke that without girls chasing him because of his hair, he could devote himself to his work, and this he did exceptionally well.

Linton entered his chief residency with high hopes and the promise of a partnership with the then chief, E. P. Richardson. However, three months before Linton finished his residency, Richardson, only 49 years of age, had a devastating stroke, and Linton was left on his own. The new chief, Edward Churchill, could offer little more than a place on the staff.

Initially, Linton's major interest was in gastrointestinal and biliary tract surgery. He greatly enjoyed pediatric surgery and continued in this field until a formal unit was established in 1960; it is of note that Linton performed the first "blue baby" operation at the MGH. In the thirties he became interested in vascular surgery which was then in its infancy. He developed strict criteria for treatment of varicose veins. His concern with postphlebitic problems led to his developing the "Linton Flap" operation. The description of him by friends and colleagues as "innovative, imaginative, boldly confident, indefatigable, and perfectionist" truly characterizes his surgical performance throughout his life. To him there was only one way, "the right way," as he often declared at conferences in the Bigelow Amphitheater. In the late thirties Linton would end a busy day by spending hours in the animal laboratory improving and testing surgical techniques. Emma recalls spending weekends in a canoe, Bob at the paddle and Emma translating the latest articles in the German literature.

Linton loved sports and took particular pleasure in skiing but had to stop late in life when he developed osteoporosis as a result of steroid therapy for asthma. Another high spot in his recreational life was the time he spent on Isle au Haut, an island off the Maine coast in Penobscot Bay. He had first spent a few months there in 1928 as a physician to a vacation colony. Each year he and Emma and, in time, their four daughters would summer at Point Lookout. In the words of Daniel Ellis, a colleague at the MGH and neighbor on Isle au Haut, Linton "took every opportunity he could to get down to Isle au Haut, which he considered a haven where he could get away from the rigors of a demanding practice and . . . be with his family. . . . Bob was at no time happier than at the helm of his sailboat." The *Sally B,* a gaff-rigged sloop built in the early years of the century, was rebuilt in 1954 and renamed the *Antiquary.* It was certainly the fastest sloop on the island. Ellis recalls parties in the Linton cottage where Bob, as host, "frequently clad in gay, if not outlandish attire supplied by his daughters, exuded warm hospitality and stimulating conversation." Yet Linton was generally a modest and private person at home.

In the developing years of vascular surgery following World War II, Linton quickly achieved a position of leadership. He provided a succession of innovative technical improvements of old procedures, such as wiring of arterial aneurysms. He designed the Linton tourniquet clamp. His early interest in portal hypertension was in the control of variceal bleeding. He developed the Linton balloon for tamponade and championed the splenorenal shunt. He was first in America to popularize the reversed saphenous vein femoral popliteal bypass. With his meticulous technique, he achieved enviable success.

Ellis provides a view of Linton in relation to his patients, to whom he was devoted: "Patients were initially awed, sometimes frightened by his direct no-nonsense approach. 'Lose forty pounds or don't come back to see me; if you don't care about your life, I have to care about mine.' (This was his observation of the hazard of obesity in any patient facing surgery.) But subsequently, his confidence was transferred to these patients who often faced limb-threatening, if not life-threatening, disease and surgery. They became devoted to him. Though a deacon of his church, he did not find it easy to sit through a Sunday service. He preferred to spend a leisurely Sunday morning making rounds on his patients because Sunday mornings were often lonely times for them."

During his life he trained many young surgeons who quickly appreciated his demanding standards. Richard Warren remembers: "His surgical skill and his emphasis on meticulous after-care produced many successes that others could not achieve. When reconstructive techniques became available, the slick operator's wisdom discerned wherein the slickness of the future would lie: meticulousness—not speed, but consummate attention to detail. The man who used to do a lumbar sympathectomy on a patient with intermittent claudication in 20 minutes now took four to six hours to do a femoral popliteal vein graft on the same person. . . . He was wonderful to work for. He never got impatient or critical, but he never failed to emphasize the firm position he was taking on certain particular points of action or technique that he believed in."

In 1973 Linton produced his monumental *Atlas of Vascular Surgery* containing 220 plates, most of them having at least three drawings. The volume has now been published in Japanese and Spanish editions. His surgical skill, as reflected in the *Atlas,* was widely recognized as shown by his many honors. He was, as might be expected, a member of the leading medical societies: American College of Surgeons, Pan-Pacific Surgical Society, American Medical Association, Society for Vascular Surgery, and the International Cardiovascular Society. He valued highly his membership in the New England Surgical Society and took great pride in helping found the New England Society for Vascular Surgery in 1973, when he served as its first president. He also was president of the Society for Vascular Surgery in 1955 and of the Boston Surgical Society in 1960. His honorary memberships in foreign societies were numerous. He treasured his membership in the Barber Surgeons of Berlin. His continued vigor and love of work made retirement unthinkable.

Note from Linton's log: "Operation: December 8 and 9, 1970. Mr. Frank Brown—resection of thoracoabdominal aneurysm from left subclavian artery to both groins with grafts to all visceral vessels; 13 anastomoses, gastrostomy—the record documents *seven* different scrub nurses, *five* different anesthetists, *three* different residents, one of whom developed phlebitis during the case, and one Dr. Linton who carried on for 23 straight hours. Patient did well and subsequently presented at the Grand Rounds as noted by Earle Wilkins, 'At the conclusion of the presentation and the ensuing discussion, something happened which was unique and unprecedented, at least in my recollection. The audience, including the usually reserved and chary surgeons present, arose and applauded. Bob Linton was 70 years old.' "

Fate dealt the Lintons a heavy blow in September 1973: On the way home from Isle au Haut, they had a serious automobile accident. Linton suffered a severe concussion and required an emergency splenectomy; after transfer to the MGH he spent many weeks in the intensive care unit. Emma suffered fractures and was home long before her husband. He was never to regain his old vitality; he assisted at operations occasionally and consulted but gradually retired. In 1978 the Lintons celebrated their fiftieth wedding anniversary, surrounded by friends and many family members.

All who knew Bob Linton mourned his passing but felt his continued presence whenever vascular surgery was debated. In 1980 the New England Society for Vascular Surgery was presented a gavel made from an oar used by Linton on his dinghy—a most appropriate memorial to this great man. (See also page 250.)

Richard H. Sweet

EARLE W. WILKINS, JR.

The name of Richard Harwood Sweet is recalled daily by all those at the MGH who visit the Sweet Room on Gray 3A, given and decorated by his family, his patients, and his friends. Many MGH surgical residents, particularly the privileged 16 who have served to date in the cardiothoracic training program, remember him for his legacy of esophageal surgery. The esophageal anastomotic technique that he perfected and preached from the early 1940s resulted in an extraordinarily low incidence of leakage and stands as a beacon for all the world to gaze on with genuine awe. It is said that at least one of his disciples never had a leaking esophagogastric anastomosis; in the more than ten years that I was privileged to assist Sweet, he had just one.

Thoracic surgery at the MGH was pioneered by E. D. Churchill and advanced, perfected, and standardized by R. H. Sweet. A graduate of Columbia University and the Harvard Medical School in 1926, he matured through two years on the East Surgical Service and his early work with Daniel Fiske Jones, the preeminent Boston surgeon of his day. Attraction to the thorax developed early and flowered in the years of World War II when he formed the first, though short-lived, thoracic surgical service at the MGH. He braved the largely uncharted regions of the chest with a knowledge of anatomy and a masterful skill of the hand that gained him reputation as the premier thoracic craftsman of his day. He always believed that thoracic surgery must be grounded on skills acquired as a general surgeon. Paraphrasing Lord Nelson, he used to say: "The battle of thoracic surgery is won on the playing fields of the pelvis." Many techniques in thoracic surgery were introduced in his room in the Baker Surgical Operating Suite. He carried out the first American esophagectomy with supra-aortic anastomosis in that room. It is not well known that he did the first splenorenal shunt at the MGH. He vied with Robert Gross from the Boston Children's Hospital for the distinction of having divided the first tracheoesophageal vascular ring. He introduced, with Edward Bland, the azygos vein–pulmonary artery shunt for patients incapacitated by the cardiac failure of mitral stenosis. All his remarkable surgical procedures are carefully described in his then pioneering textbook, *Thoracic Surgery* (W. B. Saunders Co., Philadelphia, 1950). The techniques of this self-made thoracic surgeon, delineated therein, are still up-to-date in the 1980s.

History seldom records the vignettes or word-pictures that characterize a preeminent figure. Two come to mind for Richard Sweet: One is his calm demeanor, despite the troubled pathology deep in the thorax before him, while eight South American visiting surgeons teeter precariously on the makeshift observation stand behind him in Baker Operating Room 4; the other is a completely reassuring manner at the bedside of a patient—perennial red tie suggesting cardinalesque dignity, coat parted to show the AOA key on his gold vest-pocket watch chain, the figure in the bed listening intently and unquestioningly.

Sweet retired at age 60, tragically suffered a myocardial infarction three months later, and died January 11, 1962, not yet 61 years of age. Advances in his own field of thoracic surgery, already developmental at the time, might well have prolonged his life had he incurred his MI a few years later. Churchill, his chief, in his retelling of a Kipling Hindu legend at Sweet's annual meeting of the American Association for Thoracic Surgery (he was its president at the time of his death) concluded: "I have the honor today of speaking before you, who are Masters in your craft. This brief pause in your search honors the name of one whom you chose as your president, by no means the least in your long line of seekers who have followed the quest Brahm set them—Richard H. Sweet, a Master among Masters." (See also page 247 on thoracic surgery.)

Oliver Cope

During the summer of 1981 the *Boston Globe* ran a feature on the second page— "another in a series of profiles of realistic optimists"—that began, "Dr. Oliver Cope has all the qualifications for a Grand Old Man of Medicine. He has had a distinguished career as a professor at the Harvard Medical School and a surgeon at the Massachusetts General Hospital." This extraordinarily talented surgeon is a man of imagination and humanist convictions in the tradition of the late Richard Cabot; and, like Cabot, Cope has left his indelible mark on the MGH.

Oliver Cope was born to a Quaker family in Germantown, Pennsylvania, in

1902. He learned French and German at the tender age when the learning of languages comes most easily; he started studying the piano at six, and the violin at seven. Somewhat later he went to Harvard College where he majored in chemistry. Cope's extracurricular activities as an undergraduate suggest the broad range of his youthful imagination: He sang in the glee club, was president of the liberal club, and was among the leaders of the campaign that ended the quota system for admitting Jews to Harvard. Neither maturity nor medicine forced his mind into narrow channels.

Following a brief and unsatisfactory career as a foreign correspondent, Cope entered the Harvard Medical School. As a fourth year student, in the spring of 1928, he saw a sight he would never forget: "I watched the handling in the MGH Emergency Ward of some 30 casualties burned in the Beacon Oil disaster in Everett. Staff, house officers, and surgical students were down in the EW, stripping the burns of the dead epidermis and squirting the wounds, soaking the patients in tannic acid. As the tannic acid was being applied, the patients were dying for want of attention to the developing dehydration. It was evident then that the priorities were off balance."

Cope became a house officer on the West Surgical Service in 1930. He arrived at the hospital during the period when Aub, Bauer, and Albright were at work on their studies of the parathyroids and had already shown that overactivity of these glands was responsible for certain bone diseases. "The direction that surgical treatment should take was correctly visualized by Dr. Churchill before he or I undertook an operation," Cope recalled, "and the development of the technique and the repetition of the special circumstances of the refinements became my task.

"The first step in preparation for parathyroid surgery was the development of the ability to identify parathyroid tissue grossly. At the time the parathyroid dissections were undertaken in 1931, the pathologists, Mallory, Bradley, Castleman, were no more sure of a parathyroid than I when grossly exposed. They counted on a microscope section for secure identification." Cope did more than 30 dissections that year. Castleman long carried vivid memories of Cope's presence in the morgue, baring tissues and asking for verification from the pathologists. Having learned what the parathyroid glands looked like, he next sought to determine their usual distribution and found them to be widely located from high in the neck into the anterior mediastinum. After a Moseley Travelling Fellowship in 1933–1934, during which he spent three months with Ludwig Pick in Berlin and nine months in Sir Henry Dale's laboratory in London, Cope returned to the MGH to resume his exploration of the endocrine glands, turning his attention from the parathyroid to the adrenal cortex and subsequently to the thymus and thyroid.

Around 1940 Cope joined Bradford Cannon, Francis D. Moore, and F. W. Rhinelander in studies of the physiology and treatment of burns—the spectacle of his student days having aroused a lasting concern for burn victims. They devised a treatment regimen of bland ointments, carefully protecting the blebs so that they would not rupture; the old tannic acids, dyes, and other substances were discarded following Cannon's and Cope's studies of their effects upon healing. Many of the group's findings were applied at the time of the Cocoanut Grove disaster, and, of course, much was learned about the inadequacies of burn treatment from that event. During the late forties Cope drew on the experiences of Churchill and Henry Beecher in military medicine to study the surgical excision of full-thickness burns, a practice that was demonstrated to reduce the incidence of infection and accelerate the healing of deep wounds. When the Shrine of North America was inspecting sites for a children's burns institute, their representatives were naturally attracted by the reputation of the MGH for research in this field, and it was Cope's enthusiasm, vision, and obstinacy that really won their confidence. He fought the project through to completion, overcoming the many administrative obstacles strewn in its path. (See page 298.)

This abbreviated account of Cope's work on the endocrine glands and burns falls very far short of a complete description of his contributions to surgery. As Beecher and Altschule commented in their history of the Harvard Medical School, "Oliver Cope focused a great deal of skilled attention on the education and graduate training of the surgeon. . . . It is clear that Cope is simply another one of those men of distinction who, like Edward Churchill, are truly biologists in surgical clothing." Named an associate professor of Surgery at the Medical School in 1948 and full professor in 1963, Cope evaluated advances in medicine and surgery and adopted the view—hardly fashionable among surgeons in the fifties—that "the teaching of surgical technique has less and less, indeed virtually no, place in the young doctor's education. . . . What is important for the surgeon to teach is his knowledge of the biology and pathology of the disease with which he comes in contact. In this sense he is doing the same thing as his medical counterpart."

Cope was one of the rare MGH surgeons (or physicians, for that matter) to attend seriously and respectfully to the work of his colleagues in psychiatry; he even spent three-and-a-half years in analysis under psychiatrist Grete Bibring, a Harvard professor. Although he claims to have been "unanalyzable," he developed a great appreciation for the contributions of psychiatry to medical care and became a student of the social and psychologic aspects of medicine. "It happens that most clinical teachers of medicine and surgery emphasize the quantitative, physiologic and clinical aspects of medicine," he once noted. "It is relatively easy to be sure about the metabolic aspects of thyroid disease or diabetes or the changes in the gastric content as a result of the vagus nerve activity. It is much more difficult to grapple with the emotional being of the patient or look into and identify those social aspects of the patient's life which may be leading to trouble. . . . Encouraged and sometimes needled a bit by such people as Stanley Cobb, these deficiencies in the education of clinical medicine have led me to try to pick up the pieces, to fill in the gaps. . . . In 1966 I co-sponsored and co-chaired the First Swampscott Conference on Behavioral Science in Medicine. This resulted in a monograph written by myself, *Man, Mind and Medicine*, published in 1968. Perhaps when all is considered, this monograph is the most important contribution I have been able to make."

Cope has always been willing to explore and, in the presence of persuasive evidence, to dissent from medical conventions. The refusal of a female patient to have her breast removed in 1956 led him to an examination of the results of treatments for breast cancer; his findings, which he published in a book in 1977, challenged the standard practices of his peers. Citing data from 131 breast cancer patients, Cope argued that the survival rate after limited surgery, radiation, and chemotherapy compared favorably with that for patients who had undergone mastectomies and, therefore, counseled against the removal of the breast except in advanced cases. "The reaction varied from frosty to furious," reported the *Boston Globe*, "and Cope and a colleague were even called before the ethics com-, mittee of the Massachusetts Medical Society to explain why they were not doing mastectomies." Though more recent studies lend support to Cope's position, the disagreements within the medical profession have not completely subsided.

An upstanding MGH citizen, Cope was twice acting chief of Surgery—between Churchill and Russell and, after the latter's resignation, between him and Austen. Cope stopped performing surgery in 1971, but at this writing ten years later he still sees patients and pursues further research comparing the mortality of women who have undergone mastectomies and those who have chosen an alternative, less deforming path of limited surgery, radiation, and chemotherapy. And he still plays what he refers to with characteristic simplicity as "my fiddle" nearly every day.

23. General Surgical Services, 1962–1968: The Russell Years

PAUL S. RUSSELL

At the time of Edward Churchill's retirement in June of 1962, the General Surgical Services were responsible for the care of about 80 patients situated on two floors of the White Building in the two "ward" or teaching services, East and West. Although the number of beds on the teaching services had been cut approximately in half in the early fifties, the number of operations performed each year on each service had remained nearly the same because of more rapid turnover of patients and correspondingly shorter hospital stays. The responsibility of the chief of the General Surgical Services for activities performed in the private sectors of the hospital was imperfectly defined, although it had been gradually increasing for several decades. Centralization of the surgical staff in offices within the hospital grounds in the Warren Building had progressed rapidly, although there were still several staff members who maintained offices elsewhere. General surgery was deemed to include thoracic, vascular, plastic, trauma, and gastrointestinal surgery as well as most surgical procedures for tumors of various kinds, including endocrinopathies. Open heart surgery was still in its earliest stages; transplantation had not begun.

Oliver Cope, Claude E. Welch, Marshall K. Bartlett, and Robert R. Linton were among the leaders in the department. None held a rank in the Medical School above associate professor. This pertained also to the chiefs of the surgical specialty services that fell within the Harvard Department of Surgery at the MGH, namely Urology and Neurosurgery, headed by Associate Professors Wyland Leadbetter and William Sweet, respectively. Anesthesiology also was included in Harvard's Department of Surgery at the hospital. This department was under the leadership of Henry K. Beecher, Surgery's only full professor at that time in the Medical School.

There was much discussion regarding the advisability of separating the various surgical subdisciplines into separate administrative units. This had been resisted in previous years, and considerable opinion against it remained, stemming from the feeling that further fragmentation of surgery might have deleterious consequences upon broadly based teaching of young surgeons in the important principles common to all areas of surgery. It was also feared that any interference with free communication among surgeons could retard progress. Countervailing arguments were also strong: These emphasized the possible progress that could result from further concentration upon special areas of surgery by dedicated individuals of the staff and the important dividends that can come to patients when they are treated and nursed in a specified area of the hospital.

These, then, were some of the issues confronting Paul S. Russell, Churchill's successor as chief of the MGH General Surgical Services. Russell, a 1947 graduate of the University of Chicago Medical School, had received his clinical training at the MGH; a research fellowship permitted him to study in London with

Sir Peter Medawar in 1954–1955. He returned to the hospital, completed his surgical residency in 1956, and was welcomed to the staff. He began studying problems in transplantation biology. Within a few years he accepted an invitation to pursue his work at Columbia University School of Medicine in New York, returning to the MGH in 1962 to pick up the reins of the Surgical Services.

During Russell's tenure it became apparent that there was an increasingly urgent need for operating rooms in a central location. Thus, active planning began for what was first called the North Building, (Gray) a structure that was to be devoted primarily to this objective. All operating rooms outside of this centralized area—i.e., those in Baker and Phillips House—were to be discontinued. In addition to the expanded confluent operating area in the White and North buildings, extensive space was planned for medical chemistry, bacteriology, and radiology. As the program progressed, the trustees and the director felt that this special opportunity to construct a larger building—even if it could not be finished inside—should be seized. Accordingly, plans were extended to include a much needed new blood bank and the Jackson Tower, which would provide nine floors of new laboratory space.

Centralization of the operating rooms in the new building demanded careful and thorough planning. This was undertaken by a committee under the leadership of Claude Welch and F. Thomas Gephart. Gephart, in particular, spent many hours considering the myriad of details. He traveled to many other institutions and became acquainted with all the latest developments in operating room planning. Accordingly, the newly centralized operating area functioned extremely well, even though funds did not allow the completion of all the rooms as originally conceived. One feature of the new area of particular interest to Russell was the inclusion of a surgical pathology laboratory to improve the support which Pathology could provide to operating surgeons; the new laboratory was successful and became a rich source of teaching material for all concerned.

The gradual unification of the surgical staff was abetted by the development of a voluntary group practice arrangement called the Surgical Associates. This group had been established, mainly on the urging of Marshall Bartlett, by a representative staff committee. Each member voluntarily contributed his surgical fees to the hospital and subsequently received a salary which was, in general, related to the size of his contribution. This scheme left little money for general departmental purposes, although the situation changed considerably with the advent of the new system of Harvard Medical School appointments in the mid-sixties, which included a "clinical full-time" category. The importance of this new appointment ladder to group practices rested upon a number of points, the most significant of which was probably the fact that the total remuneration of each individual in this category was limited to double the figure allowed by the academic salary at his particular level. Therefore, active practicing surgeons thus appointed might collect fees that exceeded the permitted level, and the excess funds could be used by the chairman of the department as a new resource. The growing cardiac surgical program was a particularly important source of funds.

Meanwhile the postgraduate training program in surgery remained strong. The "block system" was continued. According to this plan, interns accepted for surgical training could expect to be retained throughout the entire five years of postgraduate experience required to satisfy the American Board of Surgery. The system functioned well, especially since candidates could be continually selected from a superior portion of the national pool. As interest gained among the residents for special experiences in plastic, cardiac, and thoracic surgery, plans were undertaken to provide them. It also became apparent that some concentration of beds for patients in these and other areas would be desirable. Special management of patients with pulmonary problems was advanced greatly by the establishment of a Respiratory Intensive Care Unit in the new Gray Building in conjunction with Henning Pontopiddan of the Anesthesia Department. Close collaborative relations developed between the thoracic surgeons and anesthesiologists which persisted even though Anesthesia became a separate Medical School department about that time.

Along with these developments, Russell's six-year tenure as chief of Surgery also embraced the negotiations between the hospital and the Shrine of North America for the establishment of a burns institute for the study and treatment of burns in children, as well as the detailed planning of the new building (see Chapter 25). This was seen as an extraordinary opportunity for surgery to expand its laboratory activities since one-third of the contemplated structure was to be made up of research laboratories. This prospect meant that the hospital had to provide less space for surgical research in the new Jackson Tower; laboratory investigation had never been a strong feature of the surgical effort at the MGH, and the activities of Drs. Cope, Russell, Nardi, and McDermott were already reasonably housed in the White Building.

Thus the period of Russell's leadership coincided with the physical transformation of the hospital as well as considerable administrative and personnel changes; three different chiefs of Medicine—Drs. Bauer, Ebert, and Leaf—served during this period. Within the Surgical Services, it was a time of great developments in the fields of cardiac surgery and transplantation.

24. General Surgical Services since 1969: The Austen Years

MARSHALL K. BARTLETT, GEORGE L. NARDI,
AND W. GERALD AUSTEN

When Churchill retired in 1962, Russell was appointed to succeed him; six years later the trustees announced that Russell had asked to be relieved of his administrative responsibilities in order to devote more time to teaching and investigation. Oliver Cope became acting chief and served in that capacity until April 1, 1969, when W. Gerald Austen—who had completed his surgical residency at the MGH in 1960, received further training in England and at the National Heart Institute, and returned to the MGH in 1963 to make a major effort in cardiac surgery—was named chief.

"I was faced with some very interesting problems in 1969," Austen reflected. "The MGH General Surgical Services, to my way of thinking, had tremendous strengths, but there were some deficits, too. I felt that we had to find a way to develop emerging specialties of surgery such as cardiac, general thoracic, and plastic surgery as well as such areas as transplantation, vascular, and cancer surgery without jeopardizing the traditional strengths of general surgery.

"Another aspect that, in my view, required special efforts concerned the development of the group practice. The time had come for as many members of the General Surgical Services as possible to join together in a group practice. I believed the members would be able to achieve a greater degree of stability and productivity within the hospital environment by mutually supporting each other and the department. As noted earlier, the development of such a group practice had begun a number of years before my appointment; however, the membership in 1969 was modest. The goal—to have most of the members of the General Surgical Services participate in the group practice and to view that arrangement in a positive and happy way—represented a formidable endeavor."

Surgical Units. Continuing explosive advances in the basic understanding of pathologic physiology and equally amazing technical developments pose many challenges and opportunities for the surgeon. The efforts necessary to meet them prompted many changes in the General Surgical Services, particularly during the latter half of the period covered by this history. As Austen noted, the unified concept of general surgery could no longer be maintained, and the specialty developments which had budded during Russell's administration blossomed during the 1970s under Austen. The increasing body of knowledge, refinement of techniques, demands of certification boards and third-party payers stimulated the development of discrete surgical units within the General Surgical Services in the following areas (listed with their chiefs as of 1980): thoracic surgery (Hermes C. Grillo), cardiac surgery (Mortimer J. Buckley), plastic surgery (John P. Remensnyder), pediatric surgery (W. Hardy Hendren), vascular surgery (William M. Abbott), burn surgery (John F. Burke), gastrointestinal surgery (Ronald A. Malt), endocrine surgery (Chiu-an Wang), cancer surgery (William C. Wood and Alfred M. Cohen), transplant surgery (Paul S. Russell), and the Shriners Burns Institute (John F. Burke). Each of these units was established in response to a special need and because the personnel available fitted that need. General Surgery remains the core of the General Surgical Services.

Staff. The staff increased considerably during these exciting years, with the total professional staff reaching 215 by 1980. The clinical staff numbered 44 staff surgeons in 1969 and 57 by 1980; the resident staff increased modestly from 53 in 1969 to 63 in 1980. By 1980 approximately two-thirds of the surgical staff were full-time, in terms of the Harvard Medical School designation, and one-third part-time, representing a significant shift to the full-time Harvard category during the previous decade. For many years there had been two tenured professorships in the MGH Department of Surgery—the John Homans Professorship and one other; by 1980 that number had increased to four with the gifts from patients and friends to establish the Edward D. Churchill Professorship and the Helen Andrus Benedict Professorship.

Group Practice. The opening of five floors of the Warren Building for offices in 1957 allowed a large number of staff to be located geographically full-time at the hospital. In 1961 the MGH Surgical Associates was formed with volunteer participation of approximately 20 staff members. During Austen's tenure this association evolved and matured. Membership, which stayed relatively stable during the 1960s, expanded to well over 60 members and as of 1980 included all clinical staff members of the General Surgical Services. The group provides important financial support to the department in general as well as in its development of young surgeons and in its support of research and education. The Surgical Associates was the first attempt at group practice at the MGH and served as the prototype for the development of more than two dozen similar arrangements in the hospital.

Operating Rooms and Intensive Care Units. Successive changes in the physical plant had a major bearing on clinical activities in Surgery. As noted in the previous chapter, the multiplying activities—especially the regular increase in numbers of operations performed annually by MGH surgeons—put a tremendous strain on the facilities. Claude Welch remembered that matters had already reached a "boiling point" in the 1950s: "Operating rooms in the White Building were reserved for the ward services. Private services continued operating in the Baker and the Phillips House in facilities that even in those days had to be considered primitive." Around that time Welch sent a letter to the director of the hospital characterizing the operating rooms in the Baker and the Phillips House as "if not Neanderthal, hardly better than those of the Middle Ages." The gestation was long, but finally, in 1968, the new Gray Building was erected, housing one of the largest suites of operating rooms in the world. A long-felt need for consolidating the White, Baker, and Phillips House operating suites was realized in 1972 when the latter two units were replaced by the new facilities in the Gray Building on the third floor, connecting directly with the White operating rooms. The next year, in response to the need for improved facilities for the performance of surgical procedures on transient patients, the

Baker operating rooms were modified and, in the spring of 1974, a full-fledged surgical day care unit was initiated. The day care unit has been extremely successful, and nearly one-third of all surgery is currently performed there. (In 1982 the day care surgery unit moved into new quarters in the Ambulatory Care Center. With the aid of a generous gift from the Cabot Family Trust, the facility now consists of ten operating rooms and includes special accommodations for children and their families. The unit fulfills a vital role in the delivery of a wide range of ambulatory surgical services.)

In 1959 a small and inadequate recovery room in the White Building was replaced by a new and larger one containing 21 beds. Advances in the techniques of managing acutely ill postoperative patients have since led to the establishment of separate intensive care units for cardiac surgical patients, for thoracic and respiratory patients, and for general surgical patients on Gray 3A, and for pediatric patients on Burnham 5. There is a separate unit to accommodate adult burn patients on White 12 (shortly to be moved to new quarters on Bigelow 12) and an additional unit for transplantation patients on Phillips House 8. Austen comments that "the advantage of regionalization of critically ill patients with special problems has, of course, been clearly demonstrated in terms of better patient care. The Recovery Room facilities have also been appropriately expanded on White 3. Thus there are now 31 inpatient operating rooms and 10 surgical day care operating rooms with 30 recovery room beds, 12 cardiac surgical intensive care beds, 18 general, vascular and thoracic intensive care beds, and 7 pediatric intensive care beds. In addition there are 10 adult burn intensive care beds and 8 transplant intensive care beds. Approximately 26,000 operations are now done each year at the MGH—almost exactly double the volume in 1955. Plans are already underway for the creation of two additional operating rooms. One of these will house a linear accelerator to provide intra-operative radiation therapy."

Education. Active teaching programs continue as a major activity of the General Surgical Services at both the undergraduate and graduate levels. Great care has been taken to keep the teaching program in step with the needs and wishes of the medical students. Introduction to Clinical Medicine, coordinated for the department by Chiu-an Wang and John Head and more recently by Wang and William C. Wood, and the Core Clinical Clerkship in Surgery, run by Gordon Scannell, are both effective and rewarding and have been very well received.

At the postgraduate level the instruction of the house staff is of critical importance. The General Surgical Services has more patients in the hospital than any other service. The daily inpatient census in 1980 usually was in the range of 320 patients, and the magnitude of these clinical activities requires a large house staff—63 residents. The traditional outstanding quality of MGH surgical residents endures. The training program is generally considered to be one of the superlative programs in the world, and the MGH record of applicant acceptance to the General Surgical Residency Program is probably the highest in the country. Certainly, the surgical residents represent a crucial resource for the department, the hospital, and the community at large.

The residents' education is a careful blend of increasing individual responsibility in patient care with informal instruction through close contact with many members of the Visiting Staff as well as with more senior residents. Leslie W. Ottinger directs this program. The core of the training program has been, and still is, the presence of a large volume of patients on the East and West Surgical Services. In the more remote past these patients could not afford private hospitalization and physicians' fees; their care was provided by the Resident Staff under the supervision of the Visiting Staff. Even before 1955, increasing insurance coverage was noted as a factor tending to decrease the ratio of "ward" or "service" to "private" patients. The implementation of Medicare and Medicaid programs, aimed at providing all recipients with semiprivate care, accelerated the trend. Nevertheless, the volume of patients and operations on the East and West Surgical Services remains high.

Participation of the House Staff in the care of private patients had modest beginnings in 1930 when the Baker Memorial opened. This responsibility consisted of the admission work-up, assisting at the operation, and participation in postoperative care—all under the supervision of a member of the Visiting Staff. As the length of residency training increased, and the resident's level of knowledge and skill rose accordingly, the degree of participation in the care of the private patient also increased.

On the East and West Surgical Services, with the chief resident in the sixth year of training and eligible for certification by the American Board of Surgery, it is possible for the resident staff to enjoy a considerable degree of autonomy. Supervision remains in the hands of the Visiting Staff who make rounds with the residents but serve primarily as consultants. In recent years the chief residents have been members of the Visiting Staff, principally for administrative reasons, without change in the level of responsibility that the position has long carried. Very real efforts have been made to assure an adequate flow of patients through these services, and in large measure these efforts have succeeded.

The positions of chief resident in the specialties of cardiothoracic and plastic surgery are reserved for graduates of the general surgery program (MGH residents are given preference); these residents are all board-eligible or certified in general surgery. On completion of residency, each individual is eligible to sit for the corresponding specialty board.

Many residents choose to take an extra year or two to work in research at some point during the surgical residency program. The department encourages such options and is fortunately in a position to offer five research fellowships each year in various aspects of surgery. The fellowships bear the names of Marshall Bartlett and Claude Welch (general surgery), Robert Linton (vascular), Edward Churchill (cardiothoracic), and V. H. Kazanjian (plastic).

A large number of teaching conferences are conducted on a weekly basis. In addition to the traditional Surgical Grand Rounds which have been a Thursday morning feature for a great many years, all the specialty units as well as the East and West Services have individual weekly conferences. An active program of postgraduate courses is conducted in conjunction with the Medical School. In recent years the primary courses in general surgery have been supplemented by well attended courses in cardiac, thoracic, vascular, trauma, cancer, gastrointestinal, and microvascular surgery, and hyperalimentation. A lecture series honoring Edward P. Richardson, former professor of surgery and the first full-time chief of the West Surgical Service, began in 1949 with the aid of a generous endowment from the Richardson family. By 1981 there had been over 100 Richardson Lecturers, all of international stature.

Research. Clinical and laboratory research continues to be an integral, major part of the activities of the General Surgical Services. It is clearly impossible to document here the extensive investigative program, which extends from basic biochemical cellular studies through immunologic modifications in transplantation to innovative surgical techniques. The particular strength of surgical research lies in the ability to bridge the gap between laboratory and operating room and has certainly been successfully achieved at the MGH. These projects and accomplishments are summarized in the annual reports of the Committee on Research and, in some instances, have been alluded to elsewhere in this volume. "The research program of the General Surgical Services has expanded tremendously over the last 25 years and particularly over the last decade," Austen explains. "With the creation of the surgical research facilities in the Shriners Burns Institute as well as those for oncology surgery in the Cox Building, for pediatric surgery on Gray 5, and for vascular surgery on White 3A, our research space has improved markedly in recent years. In 1980 the research budget for the General Surgical Services approached $4 million. The funds came primarily from the National Institutes of Health but also included generous monies from the Shriners Burns Institute, gifts from patients, grants from other outside agencies, plus a substantial contribution from the Surgical Associates."

Future Clinical Facilities. "We are looking forward with great anticipation to the renovation of White 6 and 7 clinical facilities as well as the creation of new surgical facilities on Bigelow 12 and 13," Austen says. "We will maintain the same 96 beds that previously constituted the East and West Surgical Services. The much needed modernization will achieve adequate space for each patient bed, appropriate support facilities, and the elimination of 'ward-type' units which will be supplanted by single and double occupancy rooms with bathroom accommodations for each room, and so on. These facilities have been a long time in coming, and their completion in 1984 will mark a major event in the history of the General Surgical Services at the MGH."

25. Surgical Units

Plastic Unit

BRADFORD CANNON AND JOHN P. REMENSNYDER

Although an ancient art, plastic surgery did not achieve formal recognition as a surgical subspecialty at the MGH until the period currently under historic review. Over a century ago the hospital's Jonathan Mason Warren wrote several papers on surgery of the cleft palate and on the tagliacotian rhinoplastic operation in the *Boston Medical and Surgical Journal.* Yet little attention was given to the specialty in ensuing years. Much of what today is regarded as plastic surgery was done by general surgeons. Not until after World War I—because of the extraordinary contributions made by V. H. Kazanjian—did plastic and reconstructive surgery receive fitting recognition in Boston.

Born in Turkish Armenia in 1879, Kazanjian was encouraged by relatives at home and by letters from abroad to leave the land of his birth and investigate the opportunities in the new world. He came to the United States in October 1895. During the next seven years he worked intermittently in a wire mill in Worcester. In 1900 he decided to study dentistry, the alternative being a career in engineering. Endowed with natural manual dexterity, his choice of dentistry was not surprising since it gave him an opportunity for using his skill and the promise of security and a useful life.

After graduation from the Harvard Dental School in 1905, Kazanjian was associated with the Prosthetic Laboratory of the school and, in 1912, was placed in charge of this department. At that time hospital facilities for the treatment of jaw fractures were not available, and many patients went to the Dental School where they were assigned to the prosthetic department for treatment. Kazanjian treated over 400 fractures within a few years and achieved an enviable record. He was one of the first in this country to abandon the unwieldy interdental splint and to adopt the simpler method of intermaxillary wiring.

When the opportunity came in June 1915 to join the first Harvard Unit in France as dental chief, Kazanjian was singularly well qualified to serve, with his expert knowledge of prosthetic dentistry and his experience in the handling of a wide variety of jaw fractures. At that time there was no Dental Corps in the British Army, and only 15 dentists were available for all the troops. Kazanjian filled this unrecognized need and laid the foundation for one of the most remarkable services rendered in military hospitals; more than 3,000 cases of gunshot, shrapnel, and other injuries of the face and jaws passed through his skillful hands. His was the first organized dental unit of the British Expeditionary Forces in France. It continued to function under his direction, at the official request of the British War Office, until February 1919. Word of the accomplishments of the unit spread through the British Army, and more and more wounded were sent there. Medical officers were assigned as observers for two and three months for the purpose of establishing similar services elsewhere. Kazanjian was referred to by one English writer as "The Miracle Man of the Western Front." He was made an honorary Major in the Royal Army Medical Corps and decorated "Companion of St. Michael and St. George" in 1918 by King George V.

On Kazanjian's return to the United States in 1919 it was obvious that in order for him to continue with the surgery that he had so successfully carried out during the years in France, a gap in his training had to be filled. He therefore entered the Harvard Medical School in the fall of that year and received the M.D. degree in 1921. One incident in his medical school career merits mention. At one of the surgical clinics conducted by Harvey Cushing, two high-ranking officers from the Royal Army Medical Corps accompanied Cushing. On glancing up at the students, one of the officers grasped his companion's arm and pointed. They both climbed the steps and literally dragged a very reluctant student to the floor of the amphitheater. Kazanjian was introduced as the man who had taught these guests the technique that they were about to demonstrate.

The years that followed were ones of seeking recognition for plastic surgery in a professional environment traditionally reluctant to accept any of the subspecialties of general surgery. In 1922 Kazanjian was appointed to the staff of the MGH and the Massachusetts Eye and Ear Infirmary, and as head of the joint Plastic Clinic of the two institutions, a position he held until his retirement in the mid-forties. He was assigned the title of surgeon for plastic operations in 1930; this is the only mention of plastic surgery in Faxon's history. In Washburn's chronicle of earlier decades tribute is paid to Kazanjian's service in World War I as follows: "In this work of reconstruction and plastic surgery, his skill was unrivalled." Washburn mentions an "increase in plastic surgery, mainly by Dr. V. H. Kazanjian" in the mid-twenties. The special assignment to Drs. Daland and Kazanjian was formed because "a great many of the cases in the Tumor Clinic require plastic work in connection with their treatment."

Ernest M. Daland, Somers H. Sturgis, and later Bradford Cannon were associated with Kazanjian in the clinic; Edgar M. Holmes, Garret Sullivan, and Iram Roopinian represented the MEEI. Those who enjoyed the privilege of association with Kazanjian were constantly impressed with his accomplishments and his original approach to surgical problems. To the untrained observer there was an air of mystery about his work; the trained observer recognized methods based on sound principles of reconstructive surgery. The joint weekly Plastic Clinic was remarkable for the variety of disciplines represented by the staff personnel and the unique drawing power of the group for interesting and challenging patient problems. Kazanjian's ties with the Harvard Dental School furnished occasions for dental collaboration and for a broader basis in patient care.

In 1940 Kazanjian was appointed to the Board of Consultation "to continue for one year as head of the Plastic Clinic." In 1941 Bradford Cannon was appointed to succeed him as head of the clinic. The departure of many of the staff for military duty during World War II left the clinic short-handed; Kazanjian returned as head for the duration of the conflict until Cannon came back in 1947.

The New England reluctance to accept fragmentation of general surgery was reinforced by E. D. Churchill's experiences in World War II. He encountered many of the country's leading but highly specialized general surgeons who were baffled by the multiple wounds of war. His logical conclusion as chief of Surgery at the MGH was that surgical training must be very broad and as all-inclusive as possible. Not until July 1960 was there recognition of the special features of plastic surgery. At that time John D. Constable, who had served as the general surgical resident (1959), was appointed as Cannon's associate, and two surgical residents were assigned to the Plastic Clinic to work on the wards and with private patients on a two-month rotation. During the next 15 years, 23 of these surgical residents chose to specialize in plastic surgery, obtained formal training at the MGH or elsewhere, and were certified by the American Board of Plastic Surgery. Others continuing in general surgery or other surgical specialties have reported that the exposure to plastic surgical principles and methods has proven useful in their later practices.

Reflecting on the evolution of the specialty during his tenure, W. Gerald Austen observed: "The Plastic Surgery Unit is an excellent example of how a specialty area can be created in the General Surgical Services in a way that is beneficial to all concerned. When we discussed the creation of the unit and the development of a Plastic Surgical Residency in 1969, there was considerable opposition because of the concern regarding fragmentation and loss of experience for the general surgeons. Without question, the creation of the Plastic Surgery Unit in 1970 and the development of the Plastic Surgical Residency as a part of the General Surgical Services resulted in improved care of the patients, a better educational program, and significant leadership in the field."

The contributions of plastic surgery have been several. Collaboration with the late Arthur L. Watkins, chief of Physical Medicine, in the care of pressure sores in the paraplegic resulted in a better understanding of the factors important in healing and the surgical techniques for repair. Frequent consultation with the Orthopedic Service was instructive and instrumental in ensuring the earlier and safer closure of compound extremity wounds. This experience prompted reports on soft tissue repairs of the extremities, including chapters in the MGH publication *Fractures and Other Traumatic Conditions*.

Reviews of experiences with treatment of severe injuries and trauma of the hand, arms, legs, face, and neck have been published, as have those with primary and secondary cleft lip and palate surgery. The open grafting of granulating wounds was also reported—a technique that today is regularly used in the care of severe burns. A study of the late harmful effects of irradiation for benign conditions in over 150 patients confirmed the need for caution in use of this potentially dangerous therapy.

General surgical residents at the MGH who elected to specialize in plastic surgery were eager to continue their training at the MGH. Thus in 1970 a formal two-year residency program was established to make better use of the teaching opportunities on the wards, in the clinic, and in the busy Emergency Ward. The program was unusual because it was integrated with the general surgical program (one year as plastic surgical assistant resident, a second as senior on a general surgical rotation, and a final year as plastic surgical resident). This plan had the full cooperation of the chief of Surgery, Dr. Austen, and shortened by one year the eligibility requirement for dual board examination and certification.

Cannon was the first chief of the plastic surgical residency and unit, and upon his retirement in 1973 was succeeded by John P. Remensnyder. In 1977 the residency expanded to include the rich experience in cleft lip and palate surgery as well as craniofacial surgery at the Tufts-New England Medical Center.

Another dimension of plastic and reconstructive surgery became crystallized in 1968 with the opening of the Shriners Burns Institute (see Chapter 31).

Initially John Constable and then Remensnyder were the directors of the reconstructive effort at the Burns Institute. With the guidance of the entire plastic surgical division, new techniques were sought throughout the seventies for the reconstruction of the burned child, particularly the correction of the functional deformities of the burned hand and destroyed features of the burned face. Special efforts were made to dovetail early reconstructive work during the acute healing phase, reconstruction of missing thumbs in the severely burned hand, and the provision of as normal and expressive skin and tissue as possible in the burned face. With the lowered mortality associated with acute burn—especially with the survival of patients burned over 80 percent of their body surface—particularly challenging and hitherto unseen problems in the reconstruction of the burned child presented for solution.

The mid-seventies saw the virtually simultaneous introduction of successful and clinically reliable microsurgical techniques and the use of compound muscle skin flaps for repairs that had previously required tedious multistaged procedures. Under the energetic direction of James May, clinical microsurgery made its entrance on the plastic and reconstructive scene at the MGH, and May established an ongoing research program in microsurgery for small nerves and blood vessels. The direct practical benefit of these studies was a challenging influx of patients with amputated parts—including fingers, hands, arms, and legs—which have been replanted with an outstanding success rate using microsurgical techniques. Under May's careful tutelage the resident staff gained particular expertise in microsurgery.

Remensnyder added the following remarks about Cannon:

Dr. Bradford Cannon, in recent years, has been the fountainhead of the plastic and reconstructive surgical effort at the MGH. As stated above, he had a close and productive relation with Dr. Kazanjian in the Plastic Surgical Clinic and following Kazanjian's retirement continued and developed the field at the hospital.

Cannon is the son of the late Walter Bradford Cannon, who was Professor of Physiology at the Harvard Medical School and whose outstanding contributions to the field of physiology and medicine are well known, undoubtedly influencing his son in his approach to the scientific aspects of medicine. After graduating Harvard Medical School in 1933, Bradford Cannon took his surgical training at Barnes Hospital in St. Louis, Missouri. At that time St. Louis was the most active center of the United States in plastic and reconstructive surgery under the leadership of Drs. V. P. Blair and J. B. Brown. Cannon took his training in this group and brought with him new ideas and techniques on his return to Boston in 1940. He and Kazanjian ran the MGH Plastic Surgical Clinic in the forties, providing care to an increasing number of patients with deformities of all kinds. In addition, Cannon established a Crippled Children's Clinic for the treatment of cleft lip and palate deformities, based at the Mount Auburn Hospital in Cambridge, Mass. In 1942, at the time of the Cocoanut Grove fire, the task of the reconstructive and rehabilitative care of the victims of the fire, who were patients at the MGH, fell upon Cannon and his workers. He supervised the restoration of form and function of this unfortunate group of people over the months and years following the fire.

In 1943 Cannon enlisted in the Army with the initial rank of lieutenant, rising to lieutenant colonel at the time of his discharge in 1947. In the latter phases of the war the Department of the Army concentrated the reconstructive care of servicemen with facial, hand, and other traumatic deformities at several centers including Valley Forge Hospital in Phoenixville, Pennsylvania. Cannon was Chief of Plastic Surgery of this unit for two years. As St. Louis had been in the thirties, Valley Forge became a national center for the development of reconstructive techniques in the restoration of burned faces, functionless hands, and compound wounds to the lower extremities. New techniques of care, developed and reported by Cannon, served as the basis for translating these techniques into civilian practice on his return to MGH.

Back in Boston, Cannon picked up his work again in the MGH Plastic Surgical Clinic and was awarded a preceptorship for training in plastic surgery by the American Board of Plastic and Reconstructive Surgery. During the fifties and sixties, Cannon increasingly became the focus of interest in plastic and reconstructive surgery on the part of numerous surgical house officers who have subsequently become leaders in the profession in various parts of the country. John Constable, following his chief residency in general surgery, became Cannon's preceptor in 1960 and later joined him on the staff. As an increasing number of graduates of the general surgical training program in the sixties had to go elsewhere for their training in plastic and reconstructive surgery, it became obvious to Cannon that such a training program was necessary at the MGH. His thoughts and efforts in this direction resulted in the establishment of the residency in plastic and reconstructive surgery in 1970, at which time he became Chief of the Plastic Surgical Unit.

Through the years Cannon has received numerous honors and awards including presidency of the American Association of Plastic Surgeons, Founding Membership of the American Society for Surgery of the Hand, membership in the American Board of Plastic and Reconstructive Surgery and the American Surgical Association, co-editor of the *Journal of Plastic and Reconstructive Surgery,* and president of the Harvard Medical Alumni Association.

Transplantation Unit

PAUL S. RUSSELL

Following his return to the MGH from a research fellowship in London with Sir Peter Medawar in 1954–1955, Paul Russell completed his surgical residency and proceeded to set up an experimental laboratory to begin investigating problems in transplantation biology. He demonstrated with a medical student, Ruben Gittes, that parathyroid tissue in some animals appeared to be deficient in transplantation antigens and undertook several clinical trials of transplantation of parathyroid tissue to parathyroid-deficient patients. No immunosuppression was employed, and no tests for tissue compatibility were available at that time. Another early clinical effort, begun in 1957, was the program (involving Dr. Russell, Joseph McGovern, William Baker, and Leonard Atkins) to treat children with acute lymphatic leukemia with lethal doses of whole body irradiation and bone marrow transplantation. The plan in these trials was to remove bone marrow from children who were enjoying drug-induced remission of their acute leukemia and to store the marrow cells in the frozen state until such time as intractable exacerbation of the disease took place. At this time whole body irradiation was employed as a last resort to treat the leukemia, and reinfusion of the morphologically normal autologous bone marrow followed. One patient of the six treated had a spectacular response with an extended remission for many months. Uncertainties regarding the efficacy of the preservation process and failure of marrow transplants from allogenic individuals to take in those cases in which autologous marrow infusions had failed, plus Russell's move to Columbia in New York, led to a temporary discontinuation of bone marrow transplantation at the MGH in the late fifties. This had been one of the first such efforts in the world and was the first in New England by almost 20 years.

When Russell returned to the MGH in 1962 to become chief of Surgery, plans were begun to institute kidney transplantation at the hospital. Radiation had been the mainstay for immunosuppression through most of the fifties, but

Imuran—a derivative of 6-mercaptopurine—had been discovered by Burroughs-Wellcome scientists and had been employed at the Peter Bent Brigham Hospital and elsewhere with encouraging results. In those days there was no dialysis facility at the MGH, and considerable concern existed that there were more patients with renal failure than could be treated. Accordingly, a substantial research grant was secured from the NIH to cover all the patient care costs of kidney transplant recipients, and the first patient received a kidney transplant on February 27, 1963. The first few patients received transplants in the absence of any dialysis capability, but a machine was soon acquired. Lot B. Page directed early treatments; problems in infectious disease were dealt with by K. Frank Austen, and Anthony P. Monaco remained on the staff to work in the transplantation field after completing his residency training in surgery.

Russell also reactivated the research program. With the arrival of Henry J. Winn in 1965, an analysis of the immune status of transplant recipients was started, and the MGH established the first laboratory for tissue typing in the New York–New England region. The need for sharing donated organs for transplantation was recognized after a particularly dramatic episode in which a donor liver was removed at the MGH from a patient after death had been declared and transported to the Peter Bent Brigham for transplantation. Thereafter, Russell, F. D. Moore, and J. E. Murray held a number of conferences which led to the founding of the Boston Interhospital Organ Bank in 1968, with Russell as the first chairman of its board of trustees. The organization was formed with the benefit of MGH legal advice as a nonprofit corporation and has since grown to a sizeable enterprise throughout New England. Now called the New England Organ Bank, it has a central tissue-typing laboratory, 24-hour technicians on call for organ perfusion and tissue typing, and a central secretariat under the direction of B. A. Barnes.

Meanwhile a series of able young people were trained both in the laboratory and clinical aspects of transplantation. Research fellows from most European countries as well as from several African, Asian, and South American nations came to the laboratories for varying periods of time. Several individuals received Ph.D. degrees in immunology under Winn's direction, while still other scientists came to learn and participate in research projects.

One of the main objects of investigation has been the use of antibodies prepared against lymphoid cells in immunosuppression. Before this subject was taken up at the MGH in 1964, there were hints in the literature that antibodies of this kind could be immunosuppressive, but little hope had been placed in the possibility of useful clinical application. The MGH studies showed that very powerful and continuing immunosuppressive effects could be produced in animal systems by antibodies made in one species against the lymphoid cells of another. Extensive information was gathered in small animals regarding the best means of preparation of these antibodies, the methods for their fractionation and purification, and evidence related to their mechanisms of action.

During a research fellowship A. B. Cosimi built upon previous experience gained with the production of antibodies against human cells in horses and rabbits and defined optimal conditions for antibody production in the horse. Clinical trials were begun with material made and purified in the hospital, but it soon became clear that for large-scale clinical trial, collaboration with industrial concerns would be required. Accordingly, the hospital established a relationship with the Upjohn Company for serum production. This eventuated in a large-scale national trial of our antithymocyte globulin preparation, in which the MGH took the lead, and in FDA-licensing of this agent for use in transplantation.

Subsequently, with the development of monoclonal antibodies produced by hybridized cells in vitro, additional relationships were made with the Ortho Pharmaceutical Company to secure monoclonal antibodies against various T lymphocytes in order to determine the levels of these cells in the blood of patients under treatment and also to employ such antibodies in immunosuppression of kidney transplant recipients for the first time. Striking success was achieved with the use of antibodies to T cells as a means of reversing the acute rejection of kidney transplants, and the use of a new family of instruments, the flow cytometers, added a powerful diagnostic tool in which monoclonal antibodies were extraordinarily helpful. Strong collaborative relationships were developed with the Department of Pathology, with Medicine, Pediatrics, Psychiatry, Nursing, and other segments of the hospital in order to deliver optimal care to transplant patients.

With the advent of the government-financed health care plan for patients with end-stage renal disease, it was no longer necessary to support patient care from research sources. The Dialysis Unit matured under the guidance of George Baker and Nina Rubin. Extensive progress was made in the management of infectious complications of immunosuppressed patients under the guidance of Robert Rubin. Pediatric patients with renal failure have been cared for by John Herrin. A new seven-bed special unit for transplantation was established on the eighth floor of the Phillips House, and plans were made to move the Dialysis Unit to a more favorable location than its original cramped and inefficient quarters on White 12. (The unit had been placed there initially because of the natural relationship to the isolation facilities on White 12, but the growth and development of activities made it impossible to continue there.)

The number of patients receiving kidney transplants rose steadily, so that by 1980 there were more than 50 such patients, making the MGH the largest center for this type of surgery in the Northeast. By 1981 almost 450 individuals had received kidney transplants, and about one-third of the recipients had been pediatric patients. Rehabilitation has been emphasized as survival rates have steadily improved. In the early days the recipient of a kidney from an unrelated donor faced a mortality of about 25 percent in the first year after transplantation; this figure has now been reduced to lower than 10 percent. The first-year survival of transplanted kidneys in this group of patients has risen from about 50 percent to almost 80 percent, and the attrition of lives and transplants after the first year is now very small. Where living donors can be used, both transplant and patient survival are significantly higher. As many patients who are in a high-risk category because of age or such complicating factors as diabetes have been included in recent years, these improved statistics have been particularly gratifying and stand very favorably in comparison with results achieved elsewhere.

Experimental work with liver, heart, and pancreas transplantation is being actively pursued, and there is every expectation that clinical application of these treatments will begin in the relatively near future. Meanwhile, a broad range of investigative projects in cellular immunology and immunogenetics have been carried on in the laboratories.

The hospital engaged in a long and interesting debate regarding the appropriateness of entering the field of heart transplantation in 1980, having given the matter consideration on at least two previous occasions during the seventies. The trustees decided against proceeding with heart transplantation at this time mainly for logistic reasons but stated that further review of this treatment was by no means ruled out. Results with heart transplantation have improved steadily, and a number of new programs have been established in other institutions. Thus interest at the MGH persists.

As the 1980s began, the Transplantation Unit stood as an activity embracing the talents of individuals from a number of services and departments of the hospital. It was designed to be a balanced clinical and laboratory effort, using the talents of both physician and Ph.D. investigators. Each new trainee makes an individual contribution to the development of what has become an established clinical discipline closely related to a number of scientific areas, especially to the large and flourishing field of immunology which itself has been greatly stimulated by the demands of tissue and organ renewal.

Dr. Austen added this view:

Transplantation has been an area of substantial activity at the MGH and throughout the world during the last three decades. After considerable initial excitement in the fifties and early sixties, there was perhaps some deceleration of progress. This has, happily, given way to significant new advances in the late seventies, and I believe the field holds great promise for the future. The MGH unit has played a leading role in all of this. Kidney transplantation has become a major and standard activity. Investigations continue in bone marrow transplantation, pancreatic transplantation, cardiac transplantation, and liver transplantation. Clinical application appears promising in a number of these areas in the future.

Cardiac Unit

J. GORDON SCANNELL

The quarter century from 1955 to 1980 was a time of exponential growth of cardiac surgery on a national, indeed global, scale. It also saw cardiac surgery at the MGH develop into a full-time clinical specialty. This occurred within the framework of a General Surgical Service that had historically resisted compartmentalization and the designation of specialty services, and this, in turn, may account for the delayed assumption by the hospital of a leadership role on the local and national scene in cardiac surgery. That scene was a frantic one; not since the Oklahoma land rush had an area been opened, explored, and settled with the speed that characterized the development of cardiac—particularly intracardiac—surgery.

In this same period not only was an active clinical service created, but an active cardiac surgical research laboratory was also established with ample space in expanded research facilities and generous financial support. This research effort went well beyond the substantial development of the cardiac catheterization laboratory, a cooperative effort of the Medical, Radiologic, and Surgical services in place since 1948.

Finally during this 25-year period, a cardiac surgical residency of the first rank was developed. It was integrated closely with general thoracic surgery and easily conformed to, and set standards for, the external requirements of the American Board of Thoracic Surgery.

Historical Background. The history of cardiac surgery at the MGH goes back to 1928. At that time E. D. Churchill, in close collaboration with his medical colleague, Paul Dudley White, performed the first successful pericardiectomy for constrictive pericarditis to be carried out in the United States. It was a legitimate "first" based on sound clinical and laboratory preparation. Indeed, over the ensuing 15 years it continued to be a specialty of the house. It was one of the many accomplishments that projected Churchill into national prominence, but, although his interest in this particular subject persisted, in other respects cardiac surgery entered the doldrums. After this promising start, emphasis shifted to the problems of pulmonary resection, cancer of the lung, and bronchopulmonary suppuration as well as tuberculosis. A few frustrating and unsuccessful efforts were made to salvage patients dying of massive pulmonary embolus and then this program was abandoned, branded an "immediate autopsy" by Churchill. Yet it was this effort that stimulated John Gibbon, at the time a research fellow with Churchill, to initiate his laboratory studies of extracorporeal circulation, first at the MGH, later at Philadelphia. Twenty years later, in 1953, the gates of open heart surgery without limits of time were opened by Gibbon in the first successful use of a pump oxygenator in the open repair of a large atrial septal defect. In all frankness it must be said that Gibbon received relatively little support and encouragement from Churchill in this enterprise, although he did provide laboratory space for better than a year, and the two men remained close friends and professional colleagues throughout their lives. The reasons for Churchill's reluctance to embark upon the study of cardiopulmonary bypass are not clear (see Chapter 21). In the mid-forties, for example, he actively discouraged William Waddell in this endeavor, and it was not until 1953 that an active program was underway.

In the early forties a number of patients with patent ductus arteriosus were operated on by Richard Sweet following the pioneering breakthrough by Robert Gross at the Boston Children's Hospital in 1938. Sweet's technical prowess very quickly led him to a technical "first," namely the division of a complete aortic ring. This innovative procedure was done independently but contemporaneously with a similar procedure by Gross. Again, spurred on by Gross, Robert Linton undertook operations for coarctation of the aorta, and after 1947 there were a few sporadic efforts to correct tetralogy of Fallot in blue babies. But the laboratory support was not there.

Finally, in 1948 a decision was made by P. D. White and Churchill to assign the clinical development of cardiac surgery to Gordon Myers and Gordon Scannell, both recent additions to the medical and surgical staff respectively. They were soon joined by Allan Friedlich, back from two highly productive years with Taussig and Bing at Johns Hopkins. The initial priority was to establish a proper cardiac catheterization laboratory, and to this end Myers provided effective and dedicated leadership. The needed cooperation of the Department of Radiology was the responsibility of Stanley Wyman.

The catheterization laboratory pursued the study of pulmonary hypertension particularly in patients with rheumatic valvular heart disease and congenital heart disease. Both areas were about to acquire major surgical significance. Closed operations for mitral stenosis had been introduced simultaneously by Harken and Bailey in 1948. The former vigorously promoted the procedure at the Peter Bent Brigham and the Boston City. The first "closed mitral" at the MGH was done in 1951, the first of a carefully controlled series that extended over the next 15 years. The procedure is still done when the occasion presents.

Except for a modest number of Blalock shunts, patent ductus arteriosus, and coarctation with and without interposition of preserved aortic grafts, operations for congenital heart disease were deferred until the advent of safe cardiopulmonary bypass.

In the late forties 16 Bland-Sweet operations were carried out—anastomosis of a branch of the pulmonary vein to the azygos—a procedure designed to decompress the left atrium. This operation soon gave way to closed mitral valvuloplasty. In this period also Sweet and, occasionally, Scannell placed Hufnagel valves in the descending aorta for aortic regurgitation. All these operations now read like collectors' items, but at the time they were clinical challenges and acceptable pioneer attempts. Finally, in 1955 there was another national "first" at the MGH: the successful removal of an intra-atrial myxoma accomplished under the dramatic circumstances of total body hypothermia. It is interesting that 27 years later the patient is still alive and well.

By 1955 the stage was set for what was clearly in the wings, the rapid development of extracorporeal circulation and all that this implied. At this point ended Churchill's reluctance to see cardiac surgery established as more than a special assignment, a pattern that he had followed with conspicuous success in thoracic surgery in the prewar period, external and some internal pressures to the contrary.

The Years of Development, 1955–1962.

A number of important advances in cardiac surgery were made in the years from 1955 to 1962—the last seven Churchill years. The staffing, however, remained a geographic rather than an academic full-time enterprise. The latter waited the return of W. G. Austen from the NIH and the reorganization of the cardiac research laboratory. Exponential expansion of the clinical services followed. The seven-year period from 1955 to 1962 allowed the hospital, in sailing terms, to maintain a "safe leeward position" on the national scene.

In collaboration with the Department of Pathology basic studies of flow through normal and diseased valves were made by Austen, Robert Shaw, Fairfield Goodale, and Richard Kelly. Space does not permit a detailed account of these, but obvious are the imaginative genius of Shaw and the innovative ability and logical approach of Austen, then in the midst of his general surgical residency. Flow measurements were later supplemented by pulse duplicator observations by Austen and Kelly, expanding the original studies of Ian McMillan. These studies became the scientific basis for aortic valve surgery at that time. The work was recognized nationally at the Boston meeting of the American Association for Thoracic Surgery in 1959. It subsequently was the basis for a significant series of aortic valvuloplasties under direct vision carried out by Scannell at this hospital. This eventually gave way to satisfactory valve replacement by prosthetic valves.

During these interval years progress was made in the design and development of a satisfactory pump oxygenator both in the laboratory and in the operating room. In actual fact, a not inconsiderable part of this work was done by Austen and Shaw in the basement workshop of the latter's home. Among other things it was a demonstration of New England thrift. The first models were modified from the original concept of Dewall's bubble oxygenator; then sigma motor pumps gave way to DeBakey roller pumps and disc oxygenators supplanted and were in turn supplanted by disposable bubble oxygenators similar to the apparatus in current (1982) use.

The first clinical use of extracorporeal circulation at the MGH occurred in November 1956. The patient was a desperately ill infant with a ventricular septal defect. The surgeons were Scannell and Paul Russell; Shaw and Austen manned the pump, and Torkel Andersen and Phillips Hallowell conducted the anesthesia. The patient survived, but only for a matter of hours. The first successful open heart procedure with cardiopulmonary bypass at this hospital was the correction of an atrial septal defect carried out in April 1957 by Scannell and John Burke.

In the late fifties the clinical emphasis was on closed operations for mitral stenosis and the development of satisfactory mitral standby procedures, which permitted conversion of a closed to an open procedure if conditions warranted. These efforts were finally rounded off by the addition of the transventricular dilator brought back from England by Austen. Sporadic efforts, sometimes effective, were made to correct mitral regurgitation. In contrast, a series of valvuloplasties for calcific aortic stenosis had greater clinical rewards. After a formidable early mortality, more than a hundred of these taxing procedures were carried out.

By 1962 the cardiac surgical service had an operating room assigned to its use, a resident assigned from the general surgical roster, special recovery room facilities, and, perhaps most helpful of all, the special effort by the Department of Anesthesia: Briggs, Andersen, Henry Bendixen, and Hallowell. Myron B. Laver is worthy of particular mention. He joined Anesthesia in 1958, concentrating his efforts in the cardiac field from 1961 on. He added a special dimension in organizing the blood gas laboratory, bringing his considerable biochemical and physiologic talents to bear (see page 310). He left the MGH in September 1979 to return home to Switzerland; he died in 1982. His loss and the premature death of John Bland were misfortunes the department could ill afford.

By 1963 the average case load approximated three open heart procedures a week for an annual total of 150. Given the type of patient accepted for operation—usually at severe risk—and the state of the art, the operative mortality, though high, was acceptable.

The Period from 1963 to 1970.

The sixties were critical to the development of cardiac surgery as a specialty. The stage was set for the return of Austen to a full-time position in the cardiovascular laboratory and to a position of clinical responsibility after a productive clinical year in Leeds and London and two years at the National Heart Institute of the National Institutes of Health.

Austen obtained excellent funding for the tremendous expansion of the cardiac research laboratory. Major projects included studies to improve the myocardial protection of the heart, investigations related to the metabolic and physiologic changes during cardiopulmonary bypass, and the development of special bypass techniques. One of the most important projects was the early cooperative study with AVCO by Austen and Mortimer Buckley in the development of the intra-aortic balloon pump, a form of circulatory support that was to achieve major significance in the next decade, the age of the coronary bypass.

During the mid- and late-sixties a number of individuals with special interest and competence in cardiac surgery were recruited by Austen to this effort, notably Buckley, Eldred Mundth, and Willard Daggett. They were all graduates of the General Surgical Residency here; all had special qualifications and experience elsewhere. The clinical load rapidly expanded from 150 to 500 open heart procedures annually by 1970, and by 1980 it was to top 1,000 operations per year.

The clinical emphasis during the sixties was primarily on acquired valvular heart disease. Prosthetic valve replacement came into its own, but there were increasing numbers of patients with complicated congenital defects; Buckley accepted this special challenge, and Allan Goldblatt was appointed as pediatric cardiologist to help with the load carried so long and effectively by Allan Friedlich.

Just as the expansion of the cardiac surgical research laboratory led to a succession of research fellows, so too the tremendous expansion of the clinical load led to the assignment of a sufficient number of residents from the surgical roster. This culminated in 1971 with the appointment of Douglas Behrendt as the first chief resident in Cardiac Surgery.

Quite clearly the surgical effort required and received the support of the Department of Anesthesia and, equally important, the Nursing Service under Mary Macdonald, in two notable areas: the regionalization of cardiac surgical patients to Warren-Baker 12 in 1968 and the development of an adequate surgical intensive care unit specifically targeted to cardiac surgical care.

The 1970s: The Age of the C.A.B.G.*.

The decade opened with several major changes in the cardiac surgical staff. Scannell, after some 20 years of clinical involvement, gravitated back to general thoracic surgery and also to undergraduate teaching, though he continued as consultant to the now clearly defined cardiac surgical service. His efforts were recognized by election to the presidency of the American Association for Thoracic Surgery in 1978, a position formerly held by Churchill in 1949 and Sweet in 1961—as well as by Sam Robinson (1923), Wyman Whittemore (1930), and Frederick T. Lord (1932) of this hospital.

Austen, having put the cardiovascular laboratory into proper shape and led the clinical effort to its phenomenal growth, took on the responsibility, in April of 1969, of chief of the General Surgical Services and the Churchill Professorship of Surgery. Buckley and Mundth were appointed co-chiefs of the Cardiac Surgical Unit. Mundth accepted the position of chairman of Cardio-Thoracic Surgery at Hahnemann Medical School in Philadelphia in 1976, and Buckley was named chief at that time. Daggett played a major role throughout.

The impact of coronary reconstructive procedures was explosive. The clinical challenges came thick and fast: emergency revascularizations, pre- and postoperative circulatory support (the product of the earlier studies of Austen and Buckley with AVCO noted above), the management of major cardiovascular problems of thoracic aneurysms, resection of myocardial infarction and its con-

---

*C.A.B.G. stands for Coronary Artery Bypass Graft. Surgeons usually refer to these operations as "cabbages."

sequences—all this against a background of multiple valve replacements, often in patients who required coronary revascularization as well. And there was also the ongoing challenge of complicated congenital defects.

The impact of coronary reconstructive surgery required a major expansion of the cardiac catheterization laboratory, the angiography facilities, the cardiologic staff, and all surgical facilities. On the national scene, the MGH assumed a leadership role, and, in a sense, the election of Austen to the presidency of the American Heart Association in 1977–1978 was a measure of this; the position is rarely held by a surgeon.

The dedication of the resident staff at the MGH is too easily taken for granted. The development of cardiac surgery at this hospital depended upon it. For the past decade they were responsible for the day-to-day management of the patients on this unit and the education and training of assistant residents under them.

Austen contributed this additional observation:

The remarkable development of cardiac surgery at the MGH has been due to many individuals. I would like to mention particularly the outstanding efforts of Dr. Scannell in the early years—getting the whole cardiac surgical effort going in the late forties and early fifties and struggling with the early high risk cases—and doing the job with minimal resources. I would also like to emphasize the outstanding quality of the cardiac program today; under Buckley's leadership, and with the outstanding contributions of Dr. Willard Daggett, Dr. Cary Atkins, and others, the cardiac surgical unit can be justifiably proud of its national and international reputation, its excellent clinical results, and its outstanding resident education program.

Gastroenterological Unit

RONALD A. MALT

Three traditions in gastroenterological surgery at the MGH flourished simultaneously in the last decade of Churchill's tenure. First there were the great clinicians, not too different from English consultant surgeons. These were Arthur W. Allen, Leland McKittrick, and Richard H. Sweet; all maintained large practices from Beacon Hill, Back Bay, or Brookline offices, and each was always assisted by at least one board-certified graduate of the MGH surgical residency who was serving an apprenticeship for about five years until he was granted admitting privileges of his own. In addition to the early morning rounds and other visits to patients by the surgical resident assigned to his team, the private assistant made rounds morning and night, scrubbed with the senior surgeons on nearly every case, and was responsible for dealing with most telephone inquiries from postoperative patients and their families.

Because of their natural genius, their control of many surgical beds, and their capacity to work to the limit by reason of a personal assistant as well as a senior surgical resident who served as a second assistant at the operating table, the great clinicians never were slowed by the hesitancy of assisting residents who were just learning to operate. Thus Allen, McKittrick, and Sweet could gain enormous experience and rapidly examine new methods developed during this era of burgeoning techniques. Since their intuition and their command of English were superb, they distilled and disseminated the essence of this vast experience with authority and were obviously recognized figures in the national and international world of surgery.

With the opening of the Warren Building in 1956 a second group of surgeons, including Marshall K. Bartlett, Claude E. Welch, Gordon A. Donaldson, and Grant V. Rodkey, moved their offices from the Back Bay to work geographically full-time at the hospital, all without personal assistants. For the next quarter century they provided the direct role models for hundreds of residents and shaped their surgical judgment and techniques by example and direct instruction. They, too, published widely, conservatively assessing the hospital's experience with the diseases of the gastrointestinal tract. In addition, however, Bartlett, with Horatio Rogers, began the system of follow-up for end-results in patients with gastrointestinal diseases; Bartlett started the weekly gastrointestinal rounds; and he helped develop the antral exclusion-vagotomy operation for peptic ulcer, a forerunner of today's operations. Welch, Donaldson, and Rodkey were innovative in devising safe methods of gastric and colonic surgery; for example, tube duodenostomy for a safety valve in closure of the difficult duodenal stump after gastrectomy has probably saved more lives than any other adjunct to gastric surgery. Subsequently, Bartlett became vice-chairman of the American Board of Surgery, Welch president of the American Surgical Association and of the American College of Surgeons, Donaldson president of the New England Surgical Society, and Rodkey president of the Massachusetts Medical Society. Bartlett also organized the Surgical Associates, the model for all subsequent departmental group practices at the MGH.

The third movement came from younger men developed wholly under Churchill's influence. These were the forward phalanx introducing laboratory science into gastrointestinal surgery. After studying endocrine physiology with C. N. H. Long at Yale, William V. McDermott, Jr., reignited research on the mechanism of hepatic encephalopathy as a result of observing with Raymond D. Adams, chief of Neurology, that intermittent coma in a noncirrhotic patient with a portacaval shunt was exacerbated by eating meat and was associated with a high level of ammonia in the blood. Until he left in 1963 to become Cheever Professor of Surgery and chief of the Harvard Service at the Boston City Hospital and subsequently at the New England Deaconness Hospital, McDermott carried out a series of historic investigations on clinical and metabolic aspects of portasystemic shunting for the treatment of bleeding esophageal varices.

William R. Waddell, who later became chairman of the Department of Surgery at the University of Colorado, was interested in gastric physiology, surgery, and nutrition, and received his basic science training at the Harvard School of Public Health. On the one hand he was a pioneer in developing the use of fat emulsions to supplement nutrition; on the other, he worked with Bartlett in investigating antral exclusion and vagotomy for peptic ulcer. Although rare in other hospitals, this collaboration of a nominal full-time academician with a full-time practitioner in a laboratory project is commonplace at the MGH and is one of the secrets of its surgical strength.

Returning from a postgraduate year working with John Lawrence and Melvin Calvin, the Nobel Laureate at Berkeley, George L. Nardi divided his research and clinical activities among gastrointestinal, endocrine, and burn surgery. Using the radioisotope methods he learned in Berkeley, he devised methods of measuring hepatic blood flow and applied them to a number of surgical problems, including those that interested McDermott. The natural derivative of these was an interest in cardiac surgery, such that Nardi became one of the first to perform an emergency coronary endarterectomy to resuscitate a patient with an acute myocardial infarction. He subsequently became vice-president of the American Board of Surgery and of the Society for Surgery of the Alimentary Tract and president of the Collegium Internationale Chirurgiae Digestivae.

With his knowledge of epidemiology and statistics, Benjamin A. Barnes collaborated with Glenn E. Behringer, Earle W. Wilkins, Jr., and Frank C. Wheelock in some of the early studies that brought the rigor of modern day statistics to the study of common surgical diseases, such as appendicitis and hernia.

As a result of the wide scope of Churchill's system of surgical education, even a full-time vascular surgeon like Robert S. Shaw turned his attention to gastrointestinal matters. Shaw's penchant for innovation led to the discovery that acute embolism to the superior mesenteric artery need not be fatal if the embolus could be removed and blood flow to the mesenteric artery distribution restored before intestinal necrosis occurred. The same principle was later applied to the treatment of chronic mesenteric ischemia or so-called intestinal angina.

After patterns of cooperation among the geographic full-time practitioners and the academics began to be established and identification of interests began to emerge, there was a period of consolidation and progress before a younger group of surgeons was appointed to the staff. When Churchill suggested to Ronald A. Malt upon completion of his surgical residency in 1962 that he should go to MIT to learn about molecular biology, neither of them was certain what it was. Going to the MIT laboratory for two years after operating chiefly on vascular and thoracic patients at the MGH in the mornings and returning to finish hospital business in the evening, Malt came back to the MGH as a full-time clinician in 1964, while using a laboratory offered by Oliver Cope and with a long-term goal of trying to induce regeneration in mammalian organs, just as one can cause new limbs to grow in salamanders with amputated arms and legs. Although his initial model was compensatory hypertrophy of the kidney, an overall interest in regeneration naturally led to the problem of liver regeneration after partial resection and hence to studies of hepatic and colonic carcinogenesis and to a concern with the liver as a clinical subject, a point of particular concern since McDermott had just left for the City Hospital. Paul S. Russell, then chief of Surgery, appointed Malt chief of the newly constituted Liver Unit, and subsequently W. Gerald Austen extended the scope of responsibility so that the Liver Unit became the Gastroenterological Surgery Unit.

On the clinical side within that new division, Malt continued to develop the surgery of portal hypertension and to deal with increasingly frequent major hepatic resections and biliary reconstructions in an era in which the surgery was made considerably safer by reason of the advances in anesthesia, blood bank technology to provide various coagulation factors, and intensive care facilities that had not been available to an earlier generation. Stephen E. Hedberg added the new techniques of fiberoptic endoscopy to his practice of general surgery. Leslie W. Ottinger developed areas of special expertise in the surgery of hiatal hernia and the pancreas while simultaneously directing the residency education program. Ashby C. Moncure and Edwin L. Carter became known as outstanding general surgeons with considerable interest in gastrointestinal disease. The last members of the staff in general surgery trained under the Churchillian influence, all members of this group maintained active practices in vascular and oncologic surgery—and some of them in thoracic surgery as well.

Need for a continuing input of young men naturally developed as the older ones turned to clinical applications of their investigative interests. In 1970 Josef E. Fischer took up the studies of hepatic encephalopathy that had lain dormant since McDermott's departure and applied to them the new technology in neurotransmitter biochemistry. He also established the Nutritional Support Unit (Hyperalimentation), making it possible for patients who could not eat to be nourished with abundant supplies of carbohydrates, proteins, vitamins, and minerals through a large vein. After Fischer's departure to become professor and chief of Surgery at the University of Cincinnati in 1978, these activities were brought back within the general scope of the Gastroenterological Surgery Unit, and emphasis was given to using the natural intestinal tract whenever possible, reserving the use of parenteral nutrition for patients who could be nourished in no other way.

At about the same time as Fischer's appointment, Andrew L. Warshaw began his laboratory and clinical investigations of the abnormal physiology in acute pancreatitis. Although principally concentrating their efforts on oncologic surgery, William C. Wood and Alfred M. Cohen continued research and clinical activities in gastroenterologic cancer and taught effectively at gastrointestinal rounds. Michael N. Margolies combined clinical gastrointestinal surgery and teaching with studies on the chemical sequences of antibodies in the medical cardiology laboratories. Andre J. Ouellette, a biochemist, developed into a scientific leader with unique talents to head many projects on the molecular biology of regenerating organs. Nancy L. R. Bucher, the leading figure in hepatic regeneration, joined the division after closure of the Huntington Laboratories where she had worked for nearly four decades.

Not the least of the progress in gastroenterological surgery during the decade beginning in 1970 was recognition that nurses could take considerably more responsibility than they had before. The first such instance was the appointment of an enterostomal therapist. Although many English hospitals and a few in America had provided departments to help people with colostomies, ileostomies, and urostomies to manage their new conduits in a way that was compatible with a productive life, the MGH was slow to adopt this practice. Ultimately, however, permission was granted for one nurse to be trained at the Cleveland Clinic as an enterostomal therapist. As expected, the demand for a second nurse was almost instant. Patients with stomas received technical and emotional support as never before.

Thoracic Unit

HERMES C. GRILLO AND EARLE W. WILKINS, JR.

In the period between the mid-thirties and mid-fifties thoracic surgery was pioneered at the MGH most notably by Edward D. Churchill with, later, conspicuous technical contributions by Richard H. Sweet. The international community recognized Churchill for contributions such as the introduction into the

United States of pericardiectomy for constrictive pericarditis, the initial work on the concept of segmental resection (with Ronald Belsey), the excision of pulmonary metastasis (with J. Dellinger Barney), and the application of lobectomy to the problem of carcinoma of the lung. Sweet attained prominence with the successful accomplishment (with Churchill) of single-stage esophagectomy, extension to supra-aortic esophagectomy for carcinoma, azygo-pulmonary shunt (with Edward Bland) which antedated direct mitral valve surgery, and the standardization of thymectomy. J. Gordon Scannell contributed to the description of the definitive surgical anatomy of the lung (working with Boyden in Minnesota), and Edward Benedict pioneered in thoracic endoscopy.

During the years of World War II Sweet carried the clinical load of thoracic surgery. Partly as a consequence of necessity in that era of abbreviated residency training, a thoracic residency position was established in late 1943 and filled, successively, by Emerson Drake, Rodolfo Herrera, and Charles Findley. But the concept of thoracic surgery as a specialty, or even as a subdivision of general surgery, was not acceptable to Churchill, and the position was therefore abandoned upon his return from the war in 1946. It bears mentioning here only as the early forerunner of the distinct general thoracic surgical unit established a quarter century later, which eventually had its own chief surgical resident.

The decade of the fifties witnessed the achievement of national and international prominence for Sweet. Always the master of surgical technique, he was the preeminent teacher of surgery for many of the residents of the time. A founding member of the Board of Thoracic Surgery, he ultimately became its chairman. His recognition as the authority on surgery of the esophagus—perhaps worldwide—commanded attention at surgical meetings and in the operating room, which was usually filled with American and foreign visitors. In 1961 he was elected president of the American Association for Thoracic Surgery, but his death in January 1962 prevented his presiding at the annual meeting that spring. The plaque on the wall outside the Sweet Room reads, "Here are memorialized those attributes of a great surgeon: maturity of judgment, dexterity of hand, devotion in teaching and serenity in crisis."

With the departure of the two internationally acclaimed thoracic surgical giants—Churchill and Sweet—the failure of definition of the field at the MGH, and the diversion of Scannell's efforts into the development of cardiac surgery, general thoracic surgery continued a holding pattern at best. However, in the early sixties MGH surgeons (Earle Wilkins, Jr., John Head, and John Burke) demonstrated the efficacy of the excision of pulmonary metastases with cumulative survival equivalent to that achieved in the treatment of primary lung carcinoma. This was one of the earlier efforts in a trend that has now become worldwide. Wilkins, L. Henry Edmunds, Jr., and Benjamin Castleman of Pathology defined the characteristics and curability of thymoma, evaluating the factors of malignancy and myasthenia. With meticulous attention to the pre- and postoperative management of patients with myasthenia gravis, and with the help of the Respiratory Intensive Care Unit in the postoperative care of these patients, Wilkins and Head improved the technique of thymectomy for this disease, along with its management, and achieved 100 percent survival. Colon bypass for surgical replacement of the esophagus was introduced at the MGH by George Nardi and carried on with refinements in technique, including evaluation of the mesenteric arterial blood supply by arteriography by Wilkins.

The period also saw initial investigations into the anatomic possibilities for tracheal resection and reconstruction by Hermes C. Grillo. This work was carried from the laboratory into successful clinical application. The coincidental appearance of postintubation lesions of the trachea—a consequence of the success of the Respiratory Unit—led to the application of these surgical techniques to the successful treatment of such tracheal lesions. Laboratory studies by Grillo and Joel D. Cooper, then a resident in Surgery, contributed early to the definition of the etiology of these lesions and to the evolution of methods to prevent them. Henning Pontoppidan and Bennie Geffin of the Department of Anesthesia contributed to the latter studies, joining with Grillo and Cooper in the development of the low-pressure, large-volume tracheal tube cuff.

Pulmonary surgery for suppuration and tuberculosis faded during this era. Carcinoma of the lung became the dominant indication for pulmonary investigation and surgery. Treatment of carcinoma of the lung evolved selectively during these years with the introduction of surgical staging procedures and the development of close working relationships with pulmonary radiology under the direction of Reginald Greene. Scannell and Wilkins continued an ongoing and scholarly evaluation of the management of lung cancer at the MGH, begun years earlier by Churchill and Sweet. Grillo, Wilkins, and Jack Greenberg produced one of the first reports to demonstrate clearly the curability of carcinoma of the lung invading the chest wall.

General thoracic surgery was finally established as a specialized clinical unit in the General Surgical Services at Austen's direction in 1969, and Grillo was named chief of the unit. In 1975, in response to external requirements, a formal cardiothoracic surgical training program was instituted, involving the combined efforts of the Cardiac Surgical Unit and the new General Thoracic Surgical Unit. The residency program is recognized as one of the best in the United States, and in the seventies the General Thoracic Surgical Unit re-achieved the international prominence that thoracic surgery at the MGH formerly held. Residents are exceptionally well trained in breadth and depth; the annual postgraduate course run by the division has been a model for other programs; the clinical caseload has grown steadily despite constraints of beds, operating rooms, and other facilities; and once again American and foreign visitors crowd the operating room.

In addition to continuing contributions in pulmonary, esophageal, and mediastinal surgery, the MGH is recognized as the leading institution in the world for surgery of the trachea. Grillo has built upon earlier work and established techniques for the management of tracheal tumors, developed methods of reconstructing the carina following excision for neoplastic and inflammatory diseases, corrected acquired tracheal esophageal fistula, developed to a point of relative safety mediastinal exenteration and tracheostomy, and developed a single-stage technique for the management of low subglottic and upper tracheal stenosis.

The entire quarter century has been characterized by progress in the pre-, intra-, and postoperative management of thoracic surgical patients. The refinement of radiologic techniques of diagnosis, including interventional techniques, under Greene and his associates, and functional studies (Homayoun Kazemi and David J. Kanarek) have increased precision in approach. Anesthesia, under Roger Wilson and Henning Pontoppidan, has become remarkably methodical and safe.

Austen has viewed developments in the unit with satisfaction. "General thoracic surgery has indeed returned to its previous eminence at the MGH," he commented upon reading this summary. "This was accomplished in the decade of the seventies by Dr. Grillo and his associates, Drs. Scannell, Wilkins, and Ashby C. Moncure. The thoracic unit is recognized as a leader in all areas of clinical thoracic surgery and is especially prominent in surgery of the trachea as well as pre- and postoperative management of the thoracic surgical patient."

The reemerging stature of the MGH was demonstrated in the seventies by the leadership positions in professional associations held by MGH surgeons: by Scannell, first as a director of the American Board of Thoracic Surgery and then, in 1977–1978, as president of the American Association for Thoracic Surgery—the fourth from the MGH to hold this position, after Wyman Whittemore, Churchill, and Sweet; by Grillo as a director of the board and chairman of the Liaison Committee for Thoracic Surgery of the AATS; and by Wilkins who was a representative on the Advisory Council for Cardiothoracic Surgery for the American College of Surgeons.

Vascular Unit

R. CLEMENT DARLING

The Vascular Unit's ancestor, the Peripheral Vascular Clinic, was officially established at the MGH in 1928 as a special assignment for disorders of the peripheral circulation. Arthur W. Allen, then a visiting surgeon, was named its chief. It was the first clinic of its kind in the United States, unique because it was organized and run by surgeons whereas such clinics in other institutions were medical clinics with surgeons acting as consultants. Allen immediately gathered around him a group of bright and dedicated young surgeons including Leland S. McKittrick, James C. White, Reginald A. Smithwick, and Henry H. Faxon. Two years later Robert R. Linton and John B. Sears joined the clinic; Claude E. Welch became a member in 1934.

In addition to discharging clinical functions, the group conducted vascular rounds each Thursday morning from eight to nine. These started as ward rounds with bedside teaching for residents and medical students. After World War II, however, when visitors from foreign countries swelled the ranks of attendance, vascular rounds were removed to the surgical amphitheater in the White Building. There they have remained a Thursday morning ritual for the past 30 years.

Allen resigned as chief of the clinic in 1940, and leadership passed to McKittrick. (See Chapter 22 for biographic sketches.) When McKittrick resigned in 1946, Linton was appointed to the position. Without question, it was Robert Linton who led vascular surgery at the MGH to the prominent status that it enjoys in the 1980s. One of America's pioneers in blood vessel surgery, he became the premier vascular surgeon at the MGH; essentially, his professional biography comprises the development of the specialty during his 30 years as a surgeon. (An abbreviated account of his career also appears in Chapter 22.)

In the interest of historic order, however, it is instructive to step back even farther in time, if only briefly, to consider the men who preceded and influenced Linton. He drew consciously upon the examples set by Harvey Cushing and Amory Codman. Like Cushing, Linton became a creator in a new field of surgery, developed an eye for perfection, and was seriously committed to sketching his operative procedures in great detail. Like Codman, he followed in conscientious fashion all patients upon whom he had operated, a fact reflected in his multiple publications attesting to the long-term success or failure of his arterial reconstructions.

The influence of the peripatetic John Homans on Linton was more direct. Homans left the MGH to work at Johns Hopkins, fell under Cushing's spell, and settled in Boston at the Brigham in 1913. His former offices were adjacent to Linton's, and I was constantly reminded as I worked that I was sitting at John Homans' desk. Prior to Linton's 1973 *Atlas of Vascular Surgery* Homans' 1939 contribution was one of the few volumes on circulatory disease to have originated in the Boston medical community. The work contained a short paragraph that amused Linton a great deal. Homans had written: "A stiff drink of whiskey or any strong liquor is, except for the corruption of the individual, an admirable simple treatment for an intermittent limp—some even walk twice as far!" When quizzed by his students how much of this remedy one should take, his answer came back in his characteristic lisp, "Well, any damn fool knows what a stiff drink is!" As much as anybody, Homans stimulated—often through disagreement—Linton's interests and clinical applications of venous surgery.

A non-MGH surgeon similarly animated Linton in his pursuit of arterial reconstructive techniques. One Sunday morning in August 1938 Robert E. Gross, then a 33-year-old assistant, took a dying child to the operating room at the Children's Hospital, ligated a patent ductus, and changed the way surgeons approached large blood vessels. Gross's repairs of coarctation of the aorta in 1945 opened a new era in blood vessel replacement in 1949 with the introduction of arterial homografts as arterial substitutes. Though at different hospitals, Gross and Linton enjoyed a fine working relationship, and it was Linton who later applied the use of arterial homografts for peripheral reconstruction. It was not until 1958 that such homografts were abandoned in favor of the use of autogenous tissues. Of the few professional disappointments that Linton had, the ultimate discovery that atheromatous degeneration and lack of incorporation of arterial homografts occurred in the human—in contrast to findings in the animal laboratory—was his greatest. Most of these patients developed complications, and the homografts eventually had to be removed. But in typical Linton fashion, he turned this misadventure around and in the next decade became world renowned for the use of autogenous tissue with extensive aorto-iliac-femoral endarterectomy, a procedure that often took eight to ten hours to complete. He also became the leading proponent of the use of reversed autogenous saphenous vein for bypassing femoropopliteal occlusive disease.

Linton carried these rich professional influences and experiences with him into the MGH vascular clinic and shared them with colleagues and trainees. His contributions were in large part the result of interaction with these men. McKittrick's influence left its mark as well. One of his assistants, Frank C. Wheelock, followed in his mentor's steps and contributed greatly to the vascular clinic. So, too, did Robert S. Shaw. The two men produced a 5 percent mortality in aortic aneurysm resection in the first group of patients reported from the MGH—an extraordinary record. Wheelock was the first to employ the French idea of end-to-side anastomosis for bypassing occluded superficial femoral arteries. His subsequent series of femoropopliteal saphenous vein grafts in diabetics with a 98 percent success rate has never been surpassed. Both he and Shaw gave unselfishly of their time in the clinic and on vascular visits on the ward service and in all likelihood can claim equal share to the honor of having trained more general surgeons in the techniques of vascular surgery than any two individuals in New England.

The vascular clinic also had a research component. Under Linton's aegis, Fiorindo A. Simeone developed the first peripheral vascular laboratory at the MGH in the late 1940s. The laboratory was principally designed to study the effect of alteration of the sympathetic nervous system in a constant temperature room. Leadership of the laboratory passed to John J. Cranley in 1950. With his departure for Cincinnati two years later, Shaw was appointed to take charge of the laboratory while Linton continued as chief of the clinic and ran a busy private practice.

The course of research in the vascular laboratory was, however, a somewhat discontinuous one, particularly from a clinical aspect. A singular event in the late sixties altered its nature. A chance meeting between Jeffrey K. Raines, a doctoral candidate in engineering at MIT, and this author, then a junior assistant to Linton, resulted in many hours of clinical laboratory research in order to perfect what is now known as a pulse volume recorder. The results of 5,000 clinical applications were presented to the Society for Vascular Surgery in 1971. Shortly thereafter, Raines and I submitted a proposal for a clinical vascular laboratory which W. Gerald Austen, chief of the General Surgical Services, strongly supported. The facility was initially situated in quarters adjoining the Bigelow amphitheater and started with a budget of about $12,000, much of which was spent on removing a toilet, two wash basins, and other renovations. The laboratory gained popularity under the direction of Raines who by then had acquired his Ph.D. Despite many dire predictions, the laboratory had proved itself a complete success by 1975. When Raines left for the Miami Heart Institute, William M. Abbott took over the laboratory, which had become an integral part of the operation of the vascular service. Lower extremity pulse volume recordings and ankle pressure before and after exercise, venous studies to rule out deep venous thrombosis, and carotid noninvasive studies were immediate successes. Thanks to the original instrumentation developed in the 1970s, the MGH laboratory served as the prototype for a great many laboratories throughout the United States and a good share of the world. Those who had worked with Linton regretted that he had not lived to see the realization of his visions of the ever-growing field of noninvasive laboratory studies.

No chronicle of vascular surgery at the MGH would be complete without recording at least the most prominent among a series of innovations accomplished during the period under review.

Because of the large clinical load of arterial reconstructive surgery done at the MGH, a considerable number of vascular publications ensued. Linton emphasized prevention of infection, but ingenious techniques to manage well-established infections in vascular grafts were first described in this hospital. The best known is probably the use of a bypass graft through the obturator foramen in the pelvis to allow excision and drainage of infected graft in the groin. Shaw, aided by Arthur E. Baue, popularized this potentially lifesaving technique.

Both visiting as well as resident staff have a right to take great pride in the accomplishments of the vascular surgical teaching program. Though Linton and Shaw had had survivors of elective abdominal aortic aneurysmectomies, the first patient to survive a ruptured aneurysm was a 72-year-old watchman who was operated on by Jack E. Tetirick on the West Surgical Service. Despite a massive rupture and a period of respiratory and renal failure, the patient recovered and probably represents the first survivor of a ruptured aneurysm whose aneurysmectomy was performed by a surgeon in training. (assistant: Richard Cleveland; date: Sunday, June 14, 1956.)

The first successful mesenteric artery embolectomy reported was carried out by Robb H. Rutledge on October 19, 1956. This set the stage for a procedure that had been previously unsuccessful without small bowel resection. Shaw, who had published the first successful case with Rutledge, continued with his pioneer work in vascular lesions of the gastrointestinal tract and in particular the treatment of acute and chronic thrombosis of the mesenteric arteries. He performed the first mesenteric artery endarterectomy for intestinal angina.

Linton felt that all general surgery was in fact vascular surgery and this, in his mind, included cardiac surgery. On April 7, 1961, he, with this author, was the first at the MGH to implant an internal cardiac pacemaker on a patient who had a serious heart block and was awaiting surgery for an abdominal aortic aneurysm. A second successful case was carried out on September 11, 1961, on a patient who was later paraded before the surgical grand rounds where the front row was filled primarily by thoracic and cardiac surgeons. Needless to say, Linton enjoyed gently prodding E. D. Churchill a bit for not having done this sooner.

An MGH surgical resident led a historic arm replant on May 23, 1962. Ronald A. Malt coordinated the operative team responsible for the first successful reimplantation of an arm, on a 12-year-old Somerville Little League pitcher named Everett Knowles. Many were involved in this major surgical feat which demanded coordination of a team with diverse specialties in a highly complex procedure. What made this possible was the rigorous, versatile training program based on the philosophies of Churchill who commonly pointed out that "the way to handle a situation that you have never met before is to reduce it to its simplest terms and take everything in steps, conquering each step individually." The boy with the "golden arm" owed that arm to an institution, its trainees, and the personal attention of Shaw, whose technical ability made a success of the vascular anastomosis. Twenty years later, when many of his doctors had passed through their training to work in other parts of the world, Everett Knowles remains well and productive—a living symbol of what surgery in general, and vascular surgery in particular, can accomplish.

In 1972, under this author's supervision, Bruce J. Brener, then a vascular fellow, and Raines started a clinical study of autotransfusion. While hemodilution and then reinfusion of blood had been previously carried out, and while Charles E. Huggins had championed the use of frozen blood at the MGH, our team, using the Raines modification of roller pumps and a multiple filtration system, performed over 150 abdominal aortic reconstructions without the significant morbidity commonly associated with autotransfusion. The Raines modification using systemic anticoagulation proved to be a significant step forward in the management of patients undergoing aortic reconstruction. However, because of the excellence of the MGH blood bank, much of the enthusiasm was dampened; further modifications in the interest of cost effectiveness are still in process.

Austen appended the following note to this account:

Vascular surgery has had a great tradition at the MGH, and this hospital has made major contributions to the field. Linton, Shaw, and Darling have each in turn made their marks and kept the MGH at the forefront. In 1978 Dr. William Abbott was appointed chief of the newly created Vascular Surgery Unit. Drs. Abbott, Darling, David Brewster, Ashby Moncure, and others have continued to keep the vascular surgery program outstanding academically and clinically.

Burn Unit

JOHN F. BURKE

The treatment of burns at the MGH during this period was, as in all other categories of medicine, a continued building upon established methods together with the development of new modalities of treatment made possible by the ever-widening fund of biologic information available to clinicians oriented toward research as well as treatment. There was, however, a difference: Because of the unprecedented increase in information relevant to the management of acutely ill burn patients—largely due to the research support by the National Institutes of Health and specifically to the development of several methods of partial control of burn wound infections by the Army Institute of Surgical Research and by Washington University in St. Louis—the stage was set for a rapid development in the field of burn treatment. The MGH took full advantage of these opportunities by building on previous work done at the hospital, particularly that of Oliver Cope and Francis Moore in the areas of fluid resuscitation and primary excision of moderate-sized burn, to develop a different concept of treatment based on prompt removal of all dead tissue and immediate repair of the wound. These theories completely changed the philosophy and methods of burn treatment and now routinely govern the treatment of burned patients. They were, to a large extent, conceived and demonstrated effective at the MGH in the period covered by this history. Beginning in 1968 the Shriners Burns Institute (SBI), Boston Unit, played a major part in developing these modes of treatment for children (see Chapter 31). They have been widely accepted throughout the developed world as the optimal, basic management of burn injury.

Austen, who has viewed the evolution of this specialty with great satisfaction, noted that "the MGH has certainly been one of the world leaders in the development of new and more effective burn care. Fundamental research and clinical investigations have been combined to achieve tremendous advances—a major decrease in mortality, a major improvement in functional results of treatment, and a very significant reduction in hospital stay. Further progress is, of course, needed and will surely build on this remarkable period of activity."

Work directly related to the developments at the hospital began in 1957–1958 with the establishment of a laboratory investigating nonspecific host defense and methods to prevent surgical infection, under the direction of John F. Burke. The burned patient poses a remarkably difficult problem in infection prevention, and it soon became clear that control of burn wound infection was a problem of defective resistance to bacterial invasion related very largely to the burn eschar which, at that time, was allowed to remain on the patient for weeks until it separated spontaneously. This group reasoned that the only way to prevent infection was to remove the dead tissue soon after the burn injury before bacterial growth could take place. Further, it had long been recognized that immediate wound closure with skin or a skin substitute was essential to prevent an open wound. With these premises as a basis, an overall plan was evolved in 1959–1960 to develop a system of burn care based on prompt excision of necrotic tissue and immediate closure of the wound after injury for all sizes and complexities of burn injury—a development of the Cope-Moore ideas of the late 1940s. The work began with excision of small burns, concentrating on operative techniques and methods to control bleeding. Local hypothermia and CO_2 lasers were examined and discarded, and the initial work on an artificial skin started, stemming from our experience with cadaver allograft. By 1963 a clear plan of action to achieve the goal of a clinically feasible system of burn care on these bases had been developed, and the initial phases of research were well underway. At this time the MGH burn unit was on White 12, staffed by the general surgical visiting staff and the East and West surgical services.

In 1963 the program developed for burn care at the MGH evolved into a specific work plan made up of separate projects all coordinated to make burn treatment safer by reducing morbidity and mortality and more effective by shortening the hospital stay and improving the functional and cosmetic results of treatment. Since the fundamental philosophy of treatment was to be changed, new supporting methods had to be developed. The separate projects were (1) development of preoperative, operative, and postoperative techniques for prompt excision and immediate grafting for all sizes and complexities of burn injury; (2) development of a frozen skin bank to ensure a stable supply of cadaver skin allograft; (3) development of a protective environment in which the burned patient could be nursed to protect against bacterial cross-infection and reduce the risk of infection, later called the Bacteria Controlled Nursing Unit, BCNU; (4) development of a physiologically acceptable artificial skin; (5) development of a method of immunosuppression for massively burned patients to prolong skin allograft survival long enough to allow sufficient autograft donor sites to become available; and (6) exploration of the relationship between loss of host resistance and the metabolic alterations of burn injury in order to provide seriously injured burn patients the optimal nutritional support. These projects were designed to answer all the recognized problems whose solution was necessary for the successful clinical use of excision and immediate wound closure. Although they were conceived as a coordinated plan and initiated at approximately the same time, each was pursued with varying intensity depending on what was needed to solve current clinical problems as the program developed.

The present state of patient care techniques in the operative as well as the perioperative period represents a continuous process which started in the late fifties. As ability to deal with larger and larger burns progressed, further techniques were evolved. Of particular note is the "quilting" technique developed by Glenn Behringer in 1976 for stabilizing a graft on the wound bed, preventing graft loss by patient movement in the postoperative period. This allowed the back and front of a patient to be grafted at the same time and avoided the necessity of nursing the patient on his stomach when the back was grafted, making his convalescence far safer and more comfortable.

Also in the early sixties Ann Wight (later Ann Wight Phillips), working with

Cope, Raker, and Quinby, established the importance of inhalation injury to the overall problem of burn injury. Before her work the syndrome of pulmonary burn was not recognized in most treatment centers in the United States, although the basic principles had been outlined following the Cocoanut Grove fire.

The development of a skin bank had early priority because it held promise of a temporary method of wound closure allowing larger burns to be excised. The bank was also a direct outcome of research using allograft in the prevention of infection and in the early work on artificial skin. The major responsibility for this work was carried by Conrad Bondoc, who joined Burke's laboratory in 1963. Methods of harvesting split thickness skin, cryopreservation, storage, and operative technique were developed and perfected, making the first recorded viable frozen skin bank, which was ready to move into the Shriners Burns Institute when it developed a clinical load in 1969.

Artificial skin was recognized early in this period as the only efficient mechanism to solve the problems created by large deep burns with the inevitable shortage of donor sites for skin autografts. If large burns were to be treated in community hospital burn units, as well as in university centers, a physiologically acceptable artificial skin had to be developed. Work directly related to this achievement began in 1962 with the use of cadaver allograft altered in various ways and continued until the demonstration of clinical effectiveness in 1979–1980. From the beginning the goal was to create a material that would both close a burn wound and avoid scar formation, thus improving functional and cosmetic results. Peter Morris joined Burke's group in 1964 for two-and-a-half years and greatly accelerated the rate of research. Also in that year a series of experiments were carried out that established that it was possible to make a completely synthetic membrane that would successfully serve as an artificial skin; and, further, that collagen plus a glycosaminoglycan—not collagen alone—was the correct structural material. These experiments centered around the use of skin allograft in which all living cells had been eliminated by repeated freezing so that the nonliving but undenatured connective tissue matrix of the dermis remained intact. The years 1966 to 1973 saw slow progress in artificial skin research, for the major efforts in burn care focused on the planning and beginnings of clinical care in the Shriners Burns Institute as well as on perfecting the clinical methods required for prompt excision and immediate wound closure in patients with even the largest and most complex burns. However, what was accomplished during this period was a recognition that, although it was known what artificial skin should be made of, it had not yet been determined how to make a material out of it. To solve this problem we began to look for help at MIT in 1969. In December of that year Ioannis Yannas of the Mechanical Engineering Department at MIT called to say that he was also interested in biomaterials and that perhaps MIT and the MGH should talk. There followed a period of about two years during which the MGH and MIT groups exchanged ideas and taught each other. All the materials development leading to a successful artificial skin was carried out in Yannas' laboratory at MIT; biologic testing of these materials was carried out in Burke's laboratories at the SBI supported by an MIT-NIH grant through the MGH.

In early 1973 the basic construction of artificial skin as a bilayer membrane had been formulated, and attention was turned to studies continuing at MIT to gain further understanding of the material, its manufacture, and preparations for human studies. Human studies began in 1979 at the MGH and Shriners Burns Institute, and by 1980 there was ample clinical evidence that a successful artificial skin had been created.

The developments of a system of immunosuppression and temporary skin transplantation and of the protective patient environment called Bacteria Controlled Nursing Unit (BCNU) are intimately connected. Although it was always felt that artificial skin was the optimal solution to the problem of very extensive deep burns with limited donor sites, it was also recognized that this development would be slow in coming. Temporary transplantation was pursued as an interim solution until artificial skin was available. Collaboration with Benedict Cosimi and Paul Russell provided an immunosuppressive method that was successful in saving the lives of patients burned to an extent always fatal before.

The risk of infection in excisional burn treatment is an ever-present hazard. In order to reduce this risk, the BCNU was developed beginning in 1963, using concepts borrowed from NASA and germ-free animal technology. MIT engineers played a prominent role, and the work was supported by a grant from HEW. Much of the early effort was carried out in a makeshift laboratory on the fifth floor of the Cambridge Street garage then owned by the MGH. When the SBI was being designed, the nursing unit was ready to be included, and its subsequent clinical testing has demonstrated a remarkable decrease in cross-infection and the bacterial risk to seriously burned patients.

Work on the metabolic alterations of and optimal nutrition for burn patients began in the sixties and continues. The development of a mass spectrometry facility in the Shriners Burns Institute in 1972 allowed human studies both there and at the MGH to be carried out without risk. These studies have demonstrated the problems caused by providing excess glucose to seriously ill burned patients and have led to a marked improvement in nutritional management.

In July of 1974 Austen asked a group of general surgeons interested in acute burn care to take on the complete responsibility of MGH burn patients. Thus the Burn Unit in the Department of Surgery was created. This group, led by Burke and including Behringer, Bondoc, William C. Quinby, and John M. Head, has managed the Adult Burn Service since that time.

Endocrine Unit

CHIU-AN WANG

In January of 1926 a patient by the name of Captain Charles E. Martell was admitted to the MGH. Like all other patients of that era, he was registered at the admitting office, taken to the ward on Bulfinch 4, and greeted by the floor nurse and house pupils, as residents were called in those days; in short, no fanfare attended his admission. Little did these people know that the patient had an unusual disease and that he would become one of the famous MGH "firsts."

Martell had been referred to the MGH by Dr. DuBois of New York. A native of Somerville, Massachusetts, the patient had joined the U.S. Merchant Marines in 1918; at the time of his enlistment he was a strapping six feet, eleven inches tall and 22 years old. Eight years later he had lost seven inches in height and was suffering from eight fractures. He then came to the MGH where a team of physicians—Joseph Aub, Walter Bauer, and Fuller Albright—made the diagnosis of hyperparathyroidism. He was subsequently operated upon successfully by two of our great surgeons, E. D. Churchill and Oliver Cope. The captain had six neck operations, three at the MGH and three elsewhere; it was not until the seventh that he was successfully cured of the disease by resection of a mediastinal adenoma. His case was the first ever diagnosed preoperatively in this country as hyperparathyroidism and the first successful instance of mediastinal exploration in the world. The staff did not realize that they were dealing with a man who would ultimately occupy a unique page in the annals of surgery at the MGH.

Surgery of hyperparathyroidism has continued since Martell's day. During those years studies of the pathophysiology of hyperparathyroidism were pursued, and the anatomy of the parathyroid glands became better understood. In the Department of Surgery—chiefly through the insight and wisdom of Churchill and Cope—knowledge of the disease advanced greatly. Thus, surgeons at the MGH were superbly equipped to deal with the problems of this condition, and because of this ceaseless effort the MGH has been for years a principal center of referral for the treatment of hyperparathyroidism. By 1954 some 200 cases had been treated successfully at this hospital.

With this distinguished background it is perhaps not surprising that over the years many junior members of the MGH Department of Surgery developed interests in endocrine surgery: The late John Raker was deeply involved in studies of adrenal disorders, primarily the surgical management of pheochromocytoma; George Nardi, who has been interested in the pancreas particularly in relation to insulinoma, has contributed substantially to the understanding of this disease; Benjamin Barnes studied the electrolyte balance in metabolic disorder; and Charles Huggins did the first cryopreservation of parathyroid tissue in this country.

Since 1961 I have been privileged to work with Cope in the care of his patients with thyroid and parathyroid disorders. He encouraged me to study the anatomy of the parathyroid glands in the postmortem room. Accordingly, I became familiar with the anatomic basis of hyperparathyroidism. Cope stressed to me the importance of basic science research and interested me in the investigation of protein synthesis in hemorrhagic shock. Both of these projects proved to be invaluable in my subsequent surgical career.

In 1972, when Cope officially retired from his operating activities, Dr. Austen asked me to take charge of the endocrine surgical unit of the Department of Surgery. Endocrine surgery thus became officially recognized as a subspecialty of general surgery at the MGH. As mentioned elsewhere in this volume, Churchill had resisted the fragmentation of the Department of Surgery; he did not favor the division of the department into many subspecialties because he feared that the resident training program might be adversely affected. Austen, however, viewed the matter differently, as he himself, a cardiac surgeon, fully realized the importance of in-depth training in some highly specialized branch of surgery such as endocrine surgery. I accepted his offer to take charge of the unit as of that year.

From 1955 to 1980 there were approximately 800 additional cases of hyperparathyroidism treated at the MGH, making a total of over 1,000 cases since 1926. Patients have come from all parts of the world. The overall operative success rate is 98 percent. With the exception of the Mayo Clinic, we have the greatest number of cases of hyperparathyroidism treated surgically anywhere.

In 1977 we reported our experience with the use of a simple test, called the Density Test (or, in Europe, the Floatation Test), in the intraoperative differentiation of parathyroid hyperplasia from neoplasia. The test has proven of great diagnostic value and has gained wide popularity.

We have also cared for a large number of thyroid patients during this period. Although it has often been said that thyroidectomy is a vanishing art because a decreasing number of such procedures are being performed, thyroid disease has nevertheless remained prevalent and many patients still require surgery for a cure. In 1950 the late Edward Hamlin performed occasional needle biopsies in the Thyroid Clinic; they were then considered rare diagnostic feats, and only a few biopsies were done in a single year. Since 1955, however, the number of needle biopsies has greatly increased, and over 2,000 have been performed at the MGH since that time. With the increase in the use of needle biopsy, there has been a concomitant rise in the number of thyroidectomies at the hospital. A number of patients require surgery because they are found to have thyroid malignancies; other more fortunate patients have been spared surgery because needle biopsy has shown their disease to be benign. Presently, the Endocrine Unit performs approximately 150 to 175 thyroidectomies each year.

Austen, considering the work of the unit, commented that "one of the great pluses for endocrine surgery at the MGH has been the extraordinary strength of the Medical Endocrine Unit and the close relationship between the medical and surgical groups. This tradition dates back to the 1920s and has been particularly strong in recent years with Dr. John Potts as unit chief in medical endocrine and Dr. Wang as unit chief in surgical endocrine."

Pediatric Surgery Unit

SAMUEL H. KIM

The Pediatric Surgery Unit became a formal section of both General Surgery and the Children's Service with the appointment of W. Hardy Hendren III as pediatric surgeon. As mentioned in the section on the Children's Service, Hendren had trained in general surgery at the MGH and in pediatric surgery at the Children's Hospital in Boston under Robert E. Gross. With strong support tendered to him by Edward D. Churchill and sustained by Paul S. Russell and W. Gerald Austen, Hendren applied his outstanding skills as a clinician, operating surgeon, and teacher. Through his commitment to clinical excellence and unflagging devotion to his patients, he developed pediatric surgery at the MGH as a service with a reputation equal to that of other departments of the hospital. His desire to communicate with his referring clinicians generated sound relationships and a high sense of confidence in him as a caring physician. His imagination, attention to detail, and technical operating skill enabled him to carry out successfully congenital heart surgery as well as complicated general surgery and, then, to turn his attention to urology. It was in the latter field, with the encouragement of Wyland F. Leadbetter, chief of Urology, that Hendren began to understand and correct pediatric urologic problems that until then had a high morbidity and mortality. In the past only urinary diversion was offered for the seemingly hopeless situation associated with the megaureter syndrome. However, in 1964 Hendren accomplished the first successful megaureter reconstruction, which has since become a common procedure. Pediatric urology subsequently evolved into its own surgical specialty, and many of the innovative treatments are due to Hendren's ingenuity. His contributions to the treatment of patients with urinary diversion, urinary incontinence, exstrophy, and urogenital sinus are just some of the areas in which he has been successful.

The service enlarged in 1970 when Samuel H. Kim joined Hendren. The addition of a second clinical surgeon allowed for greater diversity and development of an increasingly larger, more active, clinical teaching service. Kim's interest in hypospadias repair and urinary reconstruction of patients with neurogenic bladders, particularly myelomeningocele patients, has been substantial. Because of a close working relationship with pediatric anesthesia and intensive care as well as strong ties with pediatric medicine, the Pediatric Surgery Unit thrived clinically, allowing for many people to visit and take back with them the innovations in children's surgery that they had seen demonstrated.

In 1973 Patricia K. Donahoe joined the staff and brought a balance to the service with her very strong interest in basic research. Donahoe trained in both pediatric surgery and basic research, and over the past ten years she has developed a research laboratory that has gained international recognition. Her interest in MIS (mullerian inhibiting substance) and its specific role in male-female differentiation has fostered the development of many cooperative clinical studies involving a number of other departments both in the hospital and at the Harvard Medical School. In addition to basic research, she has pursued her clinical interests with studies on Hirschsprung's disease and ambiguous genitalia in both the operating room and laboratory. The number of personnel in the laboratory increases each year with more pediatric surgeons, urologists, and residents spending part of their training working in this stimulating atmosphere.

Concomitant with the development of a formal Pediatric Surgery Unit, several areas of surgical subspecialty—in particular orthopedics, plastic surgery, and neurosurgery—also concentrated on the problems of young patients. These specialties are strong components of the Children's Service today.

Supported by Richard Kitz and under the direction of John F. Ryan, pediatric anesthesia grew as a separate subspecialty from an initial group of two to seven full-time pediatric anesthesiologists who are well recognized for their contributions to both clinical and basic research in anesthetic agents for pediatric patients. Without the support of pediatric anesthesia, pediatric intensive care, pediatric nursing, and other groups that have developed a pediatric subspecialization, pediatric surgery at the MGH could not be the strong, well-recognized department that it is today. "It has become a world renowned surgical program," Austen notes. "It is a broad and balanced service with a fine reputation in clinical work as well as research and education. The close working relationship between this unit and the Children's Service has been very enjoyable and very important in the development of this active pediatric surgical endeavor."

26. Gynecology

Joe Vincent Meigs

Death came suddenly to Joe Vincent Meigs in one of the ways he would have chosen. He had just delivered a lecture at an anniversary hospital symposium in Rochester, New York, on the subject of pelvic cancer and was hurrying home to share his 71st birthday dinner with his wife and children.

Joe Meigs was born in Lowell, Massachusetts, on October 24, 1892. Medicine was his heritage, for his father, uncle, and grandfather were also physicians. His preparation for Harvard Medical School, from which he graduated in 1919, began at the Lowell High School and was continued at Princeton. A lifetime interest in gynecology began with a service as a student house officer at the Free Hospital for Women during his last two years at medical school. This demanding job brought early contact with the operating room under the disciplined direction of the surgeon-in-chief, William P. Graves. No one who had this experience ever forgot it. After graduating from Medical School, Meigs served as house pupil, as residents were then called, on the East Surgical Service of the MGH from 1919 to 1921. After another year at the Free Hospital for Women as assistant to Graves—a superb teacher and technician but a hard taskmaster—he returned to the MGH as assistant surgeon to outpatients and began his private practice as assistant to George W. W. Brewster, an active surgeon at the hospital. In 1921 he married Elizabeth Wallace.

The years from 1922 to 1934 provided Meigs with an excellent opportunity to apply his newly acquired surgical training to the problems of gynecology in general and to genital cancer in particular. At that time gynecologic patients were treated on the general surgical service. With encouragement from Farrar Cobb and Lincoln Davis, he began to focus his attention on gynecologic problems; their efforts led to the establishment of the gynecologic Tumor Clinic. The knowledge and experience with cancer of the female pelvis acquired at the MGH and at the Collis P. Huntington made Meigs the logical choice for chief of the Gynecological Division of the Massachusetts State Hospital for Cancer, established at Pondville in 1927. He held this position for 30 years. The abundance of material available made it possible for him to develop new techniques and methods, and he soon came to be known as an authority on surgery for cancer of the female pelvis. With a solid background in pathology acquired by working with Frank B. Mallory and Frederic Parker, Jr., at the City Hospital, Meigs collected and reviewed all the pathologic material stored in the files of the MGH, related it to his experience at Pondville, and recorded his observations in clinical and pathologic detail in his first book, *Tumors of the Female Pelvic Organs*, published in 1934. This book, together with a steady stream of classic clinical papers, brought him wide recognition and led to membership at an early age in all the major American surgical and obstetric-gynecologic societies.

Meigs first came to know the Vincent Memorial Hospital during this period through Brewster. Founded in 1890 as a memorial to Mrs. J. R. Vincent, it had grown under its superintendent, Jean Cameron Fraser, to be an active women's hospital for acute illness and elective surgery. Meigs became its chief of staff in 1931, succeeding Anna G. Richardson, and continued in this capacity when the Vincent Hospital moved to the MGH as the Gynecology Service in 1942. This move was one of Meigs' greatest achievements. Initially, the Vincent's geographic identity consisted of 20 beds assigned to it on the surgical wards. When World War II was over, the original planning was carried out and the Vincent-Burnham Unit was built. New and adequate facilities became available for offices, laboratories, 43 semiprivate and ward service beds, an up-to-date cystoscopy room, and a conference room. It was then possible for Meigs to house his extensive private practice in one area, thereby enhancing his outstanding ability to communicate ideas to his junior colleagues and the successive generations of well-trained surgical residents who rounded out their education under his supervision. All who were exposed to him could not fail to develop a thoughtful approach to pelvic surgery with a strong feeling for anatomic exposure and respect for living tissues. Given laboratories, Meigs had the opportunity to foster and stimulate a research program with particular emphasis on refining and expanding techniques in cytology and in exploring endocrine and functional mechanisms peculiar to the field of gynecology.

Recognized as an outstanding spokesman for his specialty, who knew the value of basic surgical principles and the need of surgical specialties of all kinds to maintain a connection with general surgery, he was in constant demand to speak at medical society meetings throughout the country. His reputation reached international proportions, and he became the intimate of leading gynecologists all over the world. Sixteen foreign associations elected him to honorary fellowship; in his own country many associations were proud to have him as an active and contributing member. Three universities conferred honorary degrees upon him. Few physicians have received such honors—and certainly no gynecologist. Citations were also made by the American Cancer Society and the MGH House Pupils Association (on the hospital's 150th anniversary) for Meigs' contributions to science. In addition to his first book, Meigs also edited *The Surgical Treatment of Cancer of the Cervix* and *Progress in Gynecology* through four editions, with Somers Sturgis as coeditor.

In 1955, as he approached the statutory retirement age, Meigs resigned his positions as chief of staff at the Vincent Hospital and chief of Gynecology at the MGH; he was given emeritus status at the Harvard Medical School. His health was unimpaired, and from this time to the end of his life he dedicated himself with great personal satisfaction to a devoted following in private practice. With humble pleasure he followed the progress of a drive for funds to establish a Meigs professorship in gynecology at the Medical School for the chief of the Vincent Hospital, and early in 1962 he was guest of honor at the dinner which activated the chair named in his honor.

Friendship, devotion, affection—these words recur again and again in the paragraphs that were written about this remarkable physician, husband, father, and sportsman after his death. Unquestionably, his personal qualities were universally appealing. However, his real hold on his colleagues was established by the depth and sincerity of his interests. He was accorded respect without apparent effort on his own part, and many of his most distinguished confreres insisted that he exerted a major influence on their development. During his own career in gynecology Meigs gave repeated proof that this specialty must embrace all areas of medical knowledge and, in addition to surgery, must make use of developing techniques in the allied fields of physiology, endocrinology, anatomy, pathology, and radiology. The generosity of his interest was his greatest attribute and was recognized, consciously or unconsciously, by all his colleagues as his unique contribution. This man was great because he left his specialty in medicine far richer than he found it.

Adapted by the editors from a Memorial Minute, *Harvard University Gazette*, Vol. LIX, No. 38, June 6, 1964

The Gynecology Service, 1955–1976
HOWARD ULFELDER

Meigs was succeeded by Howard Ulfelder, a graduate of the Harvard Medical School and of the surgical training program of the MGH. His incumbency brought to an end the era of surgeon gynecologists; he was among the last physicians accredited in gynecology by the Board of Obstetrics and Gynecology without a requirement for training and examination in obstetrics. Although much expansion had taken place in the knowledge and scope of the combined specialty, particularly in nonsurgical areas such as endocrinology, perinatology, and the control of fertility, the old ways die hard. Under the terms of the original agreement between the MGH and the Vincent Hospital, the Gynecology Service remained under the overall jurisdiction of general surgery, and its residents were all on rotation from the surgical training program. Some benefit accrued to both parties—to gynecology because of the superb quality of this resident pool, and to surgery because the rotation offered one of the few opportunities for advanced trainees to demonstrate their leadership qualifications as a chief resident. As long as the Board of Obstetrics and Gynecology required a residency in an integrated program with time equally divided between the two disciplines, there was no alternative to consider.

But Ulfelder recognized the importance of keeping access to the Vincent clinical experience open to trainees interested in obstetrics and gynecology. In 1962 Ann Brace Barnes was approved as the first surgical resident assigned to gynecology. With the founding of subspecialty boards in gynecologic oncology and gynecologic endocrinology in 1974–1975 it became apparent that the training opportunities offered by the MGH Gynecology Service could integrate very successfully with the basic program offered by such institutions as the Boston Women's Hospital. This arrangement was, in fact, accomplished by James Nelson, Jr., who succeeded Ulfelder as chief in 1976.

The clinical programs during Ulfelder's administration can be characterized as those that place major emphasis on gynecologic surgery. Successful techniques and programs of management were developed for the treatment of vaginal hernias, stress urinary incontinence, and cancer of the cervix, corpus, vulva, and vagina. These were communicated not only to local students and residents but also, through postgraduate courses given in conjunction with the Medical School, to practicing gynecologists.

Ulfelder, with Langdon Parsons, edited two editions of a uniquely clear and complete atlas of gynecologic surgery. Parsons, previously at the MGH and later a member of the staff and professor at Boston University, authored with Sheldon C. Sommers an exhaustive text on gynecologic disease through several editions. Thomas Green, also of the Vincent staff and chief of Gynecology at Pondville State Cancer Hospital, wrote three editions of a popular text in gynecology. All staff members contributed extensively to specialty literature and medical meetings throughout the world.

In the 1960s the Josiah Macy Jr. Foundation offered fellowship support to encourage individuals in university training programs to enter academic obstetrics and gynecology. Four of the HMS fellows were surgical residents at the MGH, encouraged by Ulfelder. Three of those individuals now hold prestigious academic appointments elsewhere; the fourth, Ann Barnes, is assistant clinical professor at the Medical School and a staff member at MGH.

Meanwhile, the endocrine aspects of reproductive biology were explored and expanded in both clinic and laboratory, with many original contributions coming from Janet McArthur. With meticulous technique, using urinary assays, McArthur was the first to demonstrate the LH peak in the menstrual cycle at the time of ovulation. Subsequently she demonstrated the multiple LH peaks found in the Stein-Leventhal, or polycystic ovary, syndrome. She showed that the gonadotropic hormones were carried by specific proteins in the blood. Her pioneering work with the bonnet monkey as a good animal model of cervical mucus has recently been recognized and taken up by others.

A great strength of the Vincent under Ulfelder was productive interaction with other departments. The understanding of gynecologic pathology was significantly advanced by Robert Scully of the Pathology Department. Trainees were attracted both from pathology and gynecology to benefit from this working relationship. Radiation therapy, cytology, pediatrics, medical oncology, and social service similarly gained unique proficiency from their interaction with the Vincent. MGH gynecologists supported the pioneering primary care program in the Medical Service which has set an example for all subsequent programs in that specialty.

The kind of bounteous reward that can result from rapid intercommunication between clinical and research personnel—as well as among departments of the hospital—is well illustrated by the recognition at the MGH in 1971 of the stilbestrol disorders. Because this gynecologic service had an established reputation in oncology, all the early cases of adolescent clear cell adenocarcinoma of the vagina that occurred in this geographic area were referred to the Vincent for management. It was soon apparent that more than chance alone could be responsible for this unique eruption of what was truly a new disease entity, and a possibility raised by one of Ulfelder's patients stimulated the controlled case study that established irrefutably the association with fetal exposure to diethylstilbestrol (DES). The registry for such cases was established at the MGH and was able within three years to document the validity of the hypothesis and to define other benign effects of such exposure. In addition, the prevalence of the disorders, the behavior over time of the malignant process, and the effectiveness of treatment programs could also soon be assessed. Finally, the phenomenon rekindled careful scrutiny of the embryologic processes that could be affected or deranged, thus contributing in an important way to our understanding of the fundamental biology of the human species.

With the assistance of *Ann B. Barnes*

Obstetrics

HOWARD ULFELDER

Boston, Philadelphia, and Baltimore are cities old enough to possess hospitals organized along lines consistent with practice in the nineteenth century. At that time obstetrics and gynecology were separate, the former associated primarily with general medical practice and the latter with surgery. This certainly was true at the MGH where gynecology was included in the practice of all the general surgical staff. Although some mention is made of midwifery in Bowditch's history, it is from Washburn's volume that we learn the details. An appeal of the Harvard Medical School for obstetric teaching beds at the hospital was rejected by the trustees in 1845 on the recommendation of a special committee which opined that no decent female would come to a hospital maternity ward for delivery, particularly if it were on condition that students participate in the procedure. This decision guided the course of events until 1914 when the position of obstetrician to the hospital was created to formalize consultations requested of the nearby Lying-In Hospital on McLean Street when the occasional MGH patient's need for such opinion arose.

With the opening of the Phillips House in 1917, obstetrics made its formal appearance, and the fourth floor was set aside for this purpose. When the Baker Memorial was opened in 1930, another floor of obstetric beds became available. The care of these patients was the privilege of graduates of the hospital and a small roster of invited obstetricians, but no provision was made for obstetric house staff, training program, or students. This deficiency was much regretted, in particular by Pediatrics, Orthopedics, Anesthesia, and the nurses' training school. At least three committees appointed over the years to evaluate the need for an obstetric teaching service concluded that such a venture could prosper only at the expense of the units already in operation in Boston, and that was considered undesirable. Private obstetrics continued to be served in both the Baker Memorial and the Phillips House until after World War II. Thereafter it dwindled sharply, chiefly because the obstetricians deplored the lack of residents, specially trained nurses, and multiple practice aids which made such a marked contrast with the quality of care they could render at the Lying-In Hospital.

The final chapter in MGH obstetrics begins in 1966 when John Grover was encouraged by his chief to formalize a relationship with the Lying-In Hospital and inaugurate a pre- and postnatal ambulatory clinic for women who chose to use the MGH facilities for all aspects of their medical management and pregnancy except the actual labor and delivery which would be conducted at the BLI. If one reflects upon the fact that the MGH each day is a busy town of 10,000 inhabitants, it is obvious that there will always be a number of women who could use such a service—and this has proved to be the case. For obvious practical reasons, the fertility and family planning services of the department were combined with this function.

Remembrances

JOHN W. GROVER

When I think of the Gynecology Service at the MGH-Vincent Memorial Hospital between the years 1955 and 1980, a span of time nearly coincident with my own staff appointment, I think more of people, personalities, and philosophy than of events or accomplishments. Although I took many of my medical school rotations at the MGH, my first acquaintance with the Vincent Memorial Gynecology Service came with my internship in surgery in 1956.

At that time Joe Meigs was still the ascendant personality, even though Howard Ulfelder had become the new chief and the Meigs Professor. Meigs was still at the peak of his long surgical career. In the years leading up to this period he had personally trained virtually every gynecologist on the staff, each of whom was, like himself, trained in general surgery before subspecializing in gynecology. Ulfelder and Langdon Parsons were the most senior of the staff after Meigs, and Francis Ingersoll and Tom Green rounded out the active staff. Janet McArthur began to establish her reputation as a research endocrinologist in the new Vincent Laboratory. Celso Ramon-Garcia was developing an infertility clinic but went on to the University of Pennsylvania.

The major philosophy of those years espoused surgical excellence in the care of gynecologic patients. All the staff, with their strong surgical backgrounds, supported Meigs in this view, and the high standards of training set on the General Surgical Services were carried over for residents on the gynecologic rotation. All of us who were in training during those years remember the thrill of watching Meigs operate. His smoothly functioning team usually included a staff-level first assistant, but we all anticipated and treasured those occasions when we were fortunate—and good—enough for the first time to assist the "great man" ourselves. Weekly teaching rounds meant a huge entourage of staff, residents, medical students, and visiting physicians following Meigs or Ulfelder around on Vincent 2, discussing patients at the bedside in the grand old MGH tradition. The pathology conferences conducted by Robert E. Scully, which followed rounds, were always well attended and became models of the multidisciplinary approach to teaching and patient care so strongly advocated by Ulfelder during his tenure.

My coming to the MGH as a surgical intern represented a change in direction in some ways, since both Meigs and Ulfelder recognized that in the decades to follow, surgery alone would not be enough to allow the Vincent Memorial Hospital to continue a balanced approach in the advancement of gynecology; endocrinology, fertility, and reproductive biology and psychology were emerging as other important components of the field. Along with Churchill of Surgery and Duncan Reid of the Lying-In Hospital, they were supportive of a small but highly trained and selected group of physicians who, as Josiah Macy fellows, sought out extra study and research training in obstetrics and gynecology in preparation for teaching and academic careers. As the first of the Macy fellows to come to the MGH, I chose to emphasize the surgical and basic research component of the fellowship. Subsequent fellows, who included John L. Lewis, Jr., Arthur Herbst, and Theodore Barton, tailored their programs to their special needs, but the strong emphasis on surgery was common to us all. Ann Barnes, one of the first women to enter a field of surgery at the MGH, and David Chapin also were supported in their acquisition of strong surgical skills as a basis for their future training and work as obstetricians and gynecologists on the staff of the Vincent-MGH.

As Ulfelder noted, my appointment in 1964 (after two years in England in basic research and three at the Lying-In Hospital for obstetrics and gynecology training) represented the first time in nearly two decades that an obstetrically trained surgeon-gynecologist was appointed to the staff. A long-planned ambulatory obstetric clinic coordinated with the Lying-In Hospital was started under my direction in 1966. Herbst, Barnes, Lawrence Malone (Meigs' last junior associate), and Chapin all worked in rotation in the obstetrics and infertility clinic at various times. At the peak of activity we cared for more than 200 pregnant patients yearly.

Ulfelder succeeded Meigs in 1955 and, while committed to the surgical tradition, he continued to support the development of younger staff aiming at varied academic careers in obstetrics and gynecology. He originated and strongly espoused a combined approach to the care of cancer patients, which involved surgeons, pathologists, radiation therapists, and chemotherapists in weekly conferences long before the Cox Cancer Center appeared on the horizon.

The most spectacular development of the late sixties and early seventies was the identification of the relationship between fetal exposure to diethylstilbestrol (often given during the fifties and sixties to help a potentially failing pregnancy) and the occurrence of vaginal malignancies in young women. My personal memory of this signal event reveals how close I came to being involved in working out the relationship myself. Ulfelder suggested to me in the late sixties that there might be a relationship between the use of certain hormones in pregnancy and congenital anomalies in newborns. For reasons not now clear, I failed to pick up on his suggestion at the time. Several years later, the cluster of vaginal adenocarcinomas in young women was observed by Scully and Herbst, and the rest is history.

Other landmark experiences include testifying before the Massachusetts State Legislature in favor of birth control reform in the late sixties; Massachusetts was one of the last states to liberalize birth control legislation, and our involvement helped to bring about needed change. When the Supreme Court liberalized abortion laws, we were also involved in helping the MGH and its staff develop appropriate programs and attitudes in this complex area. I also remember the annual gynecologic postgraduate course which drew students from all over the country, and the strong support of the Vincent Club, culminating in the annual Vincent Club Show which always included the traditional "drill" and was a major fund raiser for the hospital and its programs.

During the several years leading up to his retirement in 1976, Ulfelder was a leader in facilitating the planning and development of the Cox Center, a signal and significant development in the care of all cancer patients at the MGH (see Chapter 35). At the same time it was a sign that the Vincent Memorial Hospital would focus on cancer in women in the seventies and eighties. Primary care of women, noncancer gynecology, and prenatal and obstetric care would perforce have to stand in second place; and the philosophy and direction of the Vincent determined its readiness for the next chief of Gynecology, James Nelson, whose major strength is gynecologic oncology.

For me it is important to remember how many of the physicians associated with the MGH-Vincent Memorial Hospital have gone on to significant accomplishments in the field of gynecology elsewhere. I'm sure that each of us benefited greatly from our close associations with the surgical traditions and staff at the MGH and the Vincent and carry those standards of care and skill to our work wherever we are. Not the least of the attributes that we bring to the outside world is our relevant heritage of the philosophy and teaching of Joe Vincent Meigs and Howard Ulfelder, whom we treasure both professionally and personally as surrogate parents of ourselves and of the present state of the art.

27. Neurosurgery

Development of the Neurosurgical Service

H. THOMAS BALLANTINE, JR., AND WILLIAM H. SWEET

The MGH Neurosurgical Service had an average daily census in 1980 of about 70 patients. Twenty-eight neurosurgeons, ten of whom were residents-in-training, cared for those patients. Thirteen individuals, including eight Ph.D.s, manned the Mixter Laboratories for Neurosurgical Research, and the budget for clinical and basic science investigations amounted to $1.3 million.

In 1910 there was no neurosurgical service, and the rare operations on the central nervous system were performed by general surgeons. The development of neurosurgery over a period of 70 years at the MGH mirrors in microcosm the development of the specialty, and it is in this context that the following account is submitted.

Since Faxon's volume of hospital history made but scant reference to neurosurgery, some review of the more remote past is in order. The emergence of neurologic surgery as a distinct discipline separate from general surgery began, at least in the English-speaking world, with an outstanding British neurophysiologist and surgeon, Sir Victor Horsley (1858–1916). In 1889 John W. Elliot, then visiting surgeon to the MGH, went to London for a period of study with Horsley. On returning to Boston, Elliot attempted to interest his colleagues at the MGH in this emerging specialty of surgery of the central nervous system. Fulton, in his biography of Harvey Cushing, mentioned that in 1895 Cushing, then a senior medical student at Harvard, assisted Elliot in two operations for brain tumor. Fulton speculated that it was this experience that turned Cushing toward neurologic surgery.

William Jason Mixter. Elliot's interest in neurosurgery was short-lived. But the glowing ember that he brought to Boston from London ignited the enthusiasm and interest of another general surgeon, Samuel Jason Mixter (1856–1926). S. J. Mixter never abandoned general surgery but did foster the development at the MGH of surgery of the brain and spinal cord. When his son William Jason Mixter (1880–1958) came to the hospital in 1907 he was assigned to his father's South Surgical Service, and the two worked closely to develop this new specialty. However, it was not until 1911 that a "Special Assignment in Surgery of the Central Nervous System" was given to the Mixters, at which time Jason, decided to make neurosurgery his life's work. In 1912 he spent a year with Horsley, and by 1915 he was recognized nationally for his contributions to the treatment of skull fractures, intracranial sepsis, and surgery of the spine and spinal cord. In this last endeavor he was greatly helped by collaboration with James B. Ayer, the nationally respected senior neurologist at the MGH.

World War I had a significant impact upon the development of neurosurgery at the MGH. In 1915 Jason Mixter volunteered to serve first with the American Ambulance Hospital outside Paris and later with the British Red Cross Hospital near the front lines. When the United States entered the war in 1917 he again volunteered, this time with our own forces in the MGH Unit, Base Hospital No. 6. His administrative talents recognized, he was transferred a year later to England where he served as commanding officer of two hospitals. During this period of disruption, Jason's father, Samuel, again headed neurosurgery at the MGH, and it continued to expand. The Hospital Bulletin for 1917 recorded, for example, "80–100 cases a year with the assignment steadily increasing in number."

Upon returning to civilian life, Jason Mixter resumed his position as head of the "assignment of neurological surgery." Not until 1939 did the Board of Trustees create a separate neurosurgical service at the MGH with Mixter as its chief. In addition to this administrative handicap, MGH neurosurgery had to develop in the shadow of Harvey Cushing at the Peter Bent Brigham Hospital. Cushing, ten years older than Mixter, was an acknowledged giant among neurosurgeons. A certain amount of tension always existed between the two men, slightly eased by their differing interests. Cushing concentrated mainly on the diagnosis, endocrine aspects, classification, and treatment of intracranial tumors while Mixter's interests involved the treatment of disorders of the spine and spinal cord, central nervous system trauma, pain, and disorders of the sympathetic nervous system. Cushing was seldom helpful to his younger colleague; however he did invite "young Mixter" in 1920 to join a select group of neurosurgical pioneers who were to meet in Boston to establish the Society of Neurological Surgeons.

In 1920 John Sprague Hodgson (1890–1979) began a long association with the Neurosurgical Service. A graduate of Brown and the Harvard Medical School (1915), Hodgson's surgical training at the MGH was interrupted by World War I. He served with great distinction in France and for a year after the armistice was active in combating typhus in Greece. Upon returning to Boston, Hodgson spent a year with Cushing and another year as surgical house officer at the MGH. When he joined the surgical staff, he originally divided his time equally between general surgery and neurosurgery before deciding to make a career of the latter. Hodgson was a superb surgeon, a delightful gentleman, and a humanist scholar. He had, however, little taste for research activities—unlike his younger colleague, James Clarke White (1895–1981).

White, the son of a distinguished physician and a Back Bay Bostonian by birth, was educated at Harvard College and served as a line officer in the U.S. Navy during World War I before entering HMS. In 1924 he began three years of general surgical training at the MGH. This was followed by a year of study with René Leriche of Strasbourg and A. Hovelacque of Paris where White developed his lifelong interest in pain and surgery of the sympathetic nervous system. Except for a brief period in 1933 when Tracy Putnam joined the Neurosurgical Service, Mixter, Hodgson, and White guided the evolution of the service from 1920 to 1940.

In 1933 two events of importance were recorded, the first being the presentation before the New England Surgical Society by Mixter and Joseph S. Barr of Orthopedics of a paper entitled "Rupture of the Intervertebral Disc with Involvement of the Spinal Canal." Published 11 months later in the *New England Journal of Medicine,* this paper remains a classic. The second milestone was the recognition by the hospital of the unique nature of neurosurgery. To meet the special surgical requirements, an operating room in the new Baker Memorial Building was assigned to neurosurgery. In 1936 John T. B. Carmody became the first resident to graduate from the neurosurgical program, followed by Jost J. Michelsen, William B. Scoville, Samuel Lowis, Henry Heyl, and William H. Sweet.

In 1941, having reached the mandatory retirement age of that era, Mixter handed over command of the service to his junior colleague, James White. With White's appointment as full-time with an office at the hospital, another milestone was reached.

But, as had happened a generation earlier, a world war created grave problems for this new service. White and Sweet committed themselves to the war effort, and residents were scarce. Thus from 1940 to 1945 Mixter again headed the Neurosurgical Service while serving as chief neurosurgical consultant to the Surgeon General of the Army. During this period Mixter, Hodgson, and Michelsen held the fragile service together.

White, Sweet, and H. Thomas Ballantine returned to the MGH in late 1945. With White's blessing, Ballantine, who for two-and-a-half years had performed neurosurgery in North Africa, Sicily, and Italy, went off to work with Max Peet at the University of Michigan. Sweet became full-time at the MGH and the Medical School, thus beginning his long and fruitful collaboration with White.

Under White's direction, abetted by Sweet's enthusiasm, research activities in neurosurgery grew rapidly. The year 1955 saw the formation of an informal research institute with laboratories for both neurology and neurosurgery occupying two floors of the Warren Building. Ballantine returned to the hospital in 1947 as an associate of Mixter, who was still active.

In fitting tribute to the first chief of Neurosurgery, on October 16, 1957, the Mixter Laboratories for Neurosurgical Research on Warren 4 were formally dedicated. Although then suffering from carcinoma of the lung which took his life four months later, William Jason Mixter was able to attend the ceremonies.

Mixter was a modest and self-effacing man with an abiding love for and loyalty to the MGH. While the "Cushing School" of neurosurgery was being created at the Brigham, Mixter labored to develop an MGH school which, he reckoned, might have a longer life since it was related more to an institution than to an individual. Reflecting upon Mixter's character, we note that, at a time when blatant puerile rudeness in the operating room was the fashionable prerogative of the prima donna surgeon, his behavior was precisely the opposite, and it, of course, yielded him better support from his operative team. Neurosurgical patients do not always do well. His attitude as he sought with his staff critically to determine and correct faults in management led to his service becoming known as the friendly service.

James C. White. White served as chief of Neurosurgery from 1940 until 1961. His close collaborator, William H. Sweet, succeeded him in 1961, retiring in 1977. The two men worked so closely together that the years from 1940 to 1977 can be thought of as a continuum. Before turning to the scientific work of that era, however, it is a pleasure to pause and contemplate White the man. He not only did not lose his temper, he never even became ruffled. In a day when many distinguished neurosurgeons were paragons of intemperate, even preposterous expression, especially in the operating room, Jim never visibly lost his tact or composure. White had followed Mixter's example on this score. His records of history from and examination of the patient were exhaustively complete; and his description to the patient of the risks and uncertainties of the proposed operation was equally comprehensive in an age when such emphasis was not the general custom. Regarding the extent of therapy to be pursued in those with malignant disease of the brain, he was sensitive to the wishes of those properly concerned. What to one patient seems humanitarian forebearance from the use of all therapeutic possibilities may be construed as neglect by the next. We learned from Jim how to tread the precarious path between gentleness and discretion.

Extraordinarily devoid of formality and pretense, he smoked a corncob pipe, wore reasonable quality, usually unmatching, coat and trousers likely to be of ancient vintage. He had at least one jacket with matching trousers: his naval officer's uniform, dark buttons having been substituted for the regulation brass.

Together, White and Sweet explored the realms of pain. Both were interested in the laboratory approach to understanding the mechanisms of pain and in scholarly recording of clinical observations of their new procedures as well as the standard operations. This collaboration resulted in the publication in 1955 of their classic monograph "Pain: Its Mechanism and Neurosurgical Control." Their recognition of the major role of psychiatric factors in pain prompted them to include a key chapter in the book by Stanley Cobb who had been chief of Psychiatry at the MGH. White's courageous performance of the first successful operation in man to cut the pain tracts ascending from the opposite side of the body as they lie fairly deep in the brain stem was an example of carrying into the clinic observations first made in the animal laboratory.

White's and Sweet's second, more comprehensive monograph, "Pain and the Neurosurgeon: A Forty Year Experience," was published in 1969 when White was 74 years old. He wrote more of the book than his coauthor; his unflagging industry, honesty, and scholarship, exemplified—among many other ways—by this capstone to his career, have continued to influence neurosurgeons all over the world. Hallmarks of his professional behavior included detailed descriptions of the course of illnesses in particular patients. Those with chronic pain often had had many operations and other treatments by the time they reached him, and elicitation of the clinical history frequently required two or three hours. He was rigorous in appraising his results and the causes of failure and insisted on maximal follow-ups for years of various modes of management before making any semblance of a final judgment.

Ballantine headed the Medical Acoustics Research Group which, for a period of five years, made fundamental contributions to the use of ultrasound for both diagnosis and tissue destruction. Although superseded by radiologic computerized tomography for intracranial diagnostic purposes, this work provided the basis for the development of techniques for ultrasonic extirpation of brain tumors.

William H. Sweet. Sweet succeeded White as chief of Neurosurgery in

1961. The new chief shared his predecessor's philosophy, particularly with respect to the great importance of research to improve the unsatisfactory treatment of much neural disease. Reviewing the development of neurosurgery at the MGH, he observed: "In the late forties orthopedic, urologic, and neurologic surgery had such meager appeal to the better medical students that these specialties were described as havens for mediocrity by no less an authority than the late Professor Edward D. Churchill. Our own view is that we in neurosurgery are in a strategic position to make a contribution to that most formidable of all enigmas, the mind of man, and as well are helping many with diseases afflicting the essential organ of mind, the brain. In any case, the allure of neurosurgery to some of the medical students with superior minds was evident by the mid-fifties, and we have been getting more than our fair share of such applicants."

By the late fifties it was already apparent that U.S. training centers were turning out more purely clinical neurosurgeons than the country needed. The immediate compelling attraction of helping sick people at once, and the cash associated therewith, often lured away even those whose initial bent was the more altruistic one of contributing to knowledge and improving methods of treatment. The academic posts with an opportunity to combine research and clinical work were often going begging. Hence, at the MGH dual goals for the training and investigative program became more totally basic neuroscience and more such science with potential clinical application.

These goals could be achieved if research space under the control of the Neurosurgical Service could be financed and constructed. In 1953 a small two-story wing for Pathology was in the planning stage; it was to extend out toward the Charles River Basin from the Baker Memorial. Encouraged by David Crockett, the associate director for resources and development, the Neurosurgical Service requested the authority to raise funds to construct a third floor for neurosurgical research. The facility was planned to be adjacent to the clinical neurologic and neurosurgical beds then on the third floor of the Baker. As a consequence of a $100,000 gift secured through the helpful offices of Bishop Sherrill, and of the tactful and prodigiously successful efforts on a variety of fronts by our remarkable Mr. Crockett, the deadline date set by the trustees for the raising of the necessary $250,000 was met. By the time the final plans for the structure had been completed, they had burgeoned under the Crockett magic, resulting in the 12-story Warren Building. The fourth floor became and remains wholly for neurosurgical research. With this powerful investigative support much of the clinical work has been pioneering.

Proton Beam. The MGH Neurosurgical Service initiated a major departure in the treatment of intracranial problems, the use of a high energy beam of protons to destroy specific target tissues in the head. Pioneered by Raymond Kjellberg and Sweet, the project has been brought to glorious fruition by Kjellberg and his physicist collaborators William Preston and Andreas Koehler at the Harvard cyclotron. (See page 277.)

Isotopes. Other innovative research involving close collaboration with the MGH physicist Gordon Brownell led to the recognition that positron-emitting isotopes present a peculiar advantage to achieving precise detection of radioisotopic concentrations in tissue. Brownell and Sweet developed the first clinically valuable method for the external localization of brain tumors using the positron-emitting isotope [72]Arsenic. They also worked with the chemist Albert Soloway on the new concept of treating intracranial gliomas by the special radiation that arises when one of the stable isotopes of boron, [10]boron, captures a slow neutron. Such radiation requires a powerful nuclear reactor. The necessary elaborate human operating room beneath the core of the MIT reactor was constructed through the generosity of the Rockefeller Foundation. Although work both at the MGH and by one of our trainees in Japan, Professor Hatanaka, continues on this project, it has not yet been brought to practical fruition.

Cerebral Ischemia. Another laboratory observation with far-reaching clinical significance was that of Adelbert Ames, our first full-time M.D. investigator. Using the isolated rabbit retina as a sample of brain, he demonstrated that the tissue did not die after a few minutes of deprivation of oxygen and glucose whereas a part of the human brain deprived of blood in the intact individual is likely to die that soon. Ames and his colleagues went on to show that this vulnerability is due to the clogging of blood vessels that occurs when blood flow stops and prevents reestablishment of flow when the circulation is restored. They described this as the no-reflow phenomenon, and their paper led to wide-ranging efforts to overcome the problem. By 1980 the original paper published in 1968 had been cited more than 320 times.

Hypothermia. Work in our clinical laboratory by William Lougheed demonstrated that the brain consumes less energy and hence requires less than one-third as much blood when it is cooled 10°C below the normal 37°C. In this state temporary closure of the arteries to the brain is feasible, permitting precise removal of highly vascular intracranial lesions. The first two brain operations in patients at these low temperatures were carried out by Lougheed, White, and Sweet. For a decade this remained worldwide a frequently used technique until superseded by safer methods for handling the problems of brain edema and hemorrhage.

Tissue Culture. Paul Kornblith pioneered the successful development of tissue culture techniques for the growth in the laboratory of the tumors called gliomas which appear only in the brain. He promptly exploited this success by expanding the project in so many fruitful directions that he became the full-time director of Neurosurgery's brain tumor research effort when he completed his residency in 1971. Growth of aliquots of a tumor biopsy became so standardized that assaying the effectiveness of a number of drugs in stopping that growth is feasible. The Kornblith group not only identified specific protein markers for the glial tumors but also described the characteristics of the antitumor antibodies developed by the patient to his own tumor. The importance of this work led the NIH to spirit Kornblith away from the MGH to head their Surgical Neurology Division in Bethesda.

Other contributions have involved purely clinical research.

Leucotomy. In 1954 White and Sweet began to use electrocoagulation to make lesions in the posterior inferior white matter of the frontal lobes—a leucotomy for the treatment of intractable pain. The method was soon improved by our physicist Aronow by shifting to a radiofrequency current and by incorporating a temperature-measuring unit in the electrode, which permitted precise control of the destructive heat. They have continued to use this operation mainly for the pain of advanced cancer. In 1961 Ballantine began a highly productive use of the technique, making his lesions in the higher-lying frontal white matter of the cingulum for the treatment both of psychiatric illness and of pain. By 1975 he and his colleagues had studied and carefully followed after operation

204 psychotics, principally with affective or emotional disabilities. Another 34 patients had been treated for chronic pain. The national concern over psychosurgery led to its investigation by a presidential-congressional commission, one group of which was headed by the psychologist Professor Teuber of MIT. Their exhaustive study of 34 patients on whom Ballantine had performed a cingulotomy led to a tremendous accolade for Ballantine's "human approach to these excruciatingly difficult patients" and to an unbiased appraisal that many of his results are excellent.

Tumor Surgery. Efforts to improve knowledge about and management of noninvasive intracranial tumors (acoustic neuromas and meningiomas) were coupled with a meticulous attempt to reduce the mortality and morbidity attendant upon removal of these encapsulated tumors. The major challenge of their total removal was taken up with special effectiveness by Robert Ojemann. By 1979 he had operated on 103 consecutive patients with acoustic tumors with only three postoperative deaths; 90 percent of the patients returned to their previous activities. Similarly, Sweet undertook the total removal of the tumors at the base of the brain called craniopharyngiomas. He and neuropathologist E. P. Richardson pointed out that these tumors provoke the formation of a glial connective-tissue layer around them which made radical surgery feasible in 40 of the 43 patients treated by him. A low initial surgical mortality and excellent results in the majority of the survivors ensued.

Stereotactic Surgery. Beginning in 1947 Sweet worked on the development of apparatus and methods to place a metal electrode or cannula at a desired target point in the depths of the brain. The extraordinary instrument maker Paul McPherson designed our first practically useful device. Vernon Mark and Sweet used this to make focal lesions in the thalamus to relieve pain and in the temporal lobes to stop catastrophic violence by patients with focal epilepsy. Raymond Kjellberg, returning from training in Stockholm, modified the Leksell apparatus whose use he learned there. With this he became New England's prime performer of operations for Parkinsonism and the dystonias.

The Fulltime Research Group. Following Adelbert Ames and his work on the isolated retina as a sample of normal brain, the neurophysiologists Daniel Pollen and Richard Masland have joined us and after initial tutelage from Dr. Ames have continued independent investigations of the visual system.

In the field of electron microscopy Professor Humberto Fernandez-Moran had by 1961 developed in our laboratories the highest resolution electron microscopes in the world and had begun his phenomenally successful construction of the liquid helium electron microscope operating at temperatures less than 4° above absolute zero (− 273°C).

In addition, a series of research trainees from this and other countries have come to work not only with our full-time research staff but with our clinical neurosurgical investigators as well. Several have returned home to full professorships in this country, Europe, and Japan. The same is true of our clinical trainees. In the past 45 years we have trained 72 neurosurgeons, 41 of whom achieved academic appointments. Of these, 16 became full professors.

In 1977 Nicholas T. Zervas, who had been the MGH neurosurgical resident in 1961, became the chief of Neurosurgery at the hospital where he had received the bulk of his postgraduate education. At this writing, a third generation of neurosurgeons led by Zervas now controls the destiny of the MGH service; they are achieving new levels of clinical and investigative excellence.

Recent Developments

NICHOLAS T. ZERVAS

Today the neurosurgical laboratories are busier than ever. Seven separate basic science efforts are supported by the Neurosurgical Service; financial support is supplied in part by the National Institutes of Health, the American Heart Association, private donations, and clinical activities. The core group of senior researchers is assisted by eight pre- and postdoctoral fellows in the basic sciences and five research fellows in neurosurgery.

A striking development over the past few years has been the happy cooperative intermingling of research efforts between Neurosurgery and the Neurology Service. They have combined to provide financial assistance and space to members of both departments, and the result has helped several younger scientists to begin their work. Core facilities have been developed in neuroendocrinology, tissue culture, vascular disease, and electron microscopy. Combined conferences have provided intellectual interaction in both clinical and research domains. The result has been a ferment of activity.

Clinical training of residents evolves continuously according to our perception of their needs and requirements dictated by the American Board of Neurological Surgery. Currently, our residency program, coordinated by Paul Chapman, requires six years of training. The first six months are spent on the Neurology Service under Joseph Martin, where the resident is introduced to the everyday neurologic diseases and emergencies and becomes thoroughly grounded in the examination of the neurologic patient. Time is spent in the neurophysiologic laboratories studying electromyelography and electroencephalography. During the second six-month rotation the resident is introduced to neurosurgery by the chief resident, and it is here that he begins to understand neurosurgical problems and contemporary management. He covers the Emergency Ward and assists the chief resident in surgery. Depending on his proficiency, he is allowed to carry out many minor procedures and assists at major operations. Also during this time he receives instruction in microsurgery in the laboratory under the guidance of Roberto Heros, director of vascular surgery. The third six-month period is spent with members of the attending staff and, as the resident acquires surgical skills, he is allowed to participate to a greater extent in operative procedures. He may spend a portion of this period at the Children's Hospital becoming familiar with pediatric neurosurgical problems under the guidance of Keasley Welch. The resident proceeds next to neuroradiology where he is guided in an understanding of imaging and participates in catheterization procedures. While there he has an opportunity to spend time in neuropathology to become acquainted with the gross and histologic appearance of neurosurgical lesions.

In the final two years of training the resident spends three successive six-month rotations as senior resident on the private services and ultimately becomes responsible for the care of patients on White 11. During the final six months he is given a staff appointment as assistant in neurosurgery, which gives him all the prerogatives of the attending staff. He has assigned time in the operating room and is in full charge of patients in consultation with visiting staff. In these final two years the resident begins to acquire the skills needed to deal with all the major neurosurgical procedures including the management of aneurysms, arteriovenous malformations, parasellar tumors, and posterior fossa lesions.

Research Training. The past decade witnessed a remarkable increase in basic research in neurobiology. The nervous system has become the major frontier of exploration and discovery in the biologic sciences. Paradoxically, communication between the clinician and the basic scientist has become increasingly difficult at a time when the dividends of these advances should be realized. A program, therefore, was designed to help bridge that gap.

A major goal of the neurologic and neurosurgical services at the MGH has been the training of academic neurologists and neurosurgeons. A substantial number of graduates of both residencies have continued in academic medicine, and most of them have been involved in research. The success of these efforts has been due in large part to the emphasis placed on research by Sweet and Raymond Adams, who were chiefs of the Neurosurgical and Neurology services, respectively, for almost two decades. The historic and current strengths of the program provide a unique opportunity for neurosurgery to achieve an interface with the enormous recent advances in the basic disciplines.

The goal of the new program is the preparation of a group of neurosurgeons in a basic neurobiologic discipline. To this end we select a small group of neurosurgeons based on their demonstrated interest in the basic mechanisms of neurosurgical disease and offer them an opportunity to study for two or three years with an established senior scientist in one of the basic science laboratories of Harvard University or MIT. To accomplish this, we have expanded the participation of scientists from the basic research community outside the hospital as preceptors in the training program.

Along with other advantages, sending young physicians to work in the basic science laboratories provides a flow of information from clinical neuroscience to those laboratories. Although basic neurobiologists are in general little acquainted with clinical problems, most have an active interest in the potential uses of their work. We find that our basic science colleagues welcome the opportunity to have in their groups a physician familiar with the clinical problems to which their work might be applied. Furthermore, there have been instances in which clinical observations pointed the way for major advances in fundamental neurobiology. A striking case in point is *amblyopia ex anopsia*, which led David Hubel and Torsten Wiesel to their now classic studies of plasticity in the visual system. Our trainees thus not only return their basic science experience to the clinical world but also introduce clinical problems and insights to the laboratories.

Bragg Peak Proton Therapy

RAYMOND N. KJELLBERG

Nothing, perhaps, demonstrates quite as elegantly the rewards to be reaped from dialogue between basic and clinical scientists than the story of Bragg peak proton therapy. In the spring of 1959 a luncheon occurred in a Harvard student cafeteria, attended by Raymond N. Kjellberg, MGH neurosurgeon, William M. Preston, director of the Harvard Cyclotron Laboratory (HCL), and Andreas M. Koehler, assistant director HCL; they had been assembled by William Sweet. A discussion concerning the possible use of the Bragg peak of the proton beam as a therapeutic instrument for precise focal destruction of defined brain targets such as tremors or physiologic nuclei concluded with an agreement that a joint effort to this end would be advanced by the Harvard Physics Department and MGH Neurosurgery.

A proton is a hydrogen atom, stripped of its orbital electron. Positively charged, it can be accelerated in a circular orbit at high speeds. The 160-million-electron-volt Harvard cyclotron accelerates protons to about one-half the speed of light. The tiny proton particles pass through molecules of skin, bone, and brain. Losing energy as they pass through the molecules by virtue of low-level ionization, they stop at nearly the same point in the brain. In stopping, they produce significantly greater ionization, and this burst is called the Bragg peak, after the British physicist Sir William L. Bragg. These ionizing particles are similar to x-rays in that they produce ionization, but they are not radiation because they are particles not electromagnetic rays.

In 1946 Robert Wilson, a physicist, advanced the notion that the Bragg peak or other heavy particle beams had potential for use in medical therapeutics by virtue of the concentration of ionization in a target volume such as a tumor. Later, the Lawrence Radiation Laboratory at Berkeley began the use of various particle beams to explore the potential for clinical therapeutics; they first used the Bragg peak of a particle beam on a metastatic breast cancer lesion on the skin. Professor Leksell, a neurosurgeon in Sweden, was an early advocate of focal radiation for brain disorders. He coined the term *radiosurgery* and developed a stereotactic (three-dimensional radiographically targeted) method for local radiation.

In 1959, armed with a medical foundation fellowship, Kjellberg spent several months with Leksell; in March 1960 Kjellberg studied the methods in use at Berkeley. During and following this period, design of stereotactic instrumentation was developed for experimental studies and clinical application by Kjellberg; Preston and Koehler were developing the physical characteristic of the Bragg peak of the proton beam. Experimental studies in monkeys began in May 1960. The first clinical application of Bragg peak proton therapy was performed in a 2½-year-old child with a massive inoperable optic nerve glioma in May 1961. Her initial response was sufficiently gratifying to encourage the researchers to persist in their efforts. In 1962 a patient with metastatic breast cancer and diabetes mellitus was treated to suppress normal pituitary function; both her cancer and her diabetes were ameliorated. Treatment that same year of a young woman with diabetic retinopathy improved her vision encouragingly; as a result, 178 such patients were treated, representing the first systematic application of a single session Bragg peak proton therapy to normal pituitary.

A 1962 grant from NASA led to the construction of a new treatment facility and its equipment with appropriate apparatus, greatly enhancing the treatment setting. As the sixties continued, other disorders of the pituitary responded to proton beam therapy. In 1965 a patient with arteriovenous malformation of the brain (AVM) was treated; her AVM had bled, and the prospect existed that further bleeding would cause her death. She remains alive in 1980. In 1969 Milford Schulz of the MGH Department of Radiology and Robert N. Ganz of the Children's Service advanced the idea of using Bragg peak proton therapy for ocular tumors. The first patient with ocular melanoma was treated in July 1975, and roughly 80 such patients are currently treated each year. During the past decade Bragg peak proton beam therapy has found still wider clinical applications which, nevertheless, represent only a fraction of its potential. Clinical uses can be developed for all focal (i.e., benign) neoplasms of the brain and very likely for a wider range of disturbances.

At this writing, December 1980, the MGH Neurosurgical Service has treated 1,384 patients by the Bragg peak proton method, in single therapeutic sessions normally requiring two hours or less for the procedure and seven days or less for the entire evaluation, therapy, and convalescence. With comparatively modest staffing, the MGH group has served more patients and initiated more new clinical applications to specific disease entities than any particle beam unit in the world. Single session Bragg peak proton beam therapy has an asset not always reckoned in the medical decision-making process—namely, its prominent cost effectiveness. Because hospitalizations are short, complications are few, and procedure-related mortality is not known to exist, the future of the method should be bright from the individual, social, and economic points of view.

With the assistance of *Andreas M. Koehler*

28. Orthopedic Surgery

THORNTON BROWN

By 1946 the Orthopedic Service had reached a turning point in its history. Since its beginning in 1900 it had become preeminent in patient care and had established itself as one of the leading orthopedic residency training programs. It was also recognized as an educational center to which postgraduate students and fellows came from many parts of the world. During the 17 years that Marius N. Smith-Petersen had been in charge, there had been outstanding contributions to the advancement of orthopedic surgery.

Nevertheless, in the mid-forties the Orthopedic Service at the MGH had serious weaknesses that endangered its position as a leader in the field. The chief was part-time, and there was no departmental office. In education, the service performed at a rather primitive level; there was little teaching of medical students, while in the realm of resident education the training program took the form of a preceptorship rather than a well-organized educational experience. As for research, there was some clinical investigation by the orthopedic staff but no basic science investigation of musculoskeletal problems, even though by 1946 this had become an indispensable ingredient of any preeminent academic program.

The Barr Years: 1946–1964. Such was the situation when Joseph S. Barr was appointed to succeed Smith-Petersen in December 1946 and when he became the John B. and Buckminster Brown Clinical Professor of Orthopedic Surgery at the Harvard Medical School in 1948—a title that in the past had always been held by the chief of Orthopedic Surgery at Children's Hospital. Barr had attended the HMS and received his surgical training at the Peter Bent Brigham Hospital under Harvey Cushing and his orthopedic training at the Children's Hospital and the MGH, graduating in 1929. Thereafter he had been associated with the MGH except during World War II when he was on active duty in the Navy. At the end of the war he was chief of Orthopedics at the U.S. Naval Hospital in Bethesda, Maryland.

Barr had long been aware of the weaknesses in the orthopedic program at the MGH. In January 1938 he had written Smith-Petersen as follows: "There is little or no laboratory work being done. This is an aspect of orthopedic surgery which needs more emphasis, and if our clinic is to maintain its present high position, I feel that it is imperative to establish a program of investigative work and to systematize the teaching of the house officers in the basic fields of anatomy and pathology. . . . I am willing and anxious to curtail my varied duties . . . in order to devote time to the hospital-laboratory program."

Barr had his chance in 1946, but the way was not easy. Barr's professorship was not fully endowed. There were no funds and no space. A clinically oriented residency training program is not likely to produce residents inclined toward a career in research. With no money, there was no chance of attracting a trained investigator from the outside. Thus the task of converting the Orthopedic Service into a truly academic enterprise that could provide patient care and a stimulating

280

research and educational environment for residents and medical students, consistent with the traditional ideals of the MGH and the HMS, was indeed a formidable one even for someone who could devote full-time to the project. But Barr had no such luxury since, to keep the wolf from his door, he had to maintain a busy private practice on Marlborough Street in association with Frank R. Ober, Brown Professor Emeritus. Despite these many obstacles, during the 17 years before poor health forced him to retire, Barr and his associates managed to lay the foundations for an academic department with space, funds, and personnel.

Administration. In 1951 desperately needed office space was provided by remodelling the north wing of the fifth floor of the White Building adjacent to the orthopedic wards. Thornton Brown was appointed as a geographically full-time staff member. The old conference room adjacent to the chief's new office was renovated with money contributed to the Smith-Petersen Appreciation Fund by friends and former patients. A portrait of the former chief was hung in this commodious room which came to be known as "Pete's Joint." In 1956 additional office space became available on the seventh floor of the new Warren Building, helping some members of the Orthopedic Service to alleviate the daily struggle with Boston traffic that until then had wasted so many orthopedist hours and reduced the efficiency of the staff.

Patient Care. Patient care during Barr's regime continued at a high level. Although the surgical innovations that had characterized the period of Smith-Petersen's administration were not forthcoming, many members of the staff became preeminent: Otto Aufranc in the treatment of diseases of the hip by cup arthroplasty; Barr in the treatment of low back and sciatic pain; Armin Klein in the treatment of slipping of the capital femoral epiphysis; Edwin F. Cave in the treatment of fractures and nonunions; and Carter Rowe in the treatment of shoulder problems. It might also be noted that the orthopedic staff participated in the reimplantation of Red Knowles' upper limb in 1962, the first such procedure to be performed successfully.

The Orthopedic Clinic in the basement of the outpatient department had changed little, if any, since the building was constructed in 1905. Its stall-like examining rooms, separated by partial partitions of darkening varnished oak, provided little in the way of privacy and comfort. In 1951, stimulated by a sharp drop in the patient census, the clinic was remodelled to provide more sympathetic surroundings, and scheduling changes were instituted in an effort to reduce patients' waiting time on the long, hard wooden benches in the corridor. In addition, by arrangement with the Boston Police Department, the city was regionalized so that victims of road accidents in the northern part of the city picked up by the police were brought to the MGH rather than to City Hospital.

The Fracture Clinic, which had been established in 1917, was the first such clinic in the United States. Initially it had been staffed by general surgeons, but after the First World War, members of the Orthopedic Service also participated. During Barr's tenure, Edwin F. Cave became chief in 1948, and all inpatient fracture care was provided in the orthopedic wards, while ambulatory treatment of fractures in the Emergency Room fell, in large part, to surgical residents on their orthopedic rotation. In 1938 the members of the Fracture Clinic (then both general surgeons and orthopedists) had published a textbook entitled *Experience in the Management of Fractures and Dislocations,* edited by Philip D. Wilson. This was the first volume of its kind, compiling the opinions of various authors and data from end-result studies. Twenty years later, as a result of Cave's energy and enthusiasm, a new edition was published under the title *Fractures and Other Injuries,* edited by him. Cave retired as chief of the clinic in 1965, and was succeeded by Otto Aufranc.

Physical and occupational therapy, located in the basement of the Clinics Building, had been available at the MGH since the turn of the century. Machines for mechano- and electrotherapy imported from Sweden were donated to the hospital, but these activities were terminated for reasons of economy at the outbreak of World War I. Thereafter, physical and occupational therapy apparently came on hard times. In 1929 Smith-Petersen noted that "the outstanding need of the department is the reestablishment of a Physiotherapy Department." However, little was done about the situation until 1940 when Arthur L. Watkins, who had recently completed his neurologic residency at the MGH, was appointed chief of the Physical Therapy Department which was established on the second floor of the Domestic Building. In 1945 physical and occupational therapy were combined under Watkins as the Department of Physical Medicine. With a grant of $1 million from the Baruch Foundation to the MGH and the HMS, a three-year training program in physical medicine and rehabilitation was initiated. In addition, training courses for physical therapists were developed in cooperation with Simmons College, the Children's Hospital Medical Center, and the Peter Bent Brigham Hospital. A few trainees completed their training in physical medicine and rehabilitation at the MGH, but then there were no more applicants.

In 1954, largely through the efforts of Thomas L. DeLorme, the Orthopedic Service began to play a more active role in the rehabilitation of patients in the hospital. DeLorme, who had extensive experience in physical medicine and rehabilitation during World War II and as a Baruch Fellow at the MGH, saw many patients with musculoskeletal problems on all services—especially paraplegics and quadriplegics—who were not receiving optimal care. With Barr's backing, DeLorme began to admit these patients to White 8 on the Orthopedic Service and to build up a staff of nursing and other personnel with the knowledge and equipment to provide proper care. But just as the activity was gaining momentum, the severe epidemic of poliomyelitis of 1955 diverted everyone's attention to the care of these severely paralyzed patients, many of them with paralysis of respiration and requiring respirator care. In the face of this emergency, the White 8 rehabilitation unit was allowed to wither, and all available orthopedic talent was diverted to the care of polio patients. White 9 was set up as a respirator center, and DeLorme, by then a junior member of the visiting staff, was primarily responsible for the orthopedic care of these patients, many of whom were severely disabled. There was no time for the other problems that had provided the stimulus to start the rehabilitation floor on White 8.

Gradually the polio patients recovered or were discharged to be followed on an ambulatory basis. As the census on White 9 dropped, the concept of a multiservice rehabilitation unit again surfaced. DeLorme, once more with Barr's backing, set about the task of establishing White 9 as the Rehabilitation Unit of the MGH. Through his friendship with the Pope family, DeLorme obtained funding from the Pope Foundation of Chicago. The administrative and professional staffs were developed with DeLorme as director and Leonard Cronkite of the Medical Service as internist-in-charge. William Kermond of the Orthopedic

Service was assistant director. Residents from Orthopedics now had as one of their rotations time on White 9. Other services, especially Urology, contributed to the care of these unfortunate patients. As the unit flourished, its 44 beds were filled with a variety of severely disabled patients with spinal cord injuries, persons with neurologic disease such as multiple sclerosis, and amputees. The concept of a special unit to care for them during part of their stay in a general hospital seemed amply justified.

DeLorme resigned in 1958 and was succeeded first by Irving Ackerman and later by Robert Jones, an assistant in Medicine who held the position of coordinator of rehabilitation until 1965 when he accepted an appointment elsewhere. It bears repeating that the stimulus for the formation of the White 9 rehabilitation unit had come from the Orthopedic Service, and the unit was conceived as a multiservice effort, not as part of the Physical Medicine Department.

Education. Residency training had been grossly disrupted during World War II; with the return of peace and a new chief, the program was reorganized. The orthopedic house staff now consisted of one senior resident (fifth year of training) and five assistant residents (fourth year of training), all coming to the MGH after one year at the Children's Hospital. In addition there was one third-year surgical resident and one first-year surgical intern who had rotations on the fracture and orthopedic services. In 1957 the number of residents was increased by two in response to the growing patient load at both the MGH and Children's. Resident seminars were arranged, and orthopedic and fracture rounds were combined.

Research. By all odds, the most formidable problem that faced Barr when he became chief in 1946 was the need to develop a research program. In 1934, in collaboration with W. Jason Mixter of Neurosurgery, he had been instrumental in demonstrating that low back pain and sciatica may be caused by rupture of a lumbar intervertebral disc. Because of this interest, he attempted to initiate a multidisciplinary investigation of low back pain and sciatica. With Paul Norton and Thornton Brown as the orthopedic surgeons involved, several projects were begun in collaboration with the Department of Structural Engineering at MIT, the American Mutual Liability Insurance Co., and the MGH Psychiatric Service. However, an ongoing investigation of the low back syndrome failed to materialize primarily because of lack of innovative talent. The problem clearly was to find an orthopedist investigator with the ability and motivation to start a research program of such outstanding promise that it would attract the large-scale financial help needed to build and support the work of orthopedic research laboratories at the MGH.

Happily, a solution to the research problem was in the offing. On the Surgical Service there was an assistant resident who was interested in orthopedic surgery and had impressive credentials. He had graduated from Purdue with highest honors in mechanical engineering and physics in 1946 and subsequently from the HMS magna cum laude in 1950. This young man, Melvin J. Glimcher, after two years on the General Surgical Service and following completion of his orthopedic residency in July 1956, began postdoctoral studies and a research program at MIT as a fellow of the School for Advanced Studies under the tutelage of Francis O. Schmitt, a trustee of the MGH.

Glimcher's research at MIT concerned the molecular biology of the mineralization of bone and other tissues. As the work progressed, the results were exciting, and the concept of a large basic science laboratory staffed mainly by Ph.D.s trained in the basic biologic and physical sciences evolved. The MGH trustees accepted this concept, and the efforts of all concerned turned to the raising of funds to build an addition to floors 3A and 4 of the White Building to house the laboratories. These funds came from private individuals and foundations, supplemented with matching funds from the federal government. Appropriately some of the money was the excess from the funds originally raised by Joel Goldthwait to build Ward I. The money was transferred to the building fund with his blessing; he was 93 years old at the time. In addition, funds were raised to endow a chair of orthopedic surgery at the MGH as well as to support the proposed research. Meanwhile, Glimcher and seven full-time Ph.D. investigators were established in the old Allen Street Pathology Building. Finally, on September 11, 1960, the new quarters were dedicated. They included the Chemistry Laboratory named after Robert Bayley Osgood, the Histology Laboratory named after Armin Klein, the Physical Chemistry Laboratory honoring Smith-Petersen, and the Biochemistry Laboratory named for Joel Goldthwait. Thus Barr's ideas, originally expressed in his letter of 1938, had finally borne fruit.

From 1960 until his retirement in 1964—the year of his death—Barr suffered poor health. He therefore had little time or opportunity to participate in the development of the truly gigantic research project whose origins he had engineered. But indeed his tenure as chief of the Orthopedic Service had seen great and fundamental changes. After Barr's retirement, Brown served as acting chief until Glimcher was appointed as the first Edith M. Ashley Professor and Chief of Orthopedic Surgery at the MGH on October 15, 1965.

The Glimcher Years, 1965–1970. After his return to the hospital from MIT in 1959, Glimcher had climbed the academic ladder rapidly. When he was appointed associate professor in 1962, he became the first orthopedic surgeon in the history of the HMS to hold an appointment with tenure. When he became chief of the service, he brought to that position a point of view distinctly different from that held by any of his predecessors. He was first and foremost an academician rather than a clinician, and his activities during his brief tenure reflected this interest in teaching and research.

Administration. The Ward Service was reorganized into East and West services, each with its own resident staff. The Fracture Service, which had been administratively separate, was incorporated into Orthopedics. An orthopedic resident was assigned to the Emergency Room full-time. In addition, members of the attending staff were assigned in rotation to supervise the care of patients with musculoskeletal injuries in the Emergency Room whether admitted to the hospital or not.

Donald S. Pierce, an assistant in the Orthopedic Service, was appointed director of the Rehabilitation Unit on White 9. In 1968, after Arthur L. Watkins resigned as chief of Physical Medicine, a new department of rehabilitation medicine was created with Pierce as chief; it included physical medicine, the brace shop, White 9, and the amputation clinic. This new department was to develop a team composed of physiotherapists, occupational therapists, speech therapists, rehabilitation nurses, social service workers, orthopedic surgeons, and internists. By establishing this department—with the concurrence of the Medical School—the hospital affirmed the concept that rehabilitation requires a multidisciplinary effort which, at the MGH, was to be a cooperative enterprise with an orthopedic surgeon serving as quarterback of the team.

Patient Care. Glimcher personally had had relatively little involvement in patient care since completing his residency. This circumstance may have strengthened his conviction that if the East and West services were to provide superior care, closer supervision of the residents by the visiting staff was needed. In keeping with this belief, the rotations of visits on the East and West services were modified so that there was a senior and junior visit. The fine line between too much and too little supervision of the residents is always difficult to draw.

The care of patients with injuries and deformities of the hand at the MGH was a long-standing problem finally resolved during Glimcher's regime. About 1920 it had been recognized that infections and injuries of the hand should be treated by surgeons with special interest and expertise, and a Hand Clinic was established. During World War II many young surgeons acquired vast experience in the treatment of hand injuries, and hand surgery emerged as a surgical specialty. When Edward Hamlin, a general surgeon, took over the Hand Clinic in 1946, he organized a multiservice advisory clinic which was attended by representatives from the appropriate services who could provide expertise in treatment of the skin, nerve, tendon, and bone and joint injuries that must be dealt with by the hand surgeon. The orthopedist in this group was Dr. Barr. The Hand Clinic, however, grew very little, and what hand surgery was done continued to be performed almost exclusively by general and plastic surgeons.

Orthopedic surgeons were unhappy with this arrangement. Orthopedists in other medical centers were becoming increasingly prominent in this rapidly growing specialty while hand surgery at the MGH seemed to be sidetracked and at a standstill; also, orthopedic training with no exposure to hand surgery was clearly deficient. Indeed, some experience in hand surgery was a requirement for board certification in orthopedic surgery. This situation was finally remedied during Glimcher's administration. Funds were raised to provide a junior member of the attending staff, Edward Nalebuff, with a traveling fellowship to study hand surgery in Great Britain, Switzerland, and France. When he returned, an agreement was reached with the Surgical Service that the care of patients admitted to the Emergency Ward with hand injuries would be divided equally among the General, Plastic, and Orthopedic surgical services.

Another problem in patient care was a shortage of beds and operating time in the Baker Memorial and Phillips House due, in part, to the steadily increasing number of patients with hip disease whom Dr. Aufranc and his associates treated by cup arthroplasty. These patients required four to six weeks of hospitalization after surgery and, since beds and time on the operating schedule were made available on a first-come, first-served basis, a large proportion of the beds and operating time was being devoted to them. This difficult situation was finally resolved when Aufranc and his colleagues moved their patients to another hospital in the Boston area in 1969.

Education. Unlike any of his predecessors, Glimcher involved himself in the activities of the Medical School, especially in connection with the curriculum. In the recently established second-year course in pathophysiology, he championed the need for a new section devoted to the hitherto neglected musculoskeletal system, and it was he who organized this "block"—a multidisciplinary effort in which orthopedics was deeply involved. He persuaded the curriculum committee, on a trial basis, to schedule a portion of the courses on physical diagnosis and introduction to the clinic directly in the Department of Orthopedic Surgery rather than leaving it to General Surgery to apportion the time. He also persuaded the committee to establish a four-week clinical clerkship in orthopedic surgery as a required course.

To ensure that these clinical courses were first-rate educational experiences, MGH visiting staff men were required to devote more time to medical education. The arrangement after two years resulted in the highest rating from the medical students, a turn of events that catapulted orthopedics from the bottom to the top of the students' rating list. However, as might be expected, the visiting staff found this additional teaching load a heavy burden.

Resident education was also extensively remodeled, putting more emphasis on formalized instruction and less on simple experience as gained in a preceptorship. Weekly grand rounds were changed to two-hour sessions devoted to both orthopedic and fracture problems. In addition, the traditional format in which problem cases were presented for discussion and exchange of views was superseded by a schedule of prearranged topics. A local or invited expert gave a lecture, illustrative cases were shown, and residents and visiting staff were urged to prepare in advance for the discussion and presentation of differing views. Problem-solving rounds were held in the wards or the Smith-Petersen Conference Room each week, with the chief and visitors in attendance. Other educational opportunities took the form of conferences and teaching sessions, including a basic science lecture series, on Wednesday mornings. The faculty for these lectures was drawn from experts in the Boston area. Finally, in an effort to broaden the residents' experience, rotations were arranged at outside hospitals—the Lynn and the Shattuck hospitals locally and Rancho Los Amigos Hospital in Los Angeles.

The old Children's Hospital-MGH Orthopedic Residency Program had also developed offshoots during the course of time. Toward the end of Glimcher's tenure, negotiations with the Medical School and the hospitals involved created the Combined Harvard Orthopedic Residency Program, with orthopedic professors at the MGH, Children's Hospital, and the Peter Bent and Robert Breck Brigham hospitals as well as participation of the orthopedic services at Beth Israel and the West Roxbury Veterans' Hospital. Glimcher obtained an annual grant from the Camp Corporation for a visiting professor to spend several days each year at the different hospitals in the program, making rounds with the residents and participating in conferences. Finally, the visitor delivered the Samuel Higby Camp Lecture on some orthopedic subject.

Research. It was no surprise that during Glimcher's tenure basic research concerned with the musculoskeletal system flourished. After his laboratories moved to the new quarters on White 3A and 4 in 1960, research activities expanded like gas in a vacuum. The initial group of seven Ph.D.s rapidly increased to include as many as 18 Ph.D.s and postdoctoral investigators plus three physicians. By 1968 more space was needed, and the orthopedic laboratories were moved to the tenth floor of the recently completed Jackson Tower. During this rapid growth fellows from many countries spent time working in the laboratories.

Collaborative efforts with other departments were also undertaken. Glimcher teamed with Stephen Krane of the Arthritis Unit in numerous projects and with

John Burke in General Surgery. With the financial backing of the Liberty Mutual Insurance Company Rehabilitation Center and in collaboration with engineers at MIT, a voluntarily controlled prosthesis activated by the action potentials of the muscles in the stump of the upper limb of an amputee was designed, fabricated, and demonstrated to be feasible.

During Glimcher's five-year tenure at the MGH, approximately 100 papers concerned with basic research were published—a remarkable turn of affairs. However, the happy balance of patient care, teaching, and research envisaged as the Orthopedic Laboratories were dedicated in 1960 seemed not to be materializing. In one quantum leap the service changed from a purely clinical activity to an academic and scholarly enterprise. In retrospect, it was probably too much to expect such a rapid change to come about without difficulties. In any event, in 1970 Glimcher resigned and became Peabody Professor of Orthopedic Surgery at the Children's Hospital Medical Center. Thornton Brown once again became acting chief, and another search committee was appointed to select a new chief and Ashley Professor.

In July 1972 the twin mantles fell to Henry J. Mankin. He was the first chief of Orthopedics who had not received his specialty training at the MGH. Born and raised in Pittsburgh and a graduate of the University of Pittsburgh School of Medicine, he had received his postgraduate training at the University of Chicago and the Hospital for Joint Diseases in New York City. He had then returned to Pittsburgh and joined the faculty of the medical school until 1966 when he accepted an appointment as professor and cochairman of the Department of Orthopedics at Mount Sinai School of Medicine and director of Orthopedics at the Hospital for Joint Diseases. It was from this position that he came to the MGH at the age of 44.

Needless to say, Mankin brought talents that had evolved under decidedly different circumstances than those of his predecessors. He was indeed a man of many parts. He was a seasoned administrator and clinician as well as an established investigator who had made significant contributions to the understanding of the metabolism and behavior of articular cartilage in health and disease. He was also a dedicated teacher with a passionate commitment to resident education. His qualifications therefore fitted him superbly for the job of getting the Orthopedic Service on balance with appropriate levels of effort devoted to patient care, teaching, and research. Once on the scene he began to make fundamental changes.

The Orthopedic Service since 1972

HENRY J. MANKIN

The major alteration in care-taking in orthopedics has been the institution of specialty services led by individuals with a keen interest in a specific area and directed at providing competent and skillful clinical care, high quality education, and clinical and basic research. Thus the Hip and Implant Service, ably led by William H. Harris, was established; Harris' principal responsibility is for care of patients with joint disease and, more specifically, problems about the hip. The Hand Service, led by Richard J. Smith assisted by Robert Leffert, was organized for the care of patients and education regarding hand and forearm problems. The Pediatric Orthopedic Unit, headed by Michael G. Ehrlich, is responsible for the care of children with orthopedic problems in the Burnham Children's Unit, while the Tumor Service, headed by Henry J. Mankin, is principally concerned with patients with primary bone and soft tissue tumors. The Rehabilitation Service—which includes the Upper Extremity Surgical Rehabilitation Service—based on White 9 and headed by Leffert, is concerned with restorative services to patients with primarily orthopedic (but also neurologic, cardiac, and respiratory) diseases. Robert Boyd heads the Problem Back Service, which attends principally to patients with chronic problems affecting the lower back. Dinesh Pater and Bertram Zarins run the Sports Medicine section, which deals with athletic injuries and physical conditioning, and focuses especially on problems of the knee. Carter Rowe, the senior statesman of the Orthopedic Service, serves as the guiding spirit to the sports unit. The Orthopedic Arthritis Service, headed by William Jones, has established close liaison with the arthritis unit of the Medical Service and holds joint clinic sessions with them. The Fracture Service, which had all but disappeared over the previous years, has recently been restored to full and active life under the direction of Edwin T. Wyman.

The second major change in the care-taking pattern was the "privitization" of the ward service on White 5, an event that occurred in 1972. There had formerly been a tradition whereby house officers treated the ward patients under the more or less close supervision of the visiting staff who were assigned to the unit on rotation. Since the chief residents on White 5 were board eligible, it seemed logical to appoint them to the staff and place them in the role of "visits" for care-taking purposes, thus giving them the responsibility of a private practice situation for their tenure at the hospital. The position formerly known as chief resident therefore became assistant in orthopedics, and the individual assumed responsibility for a panel of patients seen in the clinic and Emergency Ward and treated them on White 5. Over a short period of time this new system enhanced the quality of care-taking and vastly improved the educational aspects of the unit. The former visiting staff member became the consultant on the service and—since the specialty services had been developed—the assistant on White 5 was able to approach any one of the specialty groups for appropriate consultation. The system worked so well that it was subsequently adopted by other MGH services and has also been extended to our Hand Service which now has two assistants.

"Block time" for the operating room was introduced in 1972. Before that, operating time had been dealt with on a first-come, first-served basis without attention to individual schedules or concern for admitting pattern. This seemed inefficient, so the block time system was instituted; each surgeon was given priority on a specific operating time and could book cases as he wished within that sequestered period. The system was modified somewhat after 1972 and is now under the direction of the Orthopedic Service business manager. Currently we are attempting to utilize data from our operating room booking to program admissions, eventually by computer. The system should materially improve the efficiency of orthopedic admissions and surgery and has already decreased the length of stay considerably.

Since orthopedic patients tend to be long-stay and require skilled nursing and rehabilitative care, it seemed natural to establish an orthopedic service at the

Massachusetts Rehabilitation Hospital (near North Station) which could effectively serve our postoperative patients. The liaison was formed in 1973 and has substantially improved the quality of the continuing care while further reducing the length of stay—and, in fact, the orthopedic inpatient census.

Multiple changes occurred in education based principally on the total revision of the Harvard Combined Orthopedic Residency Program in 1972. Shifts were made in house officer distribution throughout the various hospital units, and the number finally established for the MGH included 15 in the three-year core and two assistants in orthopedics. A full schedule of conferences, as well as grand rounds, are held weekly for the house offices and medical students. These include basic science, hand, pathology, and trauma; other conferences, on hip and implant, sports medicine, tumor, morbidity and mortality, and problem back are held at intervals of two, three, or four weeks. Through the beneficence of Mrs. Ellen Jennings Quinn, a yearly lectureship has been established in the name of her father, Dr. Robert Bayley Osgood, one of the early chiefs of Orthopedics at the MGH.

In addition to the formal conference schedule, several of the specialty services have instituted postgraduate courses under the aegis of the HMS Continuing Medical Education Program. Also, under the direction of Howard Browne and Crawford J. Campbell, the Orthopedic Service has organized a two-week basic science course, held each summer at Salve Regina College in Newport, Rhode Island.

A biannual event of some note for the service is Thesis Day, which occurs each June and December. On this occasion the house officers who are completing the three-year orthopedic core course must present an original thesis to an audience assembled from throughout the Harvard Combined Program. Thornton Brown and J. Drennan Lowell take charge of the program, which includes a discussion by a staff member or invited guest and a luncheon.

Research activities in orthopedics are based largely on Jackson 10. There are two major divisions to the research laboratories: a biochemical unit and a biomechanical division. The former has as its central concern the structure and biochemistry and metabolism of articular cartilage in health and disease with special reference to osteoarthritis, mediator substances, and transplantation. Another project involves the evaluation of the biochemical and metabolic characteristics of chondrosarcoma. Among the investigators in this unit are Dr. Mankin, Michael G. Ehrlich, William Tomford, Louis Lippiello, and Benjamin V. Treadwell. The biomechanical unit under the direction of Dennis Carter is concerned with the structural characteristics of bone and mechanisms of fracture propagation, and, in close conjunction with William Harris, studies the engineering aspects of the normal hip and prosthetic design of implants for hip disease. The units work closely together, and numerous fellows from the residency and from outside the MGH have participated in various aspects of the research programs since their inception in 1972.

Carter R. Rowe advanced this assessment of Mankin and his guidance of the Orthopedic Service: "Few men in medical education today possess the combined abilities which characterize Henry Mankin. He is an able administrator, a superb teacher, a master surgeon, an honored scientist, with the dedicated interest of a physician in his patients and their problems. One may ask—could a man of so many talents have time and interest for hobbies? The answer is yes. Henry loves sports, especially baseball, and is an accomplished artist with watercolors and oils.

"Henry's arrival at the MGH in 1972 as chief of the Orthopedic Service was timely for, at that time, there was an urgent need for a Hand Service, a pediatric orthopedic surgeon, a director of rehabilitation, and manpower for an active, productive research department. Henry brought all of these with him from New York. This has resulted in the development of one of the strongest orthopedic residency training programs in the nation."

With the assistance of *Carter R. Rowe*

29. Oral and Maxillofacial Surgical Service

WALTER C. GURALNICK

When the Harvard Dental School—established in 1869 on Grove Street and known as the "Infirmary of the Mass. General" at a "distance of a few rods" from the main hospital—moved to Longwood Avenue in 1909, a clinic was established in the hospital, and six dentists and a dental surgeon were appointed to the staff. It became apparent, quite early, that it was not possible to provide complete dental care, and the mission of the clinic became essentially that of an oral surgical service. Kurt Thoma, an authority on oral pathology as well as oral surgery, did much to enhance the reputation of the MGH Oral Surgical Service during his tenure as its chief from 1942 to 1947.

David Weisberger, professor of oral medicine at the Harvard School of Dental Medicine, succeeded Thoma as chief. During his administration, and as a consequence of his interests, the name of the service was changed from oral surgery to oral medicine. Weisberger's work on the oral cavity as an indicator of systematic disease and the effect of oral disease on the entire body earned him renown, and he was frequently sought in consultation for diagnosis and treatment. His interest in precancerous and cancerous oral lesions and his work on salivary gland function and radiation therapy was reflected in his involvement in the Tumor Clinic. Weisberger responded to the advances being made in oral surgical training at the time and established a two-year residency program for three residents. Fellowships in oral medicine were combined with residency training to produce highly trained individuals, many of whom assumed leadership roles in oral surgery and dental medicine. He continued as chief until his death in 1966 when Walter Guralnick, a member of the staff since 1950, was selected to fill the position.

Guralnick's tenure coincided with an overall national growth in the field of oral surgery. More importantly, the position of oral surgery was redefined and redeveloped, and the name of the service was changed back to Oral Surgery. The resident training program was restructured as an integrated three-year curriculum for six residents, two new ones being selected each year. To expand the educational content, three-month rotations on anesthesia, medicine, and general surgery were established as well as exchange programs with leading European oral and maxillofacial centers. Within a very short time the applicant pool increased from a handful to well over 100 of the best and brightest competing for the two available first-year residencies.

The position of oral surgery at the MGH was also improved when the General Executive Committee was expanded to include all chiefs of service. This access provided an opportunity to educate the hospital community about oral surgery, its needs and accomplishments. The very cordial attitude of both the administration and the general surgical services, in particular, established an atmosphere in which the service flourished. In 1979 the name of the service was changed to

Oral and Maxillofacial Surgery in recognition of the scope of the specialty being practiced.

A brief review of statistics illustrates the extent of clinical activity of the service in 1980. Until the establishment of the Surgical Day Care Unit, there were approximately 800 annual in-hospital admissions to the service. Since the unit opened, house admissions have been reduced to about 650 to 700 per year, and approximately 300 more patients are operated on in the day care facility. Although the total number is relatively unchanged, the types of cases are markedly different. The majority of house admissions are now major cases of severe trauma, facial deformities, salivary gland diseases, temporomandibular joint pathology, and neoplastic disease of the oral cavity and jaws.

Much minor oral surgery has always been done on an ambulatory basis, and the busyness of the clinic is a reflection of this. No other surgical service holds as many clinic sessions, clinics being scheduled six days a week, including Saturday morning. Approximately 8,000 patients a year are treated. In addition there is an oral surgical room in the Emergency Ward where another 3,000 to 4,000 patients a year are seen. In view of the relatively small size of the resident and visiting staff, the patient load is a full one.

In 1971, as a culmination of years of studying the education of oral surgeons both here and abroad, a new residency program was introduced to function simultaneously with the traditional three-year one. This program was of five years' duration and included a year at the Harvard Medical School to finish M.D. requirements, a year-and-a-half of general surgery, and two-and-a-half years of oral surgery. The fundamental value of the program is attested to by the fact that many other training programs have increased the medical and surgical content of their curricula by as much as they can. Its value is further suggested by the respect in which graduates are held and the number of institutions that recruit them for responsible leadership positions. It has been an important and gratifying educational advancement, but unfortunately only graduates of the Harvard School of Dental Medicine can be accepted into this five-year track; the three-year residency, therefore, has continued and is offered to graduates of other dental schools. One further important improvement in the residency program occurred in 1972 when Joseph Murray and Leonard Kaban of the Peter Bent Brigham Hospital–Children's Hospital Medical Center established a joint division of plastic and oral and maxillofacial surgery on which each of our chief residents rotates for six months. This affiliation has added an important dimension to the training program, providing experience in craniofacial surgery as well as in other procedures that are done more frequently at the CHMC than at the MGH.

The service could not have grown and accomplished its teaching objectives without expanding its full-time staff. There are now five full-time staff members, two half-time, and several others who visit on a part-time basis. Significant basic and clinical research is currently in progress under the leadership of R. Bruce Donoff, a graduate of Harvard and the MGH program.

With the assistance of *R. Bruce Donoff*

30. Urology Service

Wyland F. Leadbetter

EDWARD C. PARKHURST AND SYLVESTER B. KELLEY

Wyland F. Leadbetter came to the MGH in the fall of 1954 as chief of Urology, an appointment that was to herald the development of that service into one of the leading urologic training services in this country. Over the next 15 years, under his guidance, the census in both clinic and private admissions rose prodigiously while many innovative modes of therapy, chiefly surgical, were developed.

Leadbetter arrived well prepared for leadership of the service. Born and raised in Maine, he was endowed with that straightforwardness, willingness to work indefatigably, and modesty that characterize most "down easters." He remained staunchly loyal to his home state throughout his life. Following his graduation from Bates College in Lewiston, Maine, he entered Johns Hopkins Medical School. He graduated with honors and then entered the urologic residency program at Hopkins under the direction of Hugh Hampton Young, at that time the prime source of advanced urologic theory and practice in the United States. Following a period of private practice with George Gilbert Smith, then chief of Urology at the MGH, Leadbetter entered the U.S. Army in 1941, and there honed both his surgical skills and his urologic interest. (He later collaborated on a history of the U.S. Army's urologic experience during the war.) When the war ended, he returned to Boston and engaged briefly in private practice before accepting an appointment as professor of urology at Tufts Medical School and the New England Medical Center Hospital. He served in that position from 1947 to 1954 and then accepted the appointment as clinical professor of surgery (Urology) at Harvard and chief of Urology at the MGH.

Leadbetter developed urology at the hospital into a vigorous, hard-working activity. He attended to a seemingly unending array of urologic problems that presented themselves in patients arriving from all parts of the world. He kept long hours of practice: 12- to 14-hour days were the rule, with morning rounds under way by 6 A.M. He counted Saturdays as working days, with a full schedule of office patients in the morning and, often, a full operating schedule in the afternoon. He enjoyed particularly operating Saturday afternoons and evenings because there were fewer interruptions. Sundays were reserved for paperwork and rounds, though he did find time, usually in the morning, to supervise resident teaching rounds at the South Huntington Avenue Veterans Hospital, an exercise he referred to as "teaching Sunday School."

Patients responded positively to Leadbetter's interest and attention. He possessed the innate ability to relate to his patients, to make them feel that for that moment they were his one and only concern. His surgical technique was aggressive, clever, and meticulous. He believed in finishing each case, usually supervising the last skin sutures personally. He shared postoperative care with the house staff, but he knew the patient's daily records and progress. He discussed the preoperative evaluation, the preparation of a patient for surgery, and the surgery itself equally with the resident and spared no effort to design the best possible course for each patient.

That one of Leadbetter's principal concerns was resident teaching is borne out by the fact that he brought along a dozen men, out of about 40 residents, who subsequently headed departments of urology throughout the country. He took great pride in developing his men, providing them with stimulus and support or acting as the devil's advocate to force a thorough consideration of some special problem. "Never to be forgotten is his electric stimulation while teaching," noted his colleagues. "Continually striving for perfection, not accepting complications, dogma, and current thought as foregone conclusions, he always insisted on attempting better results and thinking of new approaches. . . . Wyland always had time to discuss problems, large or small, no matter how busy he was. He had the ability to listen objectively and to get to the heart of the problem without becoming ensnared with trivia. . . . Everyone was a student to Wyland, and in his presence one always knew he was in contact with the Master." Leadbetter was often heard to comment on rounds: "You simply don't understand the situation"; or, should a patient's course not be ideal, "I cannot recall this ever happening before." He never handled any situation in a routine fashion; rather, alternatives were considered and followed to the benefit of both patient and resident.

Leadbetter was at his best at formal genitourinary rounds on Thursdays at 5. At times some of his remarks seemed a little acrimonious, but at the end of the meetings all hands were in the best of spirits. With his innate enthusiasm, he was oblivious to the passage of time. As the hours rolled on, and as certain members of the audience with personal commitments outside the hospital began to fidget, not a soul would dare to leave the room until he said—sometimes at 8:30—"Well, boys, I guess that's enough for today."

Leadbetter's residents naturally responded to his efforts to advance their education and careers, calling him frequently about professional problems. A high point in his last year as chief was a formal dinner where some 40 former residents assembled to honor him and to found the W. F. Leadbetter Society. They presented him with a silver plate inscribed with their signatures as a token of their respect and affection. He gave annual Christmas parties for the residents and their wives and delighted in seeing everyone have a good time in his spacious apartment where Mrs. Leadbetter played the role of hostess most graciously. With sufficient encouragement, he could be induced to entertain on the piano or violin, both of which he played quite well.

Innovative and aggressive surgery was Leadbetter's order of the day. Drawing on Dr. Young's instruction in urology and wartime experience in surgical techniques, he was able to put his departures from accepted urologic practice to the test. The two-stage prostatectomy was still popular, with a 25 percent mortality, when he started practice; through his efforts utilizing improved technical skills, adequate blood and antibiotic therapy as well as fluid balance, the MGH mortality dropped to less than 1 percent by the 1960s. He encouraged residents to vary their techniques for surgery, particularly prostatectomy, so that they would become proficient in several modes of therapy. He was especially enthusiastic about perineal prostatectomy and relished opportunities to demonstrate his unusual facility with the procedure.

Leadbetter's two major areas of surgical endeavor involved the management of neoplastic disease and of congenital urologic problems. His first significant contribution for patients with malignant disease involved the improvement in urinary diversion (ureterosigmoidoscopy) utilizing a tunneling of the ureters into the colon to preclude reflux, or backward flow, which led to the development of fatal chronic pyelonephritis. He also pioneered with radical retroperitoneal node dissection for testicular tumor and radical cystectomy with pelvic node dissection for malignant disease of the bladder. In another area he applied his principle of tunneling the ureters to the correction of congenital ureteral reflux, thus saving countless children the grim future of death from renal failure. His numerous contributions to urologic literature were broad in interest, carefully conceived, and skillfully presented.

Without the encouragement and support of his dedicated wife, Lois, Leadbetter never could have accomplished what he did for the development of urology. She seemed to devote her whole life to the comfort and success of her husband. Whether he got home from his evening rounds at 9 P.M. or at 1 A.M. she always had a hot meal waiting for him. In the morning it was the same story; at 5:30 she would start Wyland off with a substantial hot meal in preparation for another arduous 15-hour day. Late on a Saturday night, when he wound up a busy day of operating and realized that no special nurses were available to care for one of his sick patients, again it was Lois who scrapped plans for the weekend, donned her trained nurse's uniform, nursed that patient over the hurdle, and afforded her husband a good night's sleep. Incidents like this merely suggest the tremendous sacrifices in their family life that the Leadbetters made for subsequent generations of urologists.

Leadbetter's influence on the urologic community extended far beyond the MGH, for he was both a national and international personality. He belonged to innumerable societies, many quite selective in membership. He was also in demand as a visiting urologist-in-chief. In this role, and as secretary of the American Board of Urology, he not only inculcated his principles of urologic practice to a nationwide audience but also, as he said, kept ahead of what other centers were doing.

Once, on a trip to Tokyo to address the International Urologic Society, he was asked if he intended to take a Japanese vacation. His answer was simple and direct: "I would only take a vacation in the state of Maine." He returned the next day after delivering the paper and making rounds to several hospitals. In the year prior to his death—some years after he had stepped down as chief of Urology—he was president of both the American Urologic Association and the prestigious American Association of Genito-Urinary Surgeons, though his final illness prevented him from attending their respective annual meetings.

Characteristically, he treated others far better than himself. Although a neoplasm of the lung, picked up incidentally by a routine Medical School chest film, was cured completely by surgery, a subsequent malignancy of the cecum that presented vaguely proved fatal. He retired from his Boston practice in March of 1974 and, though he strove valiantly to maintain a urologic consultant's appointment in Millinocket, Maine, he died there in August of that year.

Urology, 1969–1980

Leadership of the Urology Service passed from Wyland F. Leadbetter to George R. Prout, Jr., on September 1, 1969. Certainly, no one could fill Leadbetter's shoes as a clinician, but he had had little time or inclination to develop research activities, and it was hoped that Prout would correct this situation. Prout, a native of Boston, was graduated from Albany Medical School and trained in urology with Victor F. Marshall at the New York Hospital and Willet F. Whitmore at Memorial Center (now Memorial-Sloan-Kettering Cancer Center). Prout had been chief of Urology at the University of Miami and, for the previous nine years, had headed the Urological Service at the Medical College of Virginia. During that time he was involved in an extensive program in renal homotransplantation in association with David M. Hume.

Upon arrival at the MGH, Prout directed his energies toward developing a further sense of responsibility among the resident staff and to organizing prospective clinical studies for patients with certain neoplastic disorders. As often happens in periods of change of leadership and familiar patterns, certain difficulties presented themselves. However, Prout held firmly to his conviction that clinical services in a teaching hospital have no excuse for being if they are not used for research and teaching, and by 1972 the policies that he might implement became clearer. A laboratory activity was started, and arrangements were made for each member of the house staff to spend six months assisting in clinical research programs. To support this effort, the service obtained funds for clinical fellowships from the American Cancer Society, and an agreement was reached with the American Board of Urology to allow each resident to participate in the program provided the individual stayed at the MGH for an extra six months, thus extending the training program to seven six-month blocks. Under this new system the extra six-month person could be board certified and appointed as an assistant in urology at the hospital and an instructor in surgery at the Harvard Medical School. Since that assistant could then care for private patients (on White 10 which was designated for this purpose), the service could support itself.

Simultaneously, both full- and part-time urologists combined to form the Urological Associates, a group practice that brought the urologists closer to each other and even closer to the house staff. The move to the new operating rooms in the Gray Building, with adjacent endoscopic rooms, ensured that a staff member was present at every endoscopic procedure. This led to improvement in patient care and a marked reduction in complications. About the same time the service acquired a conference room, residents' offices, and a residents' secretary.

When Prout arrived at the MGH, no student had elected urology in two years. The new chief sought to rectify this by appearing at each introductory session for students choosing surgery for their elective rotation. The students who elect urology may do so for five days. The service now assures that each visit spends one hour discussing a common urologic disorder such as the significance of hematuria, urinary calculi, common urologic neoplasms. The student receives a text, selected reprints, and a list of things to accomplish. The students take histories, examine patients, go on rounds with the house and visiting staff or with the chief. The service now attracts students from other schools who usually stay a month and almost always apply for a position on the resident staff.

The National Cancer Act of 1971 had a profound influence on the Urology Service since line items for comprehensive research in prostatic and bladder carcinoma were incorporated in the law. Prout was involved in the development of both research groups, a commitment that actually took years to complete. He subsequently accepted the responsibility for chairing the Administrative Center of the treatment section of the National Bladder Cancer Project, National Bladder Cancer Collaborative Group A (CGA). CGA has been conducting longitudinal studies on patients with bladder carcinoma since 1973. The MGH service has also participated in the National Prostatic Cancer Project in the conduct of a continuing search for effective cytotoxic agents. Thus far, however, no strikingly successful agent has been found. Since 1971 an analog of phenacetin, SCH 13521, has been in use; it is an antiandrogen and appears to be as effective as estrogens or orchiectomy in the treatment of prostatic carcinoma. One of its major advantages is that it maintains sexual potency; another is its exceedingly low level of toxicity.

Laboratory activities in the Urology Service have been very difficult to sustain because of intense competition for funding and a lack of space, equipment, and personnel. Nevertheless, working with Bernard Kliman and Robert McLaughlin, the service has provided biochemical explanations for why patients with prostatic carcinoma do not live. MGH researchers were the first to demonstrate the disease's biochemical heterogeneity and to provide data that demonstrated that the lethal cells of prostatic carcinoma are present at the time of diagnosis and that these cells are autonomous with regard to hormonal manipulation.

The major thrust of research in the department is in the area of genitourinary neoplasms under the National Bladder Cancer Collaborative Group A. Four protocols of the National Prostatic Cancer Project are currently being followed at the MGH; all are Phase III studies of chemotherapeutic agents used singly or in combination as compared with conventional hormonal therapy.

Prout is chairman of the American Joint Committee Task Force on the Staging and End-Results Reporting of Genito-urinary Neoplasms and chairman of the National Bladder Cancer Collaborative Group A. He is also on the board of editors of five prestigious journals.

As of January 1, 1981, the service visiting staff constituted the chief of service, one urologist, two associate urologists, four assistant urologists, and three assistants in urology, as well as an associate in biochemistry who heads the Urological Research Laboratory. All but the last are involved in patient care, most participate in clinical research, and all teach and hold appointments at the Medical School.

31. Shriners Burns Institute

Among the more visible developments of the mid-sixties was the conclusion of an affiliation agreement between the MGH and the Shriners Hospitals for Crippled Children which established the Burns Institute in its own building on Blossom Street, across from the Edwards Research Building. Judge Robert Gardiner Wilson, Jr., principal spokesman for the Shrine of North America during the negotiations—and a man who wants to make sure that historians get their facts straight—later compiled a "Complete and Authentic Chronological History" of the creation of the institute. Given the turbulence that attended the dialogue between the hospital and the Shrine, the judge found reason to commit the story to public record. This summary draws on his account.

The Shrine began sponsoring free orthopedic care for children in 1920 and by 1959 had supported 17 hospitals. During those years advances in medicine, such as the Salk vaccine, decreased childhood afflictions, and other agencies increasingly shared in the responsibility for the care and treatment of crippled children. Therefore, in the late fifties, when the Shrine's endowment funds justified further expansion of its philanthropic activities, the organization sought advice as to how it might most usefully deploy its monies. Judge Wilson related that discussions between the Shrine's General Counsel and officials of the U.S. Army Medical Research Command disclosed that "probably one of the greatest single unmet medical needs in North America, especially in this atomic age, was some facility for the specialized treatment of major burns, together with teaching and research, in what had grown to be the single greatest hazard of childhood. Not a single civilian hospital as yet existed on this continent devoted exclusively to the care of severely burned patients." The Shrine, therefore, determined to commit its funds to a children's burns center, a hospital facility equipped with research laboratories and offering training programs for doctors and other medical personnel in the treatment of burns.

Meanwhile, at MGH there existed a cluster of individuals with a long history of interest in burns. Oliver Cope of the Surgical Services was, perhaps, the most dedicated member of the group. MGH research dated back to 1940, and some of the early findings had been successfully applied to victims of the Cocoanut Grove fire in 1942. The spectacle of human suffering and loss of life caused by that tragedy made an indelible impression upon those who tended to the victims. Searches for better ways to care for burns patients had persisted through the war and into peacetime. MGH investigators had published more than 74 papers devoted to various aspects of burns treatment.

Judge Wilson, a member of the Shrine's Burns Committee, did his homework thoroughly. When the MGH's long preoccupation with burns problems came to his attention, he arranged for a conference in Cope's office at the hospital. The meeting took place on December 27, 1961. Cope listened to Shrine plans for a burns center with delight. For his part, the judge was astonished to discover the walls of Cope's office papered with maps and diagrams of a proposed burns research unit for which the doctor was hoping to raise federal grant support. Since Wilson wanted to be well prepared for a meeting of the Shrine Board of

Trustees on January 3, 1962, the two men convened again on New Year's Eve to review the arguments in favor of association with the MGH and to consider potential building sites. A few days later Wilson presented the case for Boston to his board. Though the trustees took no final action, they authorized the judge to pursue conversations with the hospital and the Harvard Medical School.

One imagines that such a fortuitous intersection of objectives would have generated an amiable atmosphere for negotiations. And, in fact, things went along smoothly for about a year. General Director John Knowles and Paul Russell, chief of surgery, expressed warm support for the proposal. The Shrine's Burns Committee, having evaluated several hospitals and medical schools, approved the MGH as the site for its first burns institute on January 22, 1963, "if satisfactory arrangements can be made"—which seemed highly probable. But during the spring, when love is supposed to bloom, the MGH-Shrine courtship ran into difficulties.

Two problems swiftly presented themselves: a building site and the structure of administrative authority. Neither issue was trivial. With respect to the first item, it must be repeated that the properties belonging to the MGH were scarce and the demands upon them intense—hence the density of building that characterizes the hospital campus. Hospital planners were already at work on the new complex now known as the Bigelow-Jackson-Gray buildings. Nevertheless, the Shrine initially received Knowles' assurance that adequate land—estimated by the architects at 25,000 square feet of ground space—would be available for the burns center. Subsequent amendments to this assurance disturbed Wilson and his committee. On May 2nd, for example, Knowles wrote suggesting that "the most ideal location for the Shrine project would be on the 4th, 5th and 6th floors of the tower of the proposed new MGH North Building." When advised by Wilson that "the Shrine Hospital building cannot be on floors or wards of another building, number one requisite is that it has to be a Shrine Hospital Building," Knowles withdrew from his position. But the issue remained a long way from settlement.

Wilson described the second source of irritation as "the continued conflict between Shrine insistence on retaining substantial autonomy in the administration of its own property, and the insistence by the MGH that coordination of operations by the two institutions must be placed in the General Director of MGH. There was a fundamental difference in approach." Moreover, as Wilson's account demonstrates, the questions of site and administrative control were linked: "It was the contention of the MGH attorney, in view of the proposed construction of the Institute on MGH land, and especially if the Shrine Hospital was to be physically an integral part of the MGH complex, that the general policies and procedures and rules and regulations of the institutions in such areas as patient care, admissions and discharges, must be uniform. There was the further claim that in such matters as staffing and housekeeping the responsibility for coordination of all operations should be with the General Director of the MGH. The only area of agreement seemed to be that medical staff appointments should be mutually satisfactory."

The carving of a path through this apparent impasse required diplomatic intelligence of the highest order. Credit for the accomplishment rests largely with a few individuals. Wilson carried almost the entire impetus for the Shrine; his confidence in Cope, in the medical excellence of the MGH, and in the HMS inspired his efforts. Had he not been unusually persistent, it is conceivable that the Shrine would have lost patience and moved the project elsewhere. On the hospital side, Cope's enthusiasm and energy animated the seemingly interminable, sometimes exasperating conversations. In addition, the hospital was fortunate at this time to have Elliot Richardson as one of its trustees. Richardson, acting as the board's attorney, put to good use the political skills that would later make him a prominent public official. David Crockett labored behind the scenes to keep various lines of communication functioning, to smooth ruffled feathers. And finally there was Jim Colbert, treasurer of the Boston Redevelopment Authority.

Architects prepared studies for sites all of which imposed one or another difficulty—in cost, in circulation, in building function. The administrative argument was at a stalemate; Knowles periodically reiterated his view that control must reside with the general director. No need to chronicle here the architects' sketches and their problems or the meetings that dragged on during the spring into the summer of 1963. However, in the first week of August, when things were looking bleak, Colbert indicated that the Redevelopment Authority might be willing to make available to the Shrine a 40,000 square foot parcel of vacant land—controlled by the BRA and the Archdiocese—across Blossom Street, opposite the MGH. "We would own the property, lock, stock, and barrel," Judge Wilson informed his committee, "and not be crowded close to the MGH, our building would certainly be far more distinguishable. . . . Best of all, Dr. Knowles, in response to my direct question, put himself squarely on the record that this . . . location would completely eliminate the problem of supervisory administration as far as he was concerned." Though the road to final agreement still held a few potholes, this alternative ultimately permitted resolution of the conflicts. The affiliation documents were signed in March 1964.

About a month later an interim operation was started in the form of a Shrine Burns Unit on the Children's Service at the hospital. Dr. Cope was named chief surgeon; John Burke, first assistant surgeon; and John Constable, assistant surgeon. This arrangement continued until the Shrine building was completed and four children transferred from the MGH to the institute on September 17, 1968.

Meanwhile, the doctors consulted with architects and Shrine representatives in developing the building program. Cope's advice helped create the character of the institute. Burke was assigned the task of developing the clinical and research facilities in the new structure. It became apparent that the Shrine's budget of $3,760,000 was insufficient to construct the necessary facilities. Fortunately, rather than reduce the scale of operations, Wilson backed Burke's pleas for research and clinical care space, for a tunnel between the institute and the Edwards Research Building, and for the evacuation of the entire basement area of the institute. The Shrine was persuaded to increase its building and equipment budget by half a million dollars. As a result, a decade after the Shrine initiated its research into a burns center, its new facility was officially inaugurated—a capacious building, well equipped to care for children burns patients, to conduct a teaching program, and to pursue research.

These events have been recorded, although in abbreviated form, in the interest of historic accuracy as well as for whatever insights they may provide into the intricacies of any large-scale undertaking at an institution as complex as the

MGH. But the bedeviled background must not overshadow the remarkable work of the institute during the dozen years since its opening.

Initially, Cope filled the role of chief of staff; Burke was named chief of surgery. They were supported by a carefully composed multidisciplinary team—representing pediatrics, orthopedics, anesthesia, plastic surgery, and psychiatry—designed to attack the full range of problems that afflict severely burned children. Burke succeeded Cope as chief of staff when the latter retired in 1969, and there have been individual changes in staff positions, but the complexion of the teams remains intact.

Cope's contribution to the psychiatric management of burn illness has been widely adopted throughout the country. The development of protective environments for patient care in the form of bacteria controlled nursing units has contributed significantly to infection control. Burke and Conrad Bondoc set up the world's first frozen skin bank at Shriners, a facility that has since been duplicated at many hospitals. Treatment regimes embodying prompt excision of burn eschar and immediate wound closure have been developed and refined. In a radical departure from past procedures, it is now possible to operate on burn victims within hours of hospitalization, to plane away charred skin, and to close the wound with skin grafts; if the patient has suffered extensive burns and a donor is not available, skin may be borrowed from the frozen skin bank or—a very recent development—artificial skin may be used. Immunosuppressive drugs prevent the patient from rejecting "borrowed" skin and carry less risk of infection than an open wound; the new manmade skin is not rejected and does not require immunosuppressives.

A ten-year progress report, written in 1978, outlined some of the dramatic advances of the decade:

Ten years ago, before the establishment of the Shriners Burns Institute, any chronicle of the sequence of events detailing the care of a burned child might be a sad saga. Organized burn care itself and knowledge of burns in children were relatively sparse. Burns of a relatively minor nature frequently caused complications and side effects which were fatal. Large-scale burns were usually fatal burns. The state of affairs is set down in a recent edition of *Encyclopaedia Britannica* describing burns: "With third degree burns only a few patients with 40% burns can be saved." Actually, there had been little change since 1902. Ten years ago one out of every two patients with burns over 40% of their bodies died. Today, in our institute, one out of every two patients with burns over 90% of their bodies will survive, and the prospects for the future are bright.

One of the key factors in early recovery and relatively shorter stays in the hospital has to do with the immediacy with which treatment can begin. The sooner new tissues can be grafted, the sooner the recovery procedure can be seen as effective. Furthermore, the longer the wait between accident and initial operative procedures, the greater the loss of skin and more extensive the number and degree of restorative operations.

The first successful treatment of massive third degree burns on a wide scale using transplantation, whether of skin or organs, has always brought with it problems of rejection. Through developments both in patient care and research, techniques have been developed which diminish this rejection and allow the body to accept the transplantation. Specifically, work accomplished at the Institute in the study of skin transplants and immunosuppression makes it possible for the Boston Unit to be the only place in which such transplants are done regularly—and successfully—in the care of the massively burned patient. Prior to March 6, 1972, no burn victim known in the New England medical community had ever survived if the burns were over 80%, 70% of which was third degree. The mortality rate to that date had been 100%. Since then, through research done in the Institute, the figure has been reduced to 36%.

The bacteria controlled nursing unit makes it possible to erect an "environment" around a patient which is free of infectious bacteria and still allows the patient to be part of the ward, rather than in lonely isolation. The unit has been adopted internationally for use in relation to a great range of maladies. It was developed at the Boston Unit of the Shriners Burns Institute for the treatment of burns. Also, the Boston Unit has pioneered the concept of identifying and storing skin to be used in grafting by developing a clinically operative frozen skin bank.

One application of research to patient care (controlled profound hypotensive anesthesia technique) has now provided a means of dramatically reducing blood loss during burn operations. The process allows for longer periods of early treatment, less loss of the patient's own skin, and fewer visits to the operating room, all of which reduce the patient's suffering and stay in the Institute. Without the direct application, the Institute would not have been able to take this kind of step.

A great deal of new knowledge concerning protein metabolism of the burn patient has been acquired at the Institute. Reconstructive surgery at the Boston Unit has adapted microvascular surgery using the operative microscope of burn surgery, enabling toes to be transplanted to make new thumbs and allowing the use of free flaps to reconstruct areas not otherwise reconstructable. In addition, reconstructive surgery has in recent years made it possible for patients to leave the hospital with "new" ears or hands, a concept which was only a wish just a few years ago. Children are not just surviving—they are being helped to resume normal, constructive lives.

The list could go on.* It is well to stop and consider that the unique combination of patient care, research and teaching related to burns was not in existence before the Shriners Burns Institute came into being. It might be said that a sense of synergetics, of interdependence, has provided discoveries and knowledge to such an extent that the result is greater than the sum of the parts. Patient care, plus research, plus teaching equals knowledge in the care of burned patients far in excess of any one of these functions acting alone.

With the assistance of *John F. Burke*

---

*The list *did* go on. In April 1981 Burke announced that the MGH-Shriners staff had achieved excellent results in treating ten severely burned patients with an artificial skin made up of layers that closely resemble those of human skin. The material had been produced as the result of a decade of collaboration between the Boston Unit and a team at MIT led by I. V. Yannas of the Department of Mechanical Engineering.

Part V. Clinical Departments

32. Anesthesia

Henry Knowles Beecher

Henry Knowles Beecher, the first Henry Isaiah Dorr Professor of Research in Anesthesia at the Harvard Medical School, was anesthetist-in-chief at the MGH from 1936 to 1969, a period that spanned roughly one-fourth the life of the specialty of anesthesia. His history as a senior student at the Medical School reads as a sequence of spectacular successes. It began with the Warren Triennial Prize, which he won in 1931 while he was the James Jackson Cabot Fellow at Harvard, for two articles published in Volume 12 of the *Journal of Clinical Investigation:* "The Measured Effect of Laparotomy on the Respiration" and "Effect of Laparotomy on Lung Volume; Demonstration of a New Type of Pulmonary Collapse." Although there is little reason to believe that Beecher fully appreciated the eventual importance of his studies on patient care (his first and last personal contributions to investigations on postoperative respiratory failure), their place in the annals of the care of the critically ill is well established.

Beecher came under the influence of Edward Churchill, chief of Surgery, early in his career when he began his journey as a house officer in surgery at the MGH. In 1935, three years into the training program, he decided to cut short his career in surgery and, at Churchill's suggestion, to consider anesthesia with the possibility of heading a new department of anesthesia at the hospital. To sharpen his physiologic skills he traveled to Copenhagen, sponsored by a Moseley Travelling Fellowship, to work in the laboratory of Professor Augustus Krogh. The reasons for Beecher's change in career have not been recorded, but it is recalled that he expressed more interest in the physiologic and pharmacologic aspects of surgery than in the technical operative side. Churchill's interest in diseases of the chest undoubtedly played a significant role in formulating this decision, as Beecher was certain to have recognized the special opportunities offered by anesthesia for physiologic research.

The MGH was without leadership in anesthesia in 1936; Beecher was offered the position of anesthetist-in-chief. Why, in the days when anesthesia afforded little professional prestige, and when he had had but limited practical experience in the field, did he accept? Perhaps the possibility of a professorship at the Medical School and the assurance of academic prominence for those interested in the specialty helped in his decision. Beyond that, however, all who knew Beecher recognized him as an honest, dedicated, controversial, critical, dogmatic, tireless, and sometimes lonely maverick. Perhaps his farsighted unconventional mind recognized a potential for a bright future when others did not.

Beecher's subsequent career was an uninterrupted series of major contributions to the science of medicine. He knew anesthesia when it had to struggle in a position subservient to the prestigious specialties. This fueled his enthusiasm and added to the importance of his early endeavors. His monograph "Physiology of Anesthesia," published in 1938, won him the Warren Triennial Prize for a second time, and in 1941, two weeks short of the five-year trial period in anesthesia, he was named the Dorr Professor.

Beecher's character as an individualist and scientist profoundly affected those who were exposed to him as students and trainees, even though they continued their professions outside anesthesia. The stamp of his influence is eminently apparent in the present practice of clinical pharmacology and the contributions made by statistics to the health sciences. Each accomplishment deserves a detailed description as to its importance for the practice of contemporary medicine. The publications generated by the laboratory he founded gained wide recognition from the basic sciences. Nevertheless, the definition of principles for ethical studies on man probably represent his greatest contribution to medicine, the epitome of accomplishment in the natural history of the scientist who graduates to an analysis of ethics, once the climax of his professional life has been reached.

There were many extraordinary aspects to Beecher that only a dedicated biographer can place in perspective with his times. The maverick qualities of his mind, the courage to come up with the unexpected, the vision to be controversial and—to the dismay of opponents—often right, the vanity to believe himself unique, the ability to anticipate, synthesize, and express concepts in a style and at a time when they could not be ignored, all criteria that must surely be considered prerequisites for greatness, were evident throughout his professional career.

Among dissenters, Beecher generated passion; among friends, unrequited loyalty. He coveted international recognition and he received it accordingly, including the Legion of Merit award for outstanding services during World War II and membership in the French Legion of Honor. The citation accompanying the latter award reads: "Dr. Henry K. Beecher, Professor of Research in Anesthesia at the Harvard Medical School has rendered invaluable services to the science of medicine by his remarkable achievements in the field of research. By his development of (the use of) synthetic agents to replace morphine, he has moreover made an eminent contribution toward the relief of pain and earned the gratitude of all peoples. France is on the front lines of those who feel called on to recognize publicly Dr. Beecher's services."

This tribute epitomizes the importance of careful clinical observation as a basis for major advance in patient care, a trait highly developed in Beecher. He was resolute in every endeavor and would not compromise with excellence. The caliber of his originality and scientific integrity accounts for both the quality and quantity of his productivity in many areas of research. Those who followed could admit with pride to membership in a once lonely specialty.

Beecher was often at odds with organized anesthesia, never hesitating to be publicly critical. He opposed the organization in its attempts to superannuate the nurse anesthetist and thereby succeeded in antagonizing all. He seldom published in anesthesia journals, for his work was of the rank that qualified for the then more prestigious scientific periodicals. As early as 1941 he wrote, "The casualness with which statistical analysis is so often undertaken does not alter the fact that it is involved, time-consuming and without value unless the fundamental laws of statistics are vigorously observed." In his subsequent career he never failed to follow his own advice. Fascination with numbers characterized his writings, from experiments in the animal laboratory to the ethics of research in human beings.

No sketch can catch Beecher all told; he was too big a man. In his case we have someone who knew the value of posturing, of serious science, of the combination of advertising and modesty, all at the same time. One of his former residents, now on the staff of one of the Harvard hospitals, wrote: "I last saw him . . . either spring or fall of 1975. I was jogging along the Charles, he dragging the other way. Each day he walked one mile, an obvious effort of the will. We did not recognize each other initially; both did a double take and then I walked with him. He wanted to know about everyone and the Department. He was content and feeling complete because he had just sent to the publisher the manuscript of his last book, *Medicine at Harvard, the First Three Hundred Years,* of which he was co-author. Before we parted he said to me, 'I am very proud of you' and I melted. I was reminded that he had told my wife at a party that he had always liked me better than I liked him, and I was sorry."

Beecher's friends and colleagues remember him with joy, tenderness, adulation, and respect for his intellectual honesty, his wide horizon; with agony for being at times a fallen idol; and most of all with love because he was a friend, like a father, a confidante for whom no personal problem was too small to deserve his audience. In science he was a Cyclops; in social life a Bacchus. He was a genial host and an enthusiastic but inept ballroom dancer. He did both with élan, so he was loved for the former and forgiven for the latter. To his peers he was an aristocrat; to his minions, a populist. Surely Beecher's most enduring legacy is a department that in his wake is probably second to none. Of over 250 trainees at least 20 have at one time or another held a post as department chairman.

After retirement in 1969, Beecher struggled with debilitating disease, his mind clear, sharp, and incisive to the very end. Typical of his style, a discussion of his case was published as a case record of the MGH in the *New England Journal of Medicine.* A final honor came within weeks before his death: In June 1976 the Institute of Society, Ethics and Life Sciences established a perpetuating award called "The Henry Knowles Beecher Award for Contribution to Ethics and the Life Sciences," in recognition that "it is unusual for a researcher in medicine to achieve international eminence in even one field. It is extraordinary when the same researcher becomes a pioneer in still another field."

Adapted from a Memorial Minute, *Harvard University Gazette,* January 1978.

Department of Anesthesia

BUCKNAM McPEEK AND JOHN HEDLEY-WHYTE

In his book *The Anesthesiologist and the Surgeon* (1975), John P. Bunker of Stanford University listed six major accomplishments of the MGH Department of Anesthesia:

It established the first research laboratory devoted exclusively to the study of anesthetics.

It was the first department of anesthesia in the world to apply the modern technology of resuscitation to the injured.

It was the first to demonstrate and use quantitative measurement of subjective responses to drugs.

Professor Henry K. Beecher, on behalf of his department, became a vigorous
proponent for human rights in science.

It was a pioneer in establishing scientific principles for the ethical study of drug
effects in man, the motivating force for the establishment of the first human
study committees at Harvard.

In the late 1960s the department became the major driving force behind the first
formal enunciation of the criteria of brain damage, a major advance in human
transplantation efforts.

From 1955 to 1980 this cosmopolitan and constantly expanding department
led an active academic life. Visitors were always coming from university centers
abroad as well as from major institutions in this country. Its own faculty members
were frequently speaking at scientific meetings, often overseas. Such an emphasis
on internationalism, such cogent criticism of anesthetic, surgical, and pharmacologic science, made the Department of Anesthesia at the MGH an object of
envy and criticism. This situation could have created problems had not the support of the Department of Surgery been so steadfast. Edward D. Churchill, late
in his career, wrote, "It has been one of the most satisfying experiences of my
professional life to observe, and in small part to assist, the development of the
art and science of anesthesia during the past four decades. As a result, anesthesia,
once the handmaiden, has become the surgeon's companion in new adventures.
To the old task of obliterating pain has been added the responsibility of maintaining life."

The pioneering efforts of Beecher laid the foundation for the performance of
the department. His early training in physiology with Augustus Krogh influenced favorably the development of the department, as its practice was always
firmly based on physiologic principles. Beecher shared Krogh's disdain for complicated equipment as well as his insistence on measurement and analytic processes.
Together with Churchill, Beecher investigated the effects of chest surgery, amass-
ing enviable results at a time when thoracic surgery was fraught with hazard.
The department's academic life was interrupted by World War II, but Beecher's
insatiable urge to make fundamental physiologic observations led to great improvement in the early management of battle casualties during the last two years
of the war. His work on the beachheads of Italy remains a monument to scholarly
observation under difficult circumstances.

After Beecher returned to the hospital he began to build up the department.
In the early fifties John P. Bunker transferred from surgery to an anesthesia
residency under Beecher. Bunker's work on the acid-base abnormalities of major
surgery was modeled on Beecher's earlier investigations of carbon dioxide ho-
meostasis in patients undergoing chest surgery. In 1961 Bunker was appointed
professor and chairman of the Department of Anesthesia at Stanford University.
Donald P. Todd joined the MGH department in 1946. He undertook with
Beecher a monumental investigation of the causes of death in over 100,000
patients undergoing surgery in university hospitals throughout North America.
The study concluded that while certain anesthetic drugs were inherently more
dangerous than others, the major cause of anesthetic morbidity and mortality
was human error and inexperience of the anesthetist. These unpalatable findings
were seized upon by many anesthetists to be a condemnation of the use of muscle
relaxants and the need for controlled ventilation. However, careful reading of

the monograph and papers resulting from the landmark study suggested the need for expansion of university-based training programs in anesthesia and an even wider scientific base for the discipline. Such an expansion began at the MGH in the mid-1950s. During the next 20 years there was a 20-fold increase in the number of physician-anesthetists at the hospital, from five to over 100. During this time the number of surgical operations only increased threefold, while the time a patient was under general anesthesia increased approximately sevenfold.

Probably Beecher's greatest scientific accomplishment was the demonstration that subjective responses are susceptible to objective measurements. Pain, nausea, thirst, and changes of affect could, he showed, be measured. The effects of narcotics, hypnotics, and other drugs on these subjective sensations could finally be quantified. To achieve these advances in pharmacology, Beecher turned for help to the Department of Statistics at Harvard. The long collaboration, spanning a quarter of a century, between the Department of Anesthesia and Frederick Mosteller, professor of mathematical statistics at Harvard, led to the introduction of sound statistical practice to the laboratories and surgical wards of the hospital.

The enormous expansion of the Department of Anesthesia was, of course, mirrored by a revolution in surgical techniques. The introduction of clinical open-heart surgery in the late fifties by J. Gordon Scannell and W. Gerald Austen; the revolution in neurosurgery by James White and William Sweet; in thoracic surgery by Richard Sweet, Earle Wilkins, and Hermes Grillo; and in peripheral vascular surgery by Robert Linton, required anesthesia of a very high order. In the late fifties interested physicians with the necessary physiologic knowledge to join the Department of Anesthesia were hard to find. In addition to drafting young, academically oriented physicians in the United States, Beecher combed the world looking for suitable recruits. Henrik H. Bendixen was enlisted from Copenhagen; he is currently professor and chairman of Anesthesiology at Columbia. Myron B. Laver was invited from Basel and was later chairman of anesthesia there. Other foreign recruits were Joachim S. Gravenstein, chairman of anesthesia at Case Western Reserve; Henning Pontoppidan who founded the respiratory intensive care unit at the Phillips House and is now professor of anesthesia at Harvard; and John Hedley-Whyte from St. Bartholomew's Hospital in London, currently chairman at the Beth Israel Hospital and professor of anesthesia and respiratory therapy at Harvard.

A major development in the latter fifties was the regular appearance of physician-anesthetists as consultants outside the operating room. In 1955, when the last of the great poliomyelitis epidemics struck New England, White 9 became an intensive care unit devoted to victims of bulbar poliomyelitis. Frequently as many as 45 or 50 patients clung to life with the aid of Drinker-type iron lungs, and physicians from the Department of Anesthesia were in constant attendance. Pontoppidan, who had had experience with similar units in Copenhagen, led the department's efforts in this area, as both anesthetists and inhalation therapists worked night and day. Much of the research interest in cardiopulmonary physiology and respiratory care that was to become the hallmark of the department in the late sixties and early seventies had its intellectual birth in 1955.

The skills developed during this great epidemic and further refined in the laboratory and on patient care floors during the later fifties laid the foundations for the development of the Respiratory Unit by the department in 1961 under Pontoppidan's leadership. Prior to the establishment of this unit, the first of its kind in the country, severely ill patients were cared for on general nursing floors of the hospital. The development of intensive care units was a major advance in the care of the critically ill. Pontoppidan's unit was quickly recognized by the hospital staff as providing the best scientific medical and nursing care available at the hospital. The unit, though firmly oriented to patient care, became an active focus for research, culminating in the publication in 1965 of a monograph on the clinical applications of the principles of respiratory physiology entitled *Respiratory Care,* by Bendixen, Egbert, Hedley-Whyte, Laver, and Pontoppidan.

The movement of the department into scientific respiratory care outside the surgical theater coincided with the flowering of cardiothoracic surgery within the operating room. Both developments occurred at a time when great advances were being made in basic cardiorespiratory physiology and catalyzed the development of Laver's blood-gas laboratory within the department's own research laboratories. Much of the original equipment was designed and built by Laver and his associates. They perfected accuracy and speed in providing serial blood gas analyses that enabled physicians to follow rapidly changing clinical situations. In his early research Laver concentrated on the effects of surgery on pulmonary gas exchange; subsequent work investigated the protection of the heart during open-heart surgery and the physiologic changes caused by acute respiratory failure.

In 1959 and 1960 the department began to form clinical teams organized around the operating room assignments of the various surgical services. For instance, a team of anesthetists, headed first by Laver and later by Edward Lowenstein, worked with the cardiac surgical unit, a similar team worked with the neurosurgical service, and teams were formed to work with each of the ward services in the White Building. Gradually this concept was extended to the Baker Memorial operating room as a special pediatric anesthesia service was formed by David Seigne to work with the pediatric surgeons. This subdivision of the clinical activities of anesthetists along lines paralleling their surgical colleagues had many administrative and educational advantages while enhancing patient care by ensuring that anesthetists took full advantage of evolving subspecialization in anesthesia. The organizational scheme was adopted throughout the department when the Baker and Phillips House operating services were transferred to the new Gray operating rooms in 1969. The organization into teams further enhanced the interplay between the clinic and the laboratory, exchanges to the enormous benefit of each.

In 1968 the MGH department joined five other Harvard teaching hospitals to form the Harvard Anesthesia Center under Bendixen's leadership. This multidisciplinary effort, funded by the National Institute of General Medical Sciences, stimulated great advances in research in anesthesia, both at Harvard and at the MGH. The contributions of the MGH department comprised approximately 70 percent of the overall effort. Anesthesia research units in respiratory care, cardiopulmonary physiology, pain and subjective responses, and neurophysiology were established at the hospital. This promising enterprise had just been established when Beecher stepped down as chief of the department in 1969.

Richard John Kitz, a distinguished anesthetist from the faculty of the Columbia Presbyterian Medical Center, was appointed anesthetist-in-chief in September 1969, and a year later Harvard's second Henry Isaiah Dorr Professor. Kitz, born in 1929 in Oshkosh, Wisconsin, took both his undergraduate and medical degrees from Marquette University in Milwaukee, trained in surgery at Columbia, and then transferred his interest to anesthesia as a resident under E. M. Papper. An able clinician, Kitz was particularly well known for his work on the uptake and distribution of anesthetic drugs and for his research in the physiology, biochemistry, and pharmacology of the neuromuscular junction. Immediately before coming to Boston, he spent a year at the Karolinska Institute in Stockholm as a visiting scientist in the Department of Toxicology with Bo Holmstedt.

On assuming the helm at the MGH, Kitz energetically set about to revitalize the staff. (Beecher had become more and more absorbed in his reflections on medical ethics and had withdrawn somewhat from administrative matters in the late sixties.) Within a year, by skillful recruitment, a number of very able new clinician-scholars arrived. Several new research laboratories opened. Kitz moved his own active laboratory from Columbia to the MGH and, joined by John Savarese, continued a number of his projects in neuromuscular pharmacology while beginning some new efforts in biochemistry. The department launched a major research effort to study the fundamental basis for anesthetic action: How do anesthetic agents produce their effect of altering consciousness and reactivity? How do anesthetic drugs act on central nervous system cells? Under the leadership of Keith W. Miller, such basic work in cellular and subcellular pharmacology represented a new direction for the department.

Kitz and the new chief of Surgery, Dr. Austen, worked closely in preparing for the opening of the new Gray Building operating, recovery, and intensive care facilities. The bed capacity of the respiratory unit was more than doubled, and associated office, conference, and laboratory space were added. The inadequate recovery room was doubled in size; for the first time anesthetists became directly responsible for the care of recovery room patients. At last the department had almost sufficient office space for senior staff. The blood-gas laboratory moved to new, larger quarters immediately above the cardiac operating rooms. The expansion of the responsibilities of the department to larger intensive care units, to the recovery room, and to more operating rooms made recruitment of superbly qualified staff Kitz's continuing concern.

The department recognized the importance of bringing technology developed in other fields to bear on problems of importance to anesthesia and its basic sciences. Kitz established a strong bioengineering research group which cemented ties with the joint Harvard-MIT program in health sciences and technology. Meanwhile, the fruitful collaboration with the Harvard Department of Statistics and the Computing Center continued, as the department, led by Bucknam McPeek, undertook studies of patient care at the hospital, looking for risk factors influencing outcome as well as the end result of intensive care. The increasing strength of the faculty was reflected in an expanding research program. At national meetings it became commonplace for reports of research from the MGH to outnumber contributions from any other institution—sometimes by a factor of two. Senior clinicians like George Battit, John M. R. Bruner, Elliott V. Miller, and John F. Ryan were in great demand as visiting professors at medical centers across the country.

All these developments acted to strengthen the educational program for residents and medical students. Within a few years of Kitz's arrival, the MGH residency in anesthesia—always coveted—became one of the most sought-after in the world. The number of residents increased, commensurate with the expanding responsibilites and educational opportunities in the department. In 1975 applicants for the residency had frequently been fully trained in another medical specialty or had a Ph.D. in one of the basic sciences. The department—even its most junior members—was becoming more mature. The program of visiting professors and lecturers was reinforced. Distinguished scientists from throughout the world visited the department and advised on overall activities as well as on specific clinical and research projects; they participated in a multifaceted teaching program that benefited students, residents, and staff alike.

The years since 1955 have, then, been years of growth and of improvement in ability to respond to the needs of the sick and injured with the best scientific medical care.

With the assistance of *Richard J. Kitz*

33. Pathology

The Castleman Years

For 19 of the 25 years encompassed by this volume—not to mention four antedating them and a spell during the Second World War—the reins of the MGH Department of Pathology rested in the capable hands of Benjamin Castleman. Remarkably, he was only the third chief since pathology became a department in 1896. James Homer Wright ran Pathology for 29 years, from 1896 to 1925; his successor, and Castleman's mentor, Tracy B. Mallory, administered for 26 years; and then the office passed to Castleman who held it (including a brief period as acting chief) from 1952 to 1974. Altogether, the record might prompt some unscientific speculation about a correlation between pathology and long productive careers. A fourth chief, Robert T. McCluskey, is currently in place and may reflect happily upon the tradition he has inherited.

Castleman grew up in Dorchester, Massachusetts, graduated from Harvard College in 1927, and entered Yale Medical School with expectations of a career in internal medicine. One or two circumstances along the way may have prepared his mind for pathology, although, of course, retrospect gives them more significance than they seemed to have at the time. For one thing, Castleman had a physician uncle who specialized in bacteriology and used to permit his nephew to tinker in his Boston City Hall laboratory. Also, Yale had a fine pathology department. One professor in particular, Milton C. Winternitz, etched himself permanently on Castleman's memory. He had a peculiar and effective—if not necessarily endearing—teaching style that forced students to probe continually deeper into the subject matter, and Castleman liked his classes.

Then in the summer of 1930, between his third and fourth years of medical school, Castleman found work as a clinical clerk in the laboratories of the MGH Department of Pathology. He was the only student in the lab that summer, and Mallory, eager to recruit young talent to the specialty, spent a great deal of time with him. Mallory was a quiet gentle man who, as Castleman recalled, "didn't throw his weight around" or act like a boss. Half a century later Castleman paid tribute to Mallory's influence by observing: "He instilled in me certain principles of conservatism in pathology—being sure that when you say something, you're *sure* of it; if you're not, to *say* so, and always to act conservatively, in the interest of the patient. . . . Because at the end of that slide is what the physician or surgeon is going to *do* to that patient."

Toward the end of the summer Castleman asked Mallory if he would accept him as an intern in pathology after completing his studies at Yale—in part because he had enjoyed working in the lab, in part because he had developed a tremendous respect for the MGH, and in part because such an arrangement would relieve him of the necessity and anxiety of formal applications for internship. Though still aiming for internal medicine, he thought a year in pathology would be a useful and compelling detour, never realizing that for him, pathology would be the main road. Mallory readily agreed to this proposal.

Simultaneously with his graduation from Yale in 1931, Castleman came down with rheumatic fever; fortunately, Mallory held his slot open, and Castleman joined the MGH house staff in October. And so began the long and mutually satisfying relationship between Ben Castleman and the MGH. He rose steadily through the ranks of Pathology to become, after Mallory died in 1951, its chief in 1953. His career at the Harvard Medical School traveled along the same ascending curve, ending as Shattuck Professor of Pathological Anatomy.

Castleman took a serious view of his responsibilities as a citizen of the hospital at large. As chief of Pathology he sat on the General Executive Committee—in the days when it wielded considerable power, before John Knowles expanded the membership. Between Knowles' departure and Sanders' appointment, from January through August 1972, Castleman served as acting general director while continuing to run his own department (see page 26). "I really enjoyed it," he said later, while admitting, "I wouldn't have wanted to do it for the rest of my life." Thereafter, the MGH community affectionately adopted him as one of its "senior statesmen." Recognizing the mutual dependence of medicine, science, education, and the soundness of the institution in which they are practiced, Castleman carefully distributed his energies. Fortunately, those energies were prodigious.

Castleman the scientist appeared in the pages of Washburn's history wherein it was noted that "the remarkable material offered for the study of parathyroid disease was utilized by Drs. Castleman and Mallory for an extensive study of the pathology of hyperparathyroidism, which served to round out the clinical study of the Medical and Surgical Departments." The latter study, instigated by the work of Albright and Aub (and Oliver Cope who haunted the autopsy room for almost two years getting a surgical fix on the parathyroids), resulted in a paper still considered a classic in the annals of pathology.

In 1961 a committee of distinguished colleagues summarized his research efforts:

Dr. Castleman's scientific contributions to pathology lie in the recognition of new disease states (e.g., pulmonary alveolar proteinosis and mediastinal lymph node hyperplasia, known as Castleman's Disease), the careful clinical-pathological correlation of problems of current importance, and the imaginative utilization of the rich opportunity gained from working in a large general hospital where clinical advances of importance are so numerous. His study of the relationship of vascular disease to the hypertensive state, based upon a study of renal biopsies removed from 1000 hypertensive patients during sympathectomies by Dr. R. H. Smithwick, is a landmark in the field of hypertension. He has written authoritatively on the thymus gland and he is being increasingly recognized for his comprehensive knowledge of surgical pathology in general.

Richard Schatzki, an eminent radiologist, remembered:

I first met Ben when he was a resident and came to the Radiological Conferences at the MGH to present the pathological side of the cases which were discussed, and showed specimens if available. He contributed greatly to the conferences by being factual, to the point, helpful, and not opinionated. He showed then, already, what I believe is his greatest strength—namely, an interest in the whole patient and the whole abnormal process, not restricted solely to the pathological findings. . . . Although principally trained as a morphologic pathologist, his interest in other phases of pathology, e.g., chemo-pathology and immunology became even stronger. He grasped their importance and supported their development in his department. His interest in clinical problems, however, always supervened.

The ad hoc committee for his appointment as professor similarly remarked that "his taxing duties in teaching and hospital service have left little time for the use by Dr. Castleman, himself, of newer technics brought into pathology from the various sciences basic to medicine. His recognition of their importance, however, is attested to by his excellent choice of younger men to work with these tools in the laboratories that have been created at the MGH by his enthusiasm, his broad knowledge of the important developments of medical research, and his administrative skill."

Castleman's alertness to those developments permitted him to avoid the intellectual paralysis that is a very real hazard of long governance in a fast-moving discipline. He outlined his concepts of an appropriate balance of activities in his 1966 annual report as follows:

Although in recent years the emphasis in many university pathology departments has been on the biochemical and molecular biologic aspects of disease, it is important to bear in mind the fact that hospital pathology laboratories have, in addition, the responsibility of patient care and thus the necessity of expert knowledge of anatomic pathology. Fortunately, our department is large enough to permit a balance of the research effort with the patient-care activities so that neither discipline suffers in the training of our residents—a situation that is not prevalent in many university pathology departments. . . . Proof of the great need for experts in the field of anatomic pathology is to be found in the increasing volume of consultations that come into our laboratory from all parts of this country and abroad and in the large number of invitations to our staff members to speak at universities and medical meetings.

Reflection upon Castleman's character prompted Schatzki, who has been his friend for decades, to remark that "success did not make him conceited. In his younger years, his drive and desire not to waste time at times offended people. With the years, he became more and more settled, self-assured, thinking of others."

Benjamin Castleman, of course, is also Castleman of the CPCs which is about as close as one can get to a household word in the universe of medicine. CPCs are the reports of clinicopathologic conferences that appear weekly in the *New England Journal* describing interesting clinical cases at the MGH that are resolved in the Department of Pathology. English- (and Spanish- and Japanese-) speaking physicians, dentists, psychiatrists, surgeons, pathologists, and so forth read them with the same kind of fascination that detective fiction devotees derive from a Simenon mystery.

"It is hard enough, many a vexed author or consortium of authors would testify, to prepare a single article for a medical journal—what with the original preparation, revisions, and the editorial idiosyncrasies to be complied with," wrote Franz Ingelfinger, editor of the *Journal,* about Castleman's work. "Imagine, then, the gargantuan task of preparing manuscripts, week by week with chronographic regularity, and submitting them without fail and on time over a period of 23 years—a total of about 1200 manuscripts comprising about 2000 case reports. But this is an achievement that, among his many other accomplishments, Benjamin Castleman can look back upon as he retires this summer from the position of chief of the Pathology Department at the Massachusetts General Hospital, and hence, concurrently, from that of editor of the Case Records of that institution. 'Editing,' however, is an inadequate word for what Ben did. Although he has had the stout and indispensable support of Robert E. Scully as associate editor, and of Betty U. McNeely as assistant editor, the CPCs published by the *Journal* during the Castleman regime have been ineluctably marked by the man's stamp. It was he who selected the cases and the discussor, who trimmed off the fat, and who, often as not, delivered the devastating dénouement. Moreover, he insisted that the published cases conform to a precise format. Woe to the *Journal*'s editors if a figure illustrating a pathologic finding was printed before the reader came to the pertinent text. About such matters Castleman was adamant. His has been a performance combining the qualities of a virtuoso and a martinet."

Said Castleman, "I enjoyed doing it because I thought it was an important and valuable way of teaching students and doctors. It showed how medicine was being practiced at the MGH. . . . I learned a lot of medicine doing them."

Castleman invested the same kind of personal, scrupulous attention in administering the Department of Pathology and in training young pathologists as he put into the CPCs. "I personally believe that contact with one's Chief of Service is very important and I give almost two hours a day to actual participation with my staff," he explained to the General Executive Committee in 1961. "The entire staff meets every morning at 8:15 and for up to one hour I personally check all the gross material of the autopsies of the day before. This is a very popular exercise and almost every morning various members of the clinical staff, both house and members of visiting staff, appear to take part when their case is coming up. Every afternoon from 2 to 3, I personally check the interesting and problem microscopic slides of the surgical pathology specimens that have come through that day. These two hours each day give me an opportunity to actually know what is going on in the department and also give an opportunity to the various members of the department, who are working on research problems or who are assigned to bacteriology, hematology, or chemistry to return to the laboratory each day in the morning before they start their regular work and right after lunch before they start their afternoon's work. This personal teaching of the house staff has paid off in that applications for appointments come in in droves."

In 1972, the year of his theoretical retirement as chief, Castleman surveyed the history of the department during his tenure. (He would, in fact, continue to administer for another two years until McCluskey took charge.) That report is quoted at length below.

Over the past 20 years the patient care activities and the teaching program have greatly increased, and with our move into the Warren Building the research done in the department was expanded in many directions. Probably very few members of the staff realize that the Pathology Department is closely interwoven with the other departments in the hospital. This interrelation, begun during Dr. Mallory's regime, has continued and broadened in scope. At the present time members of the pathology staff attend a wide variety of service and specialty-unit staff meetings, demonstrating gross and microscopical material with clinicopathological correlation. Each week there are 15 to 20 such meetings. Three units with which the laboratory has a close affiliation are the Neurology and Dermatology services and the Otolaryngological Department of the Massachusetts Eye and Ear Infirmary.

The neuropathology laboratory, established within the Department of Pathology in 1926 under Dr. Charles S. Kubik and supervised since his retirement in 1951 by Dr. Edward P. Richardson, Jr., was officially named the Charles S. Kubik Laboratory for Neuropathology in 1961. Its major activity has been to define pathologic processes in the nervous system, to relate the tissue changes to clinical phenomena and to use the insights thus gained in the teaching of residents and fellows in the neurological sciences as well as in pathology.

Although dermatopathology had been emphasized in the department in the 1940s by Dr. Walter Lever, a former member of the Dermatology Service, it became a more specialized unit in 1962 with the arrival of Dr. Wallace H. Clark, formerly professor of pathology at Tulane University, and a closer liaison with the Dermatology Service was effected. The unit has recently been expanded under Dr. Martin C. Mihm, a graduate of both the Dermatology and the Pathology services. This unit now provides teaching, consultative service and opportunities for research to residents in both dermatology and pathology as well as to residents in the Harvard-affiliated hospitals.

In 1962, on the retirement of the pathologist for the Otolaryngological Service of the Massachusetts Eye and Ear Infirmary, arrangements were made for our laboratory to process their surgical specimens, and one of our staff, Dr. Karoly Balogh, became the pathologist for the MEEI. This liaison has been well coordinated and provides an opportunity for our resident staff to be exposed to this type of pathological material. Balogh resigned in 1968 to become pathologist to the University Hospital and was succeeded by Dr. Max Goodman.

In 1942 Dr. Joe V. Meigs and Dr. Maurice Fremont-Smith set up an exfoliative cytology laboratory under the direction of Ruth M. Graham in the Gynecology Service. In 1950 the Cytology Laboratory became incorporated in the Department of Pathology, although it remained physically in the Vincent Building until January 1957. At that time Dr. Priscilla D. Taft became its director, and the Cytology Laboratory joined the rest of Pathology in the Warren Building. . . .

In 1957 Dr. Leonard Atkins, under a grant from the Atomic Energy Commission, originated a bone-marrow bank for use in the event of atomic bomb casualties, and the bank was later used for storage of autologous marrow, obtained during remission, for treatment of leukemic patients. This involved bone-marrow culture and led to chromosome preparations and ultimately in 1959 to the establishment of the Cytogenetics Laboratory. This unit now has a larger volume of specimens to study than any such laboratory in the state, providing service not only for the MGH, but also for most of the hospitals in metropolitan Boston. The definitive diagnosis of mongolism, the detection of translocation carriers and the finding of chromosome abnormalities associated with congenital abnormalities have been among the practical aspects of the work in the laboratory. In collaboration with the Fernald School the Cytogenetics Laboratory has participated in a study of amniocentesis fluids for prenatal detection of chromosome abnormalities.

Included in the category of patient-care activities is our service to numerous community hospitals. Pathology was one of the first departments in the hospital to establish an association with a community hospital. In 1941 I became the pathologist to the Emerson Hospital, in Concord, a post that I held for over 20 years. In 1946 we undertook the pathological examinations for the Brockton Hospital and continued that service until 1959. In 1949 a close affiliation with the Memorial Hospital in Worcester began when Dr. Ronald Sniffen, one of our graduates, was appointed pathologist there, where for many years we had rotated members of our resident staff. The three full-time pathologists now at the Memorial Hospital are all MGH alumni. During the war we helped a few small community hospitals. Several of our alumni, now in community hospitals, continue their association with the laboratory as clinical assistants or clinical associates. This interrelation is helpful to the community hospitals because these young pathologists bring their problems to our large staff of experts, and the MGH gains from the association because the problem cases are often referred to members of our clinical staff. Our neuropathology unit has affiliations with the Fernald, Paul Dever and Wrentham State Hospitals.

Teaching: Teaching of the pathology house staff and fellows in training was augmented considerably during this 20-year period. In 1952 training in clinical pathology was made available by rotation through the Chemistry, Bacteriology and Hematology Laboratories, enabling these residents to be eligible for Board certification in Clinical as well as Anatomic Pathology and later for positions in hospital laboratories. . . . In 1956 the post-sophomore fellowship was introduced, and until the recent change in the HMS curriculum two to four students spent a year between their third and fourth years in the laboratory, dividing their time between patient-care pathology and research. This program has been one of the best methods of recruiting medical students to the field of pathology. Of the 18 students who joined this program, currently six are pathologists, 9 are in academic institutions, and two are professors and chairmen of departments of pathology.

With the introduction of the block system in the teaching of pathology at the Medical School all members of our staff and many of our house staff have participated in teaching at the HMS. A recent survey has shown that annually about 2000 hours of teaching students are supplied by our full-time staff, with our house staff contributing approximately the same amount of time.

The members of the staff participate in the many postgraduate courses given in the hospital by various clinical services. In 1964 we introduced a course on the Pathology of the Endocrine Glands. . . . Another aspect of our postgraduate teaching is the large number of lectures and slide seminars that our staff members are asked to conduct at medical schools and national meetings in both the United States and in foreign countries. This is especially true of Dr. Robert E. Scully, whose clinicopathological investigations and talents in gynecological pathology are being acknowledged by the many invitations he receives throughout the world. A corollary of our lecture tours and visiting professorships in various foreign medical schools has been to provide an opportunity in our laboratory for trained pathologists from foreign universities to learn our methods of training in patient-care pathology, teaching and research. A few of these fellows became members of the resident staff, and several now hold university chairs.

Perhaps the greatest impact of the laboratory on medical teaching throughout the world has been effected by the clinicopathological conferences published weekly in the *New England Journal of Medicine.* Since these exercises are used for teaching by many medical schools, hospitals and other medical organizations throughout the world, in 1954 we introduced a lantern-slide service providing 35-mm slides of pertinent x-rays, electrocardiograms, gross specimens and photomicrographs of the cases published each week to those interested in conducting conferences similar to ours. This project continues to be popular, and each of the current 160 subscribers receives over 600 lantern slides per year which can be added to their permanent teaching file. A final spin-off of the Case Records was the publication by Little, Brown and Co. of five volumes of selected specialized cases, 50 cases to a volume, re-edited and amplified with more photographs and addenda. These volumes, published between 1960 and 1972, are collections of medical, surgical, bone and joint, neurologic and, most recently, cardiac cases presented over a span of several decades.

Research: Before we moved into the Warren Building in 1956 the research carried on in the old Allen Street Building was primarily clinicopathological correlations and was not supported by outside funds. Nevertheless, important papers dealing with the pathology of the parathyroid and thymus glands, renal biopsies in hypertension, malignant lymphoma, aortic dissection, pulmonary embolism and infarction, and Mikulicz's disease were published. This type of clinical research, based on careful observations and often with new technics, has continued, with the emergence over the years of new clinicopathological entities, such as pulmonary alveolar proteinosis, mediastinal lymph-node hyperplasia, several distinctive ovarian and testicular tumors, chemodectoma of the lung and clear-cell carcinoma of the vagina arising in young women who had been exposed to stilbestrol in utero. In 1967 Dr. Gerald Nash and Dr. Blennerhassett, in collaboration with Dr. Henning Pontoppidan of the Department of Anesthesia, demonstrated that many patients who died after mechanical ventilation had pulmonary lesions consistent with oxygen toxicity, and partly as a consequence it is now standard practice throughout the world to monitor closely the dose of oxygen during mechanical ventilation.

With the move into the Warren Building, space for more sophisticated research became available, and outside support was obtained. . . . An important addition to the research facilities was the establishment of the Edwin S. Webster Laboratory to house the first electron microscopy laboratory for human pathology in New England, under the direction of Dr. David Spiro. . . . During his five-year tenure before resigning to become a professor at Columbia University many of our residents and fellows were trained in this new technic. Dr. James B. Caulfield took over the direction of this unit in 1961 and demonstrated renal glomerular changes in prediabetic patients and further noted that dermal elastic tissue of prediabetics and diabetics is severely altered. Continuing work on cardiac diseases, Caulfield has defined the major cause of cardiogenic shock and the secondary myocardial lesions induced by this syndrome. Recently, he moved his laboratory to the Shriners building, where he is investigating ground substance in wound healing. Dr. Ronald S. Weinstein and Dr. N. Scott McNutt, pathology research trainees, using the equipment in the Mixter Neurosurgical Laboratory, applied high resolution electron microscopy technics to the study of normal and neoplastic cell membranes.

The chance finding by Dr. Kilmer S. McCully at autopsy of accelerated arteriosclerosis in two patients with homocystinuria resulting from two different enzymatic disorders led to the experimental production of arteriosclerosis in animals given homocysteine derivatives. Cell cultures from other patients with one of these types of homocystinuria were then found to elaborate an abnormal highly sulfated matrix, accounting for the prominent accumulation of matrix in the walls of arteries involved by early arteriosclerosis. Investigation of these cell cultures led to the discovery of a new metabolic pathway for sulfate ester synthesis from homocysteine, requiring ascorbic acid and controlled by pyridoxine.

Recognizing the increasing importance of immunologic thought and technology in the understanding and treatment of many diseases, I established in 1959 an Immunopathology Unit within our department, designed to serve as a focus of teaching, research and diagnostic expertise in this field. Under the able direction of Dr. Martin H. Flax this unit formed close liaisons with clinicians in other units, such as the Renal Transplant Unit, with improved patient care as a consequence. In addition, Flax made fundamental contributions toward an understanding of the pathogenesis of autoimmune thyroiditis. His investigative activities created a tradition of intellectual excitement that was passed on to his successor, Dr. Harold Dvorak, when Flax became professor and chairman of the Department of Pathology at Tufts University Medical School in 1970. Dvorak's research has been concerned with the morphology and pathogenesis of cellular hypersensitivity. He has described a new form of lymphocyte-mediated immunologic response characterized by the presence of large numbers of basophilic leukocytes, which apparently have a prominent role in such diverse entities as viral infection, contact allergy, and tumor and graft rejection in both animals and patients.

Since 1958 we have been very fortunate in having an NIH research training grant to support four trainees per year. Its recipients obtain a basic training in anatomic pathology and in addition join one of the research units in the department or one of the investigators in another hospital laboratory. The purpose of this grant is to train academic pathologists. It is of interest to compare this small group of trainees with the entire group of residents over this period; 80% of the 30 research trainees are now in academic pathology, whereas 53% of the regular house staff are in academic pathology. We are, of course, very proud of the fact that 26 of our alumni of the last 25 years were appointed to full professorial chairs, and that 15 of them are or were chairmen of departments at their universities.

Castleman actually did retire two years after composing this synopsis—if "retirement" can be used to describe a life that came to consist of far-flung speaking engagements, consultations, and various services in behalf of the MGH. He was, among other things, an editor of this volume; he did a prodigious quantity of editing during the spring of 1982, working until a few weeks before his death in June of that year. The honors that came to him over the years, both national and international, are simply too numerous to list here. Two tributes, however, deserve special notice. In 1977 the Harvard Corporation voted to establish a professorship in his name at the Medical School; fortunately, Castleman was able to attend the celebration of the activation of that chair in early June 1982 and to enjoy the accolades of friends and colleagues. And in 1980 his former trainees and co-workers established through the MGH the annual Benjamin Castleman award to be given to a young pathologist who during the previous year has published an outstanding article in the field of human pathology. Both the professorship and the award will perpetuate Castleman's name in pathology—whatever path the science may take—and in the hospital that was his professional home for half a century.

With the assistance of *Richard Schatzki*

1975–1980

The MGH found a successor to Castleman in the person of Robert T. McCluskey, an alumnus of Yale and New York University School of Medicine. McCluskey had been a professor of pathology at NYU in the early sixties and then accepted the position of professor and chairman of the Department of Pathology at the State University of New York at Buffalo. He moved to the Boston area in 1971 as a professor at the Harvard Medical School and pathologist-in-chief at the Children's Hospital Medical Center. Though officially appointed chief of the MGH Pathology Department in July 1974, McCluskey was obliged to share his time with the Children's Hospital until January 1975. He used the occasion of his fifth year in office to reflect upon the evolution of his domain, and the following remarks were adapted from his annual report for 1980.

The Department has 31 full-time staff pathologists and 12 clinical associates or part-time staff. Most of the salary support for the staff comes from general operating funds of the hospital or research grants (mostly NIH). Harvard Medical School provides a negligible sum, and consultative services and postgraduate courses bring in a relatively small amount of revenue. Largely because of a lack of grateful patients, the department has only modest endowment funds. Furthermore, our department—unlike most departments of pathology—does not supervise the clinical laboratories and we, therefore, cannot draw directly on this abundant source of funds. Despite these considerations, the department is well supported by the hospital (for which we are grateful).

The department is responsible for diagnostic services in anatomic pathology (surgical and autopsy), cytology, and cytogenetics. The number of surgical pathology specimens received annually has risen from about 21,500 in 1975 to 28,000 in 1980. In addition, certain special procedures have increased at an even faster rate. For example, the number of frozen sections and operating room consultations jumped considerably in 1975 and 1976 following the establishment of the pathology laboratory on Gray 3. In addition, the use of sophisticated procedures such as electron microscopic and immunofluorescence studies has expanded appreciably.

Surgical pathology, like other branches of medicine, has become increasingly subspecialized. Almost all the staff have developed special expertise. There are several units to which surgical specimens are generally sent directly—dermatopathology, gynecologic pathology, neuropathology, immunopathology, renal pathology, and some bone and lung specimens. Other specimens are initially reviewed by the resident and the staff pathologist on sign-out rotation and then referred as indicated to the appropriate specialist. Despite increasing subspecialization, we have not found it feasible to establish autonomous units with individual cost centers, in large part because of the continued overlapping responsibilities of staff pathologists and also because of the reliance on common services, notably technical, secretarial, computer, and administrative functions. Moreover, the general surgical pathologists and residents have resisted further subdivision because of anticipated logistical difficulties and adverse effects on resident training.

In 1976 a computerized system known as CAPER (Computer Assisted Pathology Encoding and Reporting System) was introduced for use in surgical pathology, largely through the efforts of Stanley Robboy and members of the Laboratory of Computer Science. CAPER automatically records for each specimen the patient's number, consolidates information on different specimens from the same patient received at different times, and provides information concerning the reporting status. CAPER was the first comprehensive computer system developed for a pathology department in this country.

The Cytology Laboratory, under the direction of Priscilla Taft, reported slight increases in the number of specimens from 1975 to 1979 and a slight decline thereafter. The Cytogenetics Laboratory, directed by Leonard Atkins, serves outlying hospitals and private physicians as well as the MGH. Approximately 80 percent of the specimens (including prenatal specimens) are submitted from outside, many of them passing through the prenatal laboratory of the MGH pediatric genetics unit. In 1980 the Cytogenetics Laboratory handled 1467 specimens, which is about as many as are processed in any such laboratory in the country.

The MGH has shared in the decline in the autopsy rate that has occurred throughout the nation. Since the 1950s the rate here has declined from about 60 to about 48 percent. In many comparable teaching hospitals, however, autopsy rates have declined to 10 to 20 percent. Explanations that have been offered for this phenomenon include the removal of the requirement by the hospital-accrediting agencies for a specified percentage of consents for autopsies, the belief that major advances in clinical diagnostic techniques have rendered autopsies unnecessary, fear of information being uncovered that might be damaging in malpractice suits, and a decline in emphasis on the teaching of pathology in medical schools. Nevertheless, I believe autopsies continue to provide important information concerning the quality of patient care, including findings that are useful in the evaluation of the effectiveness and hazards of new forms of therapy. In addition, autopsies are necessary for the training of pathology residents.

Education. The department is very active in house staff training, medical school education, and postgraduate courses. A substantial number of the staff and some of the residents teach in the general pathology course and the pathophysiology courses at the Medical School. In addition, an elective course for medical students in pathology is given at the MGH. Three postgraduate courses have been introduced in recent years—in surgical, gynecologic, and dermatopathology. Members of the department also conduct a two-day biannual course in Immunopathology at the International Academy of Pathology. However, probably our most demanding teaching exercise is the CPC, which is now in the capable hands of Robert Scully as editor. Despite extensive commitments in other areas, he consistently provides excellent selection (with the help of the chief resident) and editorial review of the cases.

Training in pathology leading to board certification generally follows one of two tracks: One requires three years of training in anatomic pathology and the other two years in anatomic pathology and two years in clinical pathology (i.e., clinical chemistry, hematology, blood bank, bacteriology, and clinical immunology). The first track is usually followed by individuals who want to develop subspecialty or research skills and who plan a career in large teaching hospitals or medical schools. The second is taken by residents who expect to practice pathology in a community hospital, as well as by some who hope to have an academic career but nevertheless want accreditation in clinical pathology as an "insurance policy." Lately, an increasing percentage of residents have requested training in both clinical and anatomic pathology, which appears to reflect a growing reluctance of young pathologists to pursue a career in research or academic medicine. The MGH department has responded to the aspirations of this latter group by improving the training program for residents in clinical pathology. The staffs of the clinical laboratories have been most cooperative in this effort.

The American Board of Pathology has stiffened its requirements not only in clinical pathology but also in anatomic pathology by increasing requirements in forensic pathology, cytology, cytogenetics, neuropathology, immunopathology, and electron microscopy. In order to comply with these standards, we have had to increase the number of required assignments in anatomic pathology. There are 23 pathology residents, including one assigned to dermatopathology and another to neuropathology. In addition, residents rotate through the Boston Hospital for Women for training in obstetric and perinatal pathology. The department can continue to say with pride that the MGH program is considered one of the busiest—and one of the best—in the country.

Research. In 1976 major new research (and diagnostic) facilities were completed in the Cox Building. The principal programs located there are in the fields of immunology and immunopathology. The past decade has seen an explosion of knowledge about the immune system; it is now possible to study, in ways that were not foreseen even a few years ago, the various cells that govern immune response in a variety of human diseases. We are making use of the monoclonal antibodies against T cell subsets in two major ways: one, through identification of T cell subsets in tissue sections by immunofluorescence or immunoperoxidase techniques; and two, through identification of cells in suspensions by flow cytometry.

Drs. Atul Bhan and McCluskey, in collaboration with Drs. Schlossman and Reinherz, have studied the distribution of T cell subsets in normal human thymus and lymph nodes. Studies on lymphomas and various inflammatory infiltrates, such as contact reactions, rejecting renal allografts, and in association with tumors, are being performed by Nancy Harris, Martin Mihm, Terence Harrison and others in the department; they will employ not only antibodies specific for T cell subsets but also monoclonal antibodies against B cell subsets and mononuclear phagocytes.

The identification of cells in suspension depends upon new technology, flow cytometry, which can measure surface components of cells in suspension through excitation of light from fluorescein labeled antibodies with a laser beam. This technique can detect as few as 3,000 molecules per cell and can be used to separate individual cell populations from complex mixtures. The Flow Cytometry Laboratory is under the direction of Robert Colvin, who has found, in collaboration with Paul Russell, Benedict Cosimi, and others in the Transplant Unit, marked changes in the ratios of circulating suppressor/cytotoxic and helper T cells in renal allograft recipients. It already appears that this information is useful in predicting which patients are at particular risk for rejection or infection. James

Kurnick, who joined the department in July 1980, has developed an approach that should prove useful in the development of new monoclonal antibodies against human T cell subsets. His techniques make it possible to maintain and clone human T cells in vitro; the cultured cells maintain their functional properties.

Other studies on Cox 5 concern immunopathogenetic mechanisms in experimental renal disease. Bhan, Bernard Collins, Eveline Schneeberger, and McCluskey have obtained evidence that delayed hypersensitivity reactions can be triggered in glomeruli and produce hypercellularity and damage. Colvin and Alan Brown have shown in a model of autoimmune tubulointerstitial nephritis that anti-idiotype antibodies can markedly suppress the autoantibody response and reduce the renal damage. This may provide an approach for suppression of other autoimmune diseases.

Schneeberger is engaged in investigations on the regulation of solvent transport across epithelial and endothelial surfaces in the lung. She has demonstrated the importance of tight junctions and pinocytotic vesicles in transport.

There are three laboratories at the Shriners Burns Institute that are involved in studies investigating the connective tissues and their role in normal growth and development and in pathologic problems such as scar formation. These are the Experimental Pathology Laboratory, directed by Robert L. Trelstad; the Wound Healing Laboratory, led by H. Paul Ehrlich; and the Physical Biochemistry Laboratory, directed by Fred H. Silver. These laboratories, which were established through Trelstad's efforts, have taken a number of different but complementary approaches to the study of connective tissues.

The gynecologic and dermatologic pathology units carry out extensive research programs in the Warren Building. The gynecologic pathology group is actively engaged in continuing studies on the effects of intrauterine exposure to diethylstilbestrol (DES). In 1974 the National Cancer Institute commissioned a national collaborative project to study the non-neoplastic lesions associated with intrauterine exposure to DES. Ann Barnes and Stanley Robboy are the co-principal investigators. The first major report from the project indicated that the frequency of the cancer was low, that non-neoplastic changes in the vagina occurred in one-third of women rather than the 90 + percent suggested by others, and that the abnormalities might be self-limited.

The dermatopathology group, under the direction of Mihm, is involved in several important investigations. Of particular interest are studies on malignant melanoma aimed at identifying or elucidating precursor lesions, risk factors, and prognostic indicators. Other investigations are directed at identification of T cell subsets in infiltrates surrounding melanomas and other cutaneous neoplasms and in various inflammatory conditions.

34. Radiology

The Robbins Years

Though the words *growth* and *development* apply to practically every facet of the MGH during the past 25 years, there is no more dramatic instance of those dynamics than the Department of Radiology which recorded phenomenal increases in clinical responsibilities coupled with an accelerated rate of scientific and technological evolution. Laurence L. Robbins, who had been appointed radiologist-in-chief shortly after the war, in 1946, presided over this exuberant activity until 1971 when he retired from administration to, as he put it, "do an honest day's work by reading a few films and devoting more time to teaching the residents and medical students."

Robbins was born in Burlington, Vermont, in 1911, the only child of a Methodist minister. He did his undergraduate work at Ohio Wesleyan College and the University of Vermont, acquired his medical degree from the University of Vermont in 1937, and spent the next two years in radiology at the Mary Fletcher Hospital in Burlington; he completed his residency under the supervision of George W. Holmes at the MGH and was appointed to the staff in 1941. The war, of course, depleted the ranks and precipitated staff upheavals in Radiology as it did elsewhere in the hospital. Holmes retired as chief in 1941 and was succeeded by Aubrey O. Hampton; but when Hampton was summoned to Washington to serve as chief of Radiology at Walter Reed Hospital, in 1942, Holmes returned to run the department. Robbins' assistance to him during those short-handed, chaotic years proved invaluable. After the war a number of senior staff—including Hampton—departed, and Holmes retired with finality, leaving a core of younger men to carry on the work of the department. Robbins emerged from this group as chief.

Robbins was the fourth chief of Radiology at the hospital and the first to hold the title of professor of radiology at the Harvard Medical School. Like his predecessors (Walter J. Dodd, Holmes, and Hampton), he was both an academic and clinical radiologist. More than 90 publications—addressing various aspects of radiotherapy, clinical diagnosis, radiation protection, radiologic education, and the delivery of professional services—attested to his broad clinical and scientific interests. His single most stunning contribution to diagnostic radiology was contained in a series of articles on the roentgen appearance of lobar and segmental collapse of the lung. His bibliography included a volume, written with Holmes, entitled *Roentgen Interpretation,* which for many years served as the basic text in diagnostic radiology; it went through eight editions. Robbins combined backgrounds in medicine and pathology with an uncanny eye for an abnormal x-ray pattern and established a reputation for diagnostic accuracy that made him a legend in his own department. He could dazzle staff conferences by spotting the pathology from a distance of 15 feet at a 45-degree angle to the view box and then finish his bravura performance by referring to similar cases he had seen ten or 15 years earlier—even remembering the names of patients.

While Robbins' professional talents earned the respect of his peers, his personal qualities won the hearts of his staff and students. He was for them a source of intellectual honesty, kindness, understanding, and support. He kept the door to his office open and received people without appointments. A true father figure, he attended with sympathy to the personal or professional problems of innumerable residents and staff. He possessed an uncommon ability to listen, to identify alternatives, and to so direct a conversation that the person in trouble never felt that he or she was being handed a solution but, rather, was evolving one independently. His blend of professional excellence and loyalty to his staff generated an atmosphere of friendliness, cohesiveness, and mutual support in the department. Two concerns dominated Robbins' stewardship: to provide the best possible patient care and to develop young people in the field of radiology. He never promoted himself in public or private life but stepped out of the limelight so that the junior staff could develop expertise and reputation. He found his greatest satisfaction in seeing those he had trained achieve recognition for their own accomplishments in academic radiology or in private practice.

Robbins' years in office were marked by the prodigious increase in the utilization of radiology as well as advances in both diagnostic and therapeutic techniques and equipment. Though all that ferment was exciting, it created a progressively heavier administrative load. Robbins, having borne it for more than two decades, was ready to relinquish it. He had, by then, become a leading figure in American radiology; he held numerous high offices in professional societies and received American radiology's highest awards—the gold medals of the Radiological Society of North America and of the American College of Radiology.

During the early years of his tenure, Robbins was assisted by Milford D. Schulz and Stanley M. Wyman. They were joined by Joseph Hanelin, James J. McCort, Jack R. Dreyfuss, and William R. Eyler and somewhat later by John D. Reeves. By the time of Robbins' retirement, the department had a staff of 28 radiologists, one clinical fellow, and three physicists to uphold the high standards in radiologic education and clinical investigation for which it had gained international renown. The department attained and sustained excellence in spite of plaguing deficiencies in equipment and space. This want was felt not only in the thwarted development and expansion of new areas in research but also in clinical radiology for the routine care of patients. Holmes had commented in 1940, after the opening of the White Building, that for the first time in the department's history the space was comfortable and the equipment adequate. During that year 31,500 examinations were performed. In 1957, 78,000 examinations were undertaken in the same physical space augmented only by one room for special cardiovascular procedures. An additional division, equipped to handle ambulatory patients referred by private physicians, failed to alleviate the overcrowded facilities of the general hospital. By 1963, when the White 1 unit opened to serve the Emergency Ward, the annual number of examinations had risen to 146,500. This unit helped relieve conditions in the routine diagnostic areas but did nothing toward supplying space so badly needed for special studies in neuroradiology and the rapidly expanding field of angiography. It was not until 1970—when the annual tally of examinations had reached almost 160,000—that these needs were partially met by the provision of some space in the new Gray Building.

Though Robbins' own interests centered on diagnosis, he often stressed the needs of radiation therapy. When Milford D. Schulz came to the MGH from Huntington Memorial Hospital, he brought a vast experience in the use of supervoltage radiation for treating malignant disease. A one-million-volt machine had been installed in 1940 and a 2-Mev Van de Graff generator in 1949; during this period the annual rate of treatments had climbed from 2,000 to over 12,000. A Cobalt-60 therapy unit displaced the older supervoltage machine in 1956, but the radiation therapy division did not gain any space, and by 1970 36,800 treatments were registered. (For more extensive background and further developments in therapy, see Chapter 35, Radiation Medicine.)

In 1953, after many years of need, the department was able to appoint a physicist in the person of Edward W. Webster. His services to all divisions and his assistance in the teaching program for residents and technicians were invaluable. He earned international recognition for his contributions to the field of radiation physics, particularly those in radiation protection and dosage. In addition to serving in numerous national offices, he was a consultant to the International Atomic Energy Agency and to the Bureau of Radiation Health.

Shortly after radioactive isotopes became available, the department began to use them in radiation therapy, and in 1946 Robbins instigated the formation of an Isotope Committee for controlling and expanding the use of radioactive materials in diagnosis, therapy, and research. However, the development of the use of these isotopes remained rather diffuse because each service promoted only the isotopes or tests pertinent to its particular interests rather than allowing these activities to become concentrated in a single department. These circumstances left some gaps in the radiology training program, so the department arranged for the Atomic Energy Commission to receive each resident for three months of training in the use of radioisotopes at the nuclear facility in Oak Ridge, Tennessee. Majic S. Potsaid, who joined the staff in 1957, was responsible for the infusion of many new ideas into the department, but his work with cine-radiology and with television were particularly noteworthy. He became interested in expanding the use of isotopes in the department. While continuing his many research projects, he was able to promote the diagnostic use of isotopes to the point that he could also assume the responsibility for that portion of the residency previously obtained at Oak Ridge, and by 1968 he had succeeded in making nuclear medicine an important activity in the department. Two years later Nuclear Medicine and Radiation Physics acquired quarters of their own in the Gray Building.

When Robbins became radiologist-in-chief the department had three residents, one being accepted each year for a three-year program; that year it was decided to accept two new residents each year, and a fourth year chief resident was added in 1966. In early 1970 there were 30 residents, and 12 new residents were accepted in July 1971. The regular program remained three years long, but an NIH training grant program provided for applicants interested in an additional year of basic laboratory research. The department produced a number of graduates who entered academic radiology, many to become department heads and professors. Four former radiology residents were awarded the Advanced Fellowship in Academic Radiology by the James Picker Foundation; one of them, Gerald W. Kolodny was also designated a scholar in radiological research by the Picker Foundation for the purpose of studying molecular events basic to radiation response in cultured cells. In 1965 Lucy Squire of New York City, a talented teacher, began to participate in the instruction of medical students. The interest generated by this program was reflected in an increase in the number of students choosing the elective in radiology at the MGH as well as in the number of applications for radiology residencies received from Harvard graduates exposed to Squire's lectures.

In the pioneer days of radiology the training and supervision of x-ray technicians was largely by apprenticeship, but it gradually developed into a more formal course. Many early technicians were nurses, particularly during World War I when many men from the department were called to military service. By 1970, however, there were almost no nurse-technicians in the hospital except for some assistants in radiation therapy. By that time most x-ray technologists, as they came to be called, entered training directly from high school. In 1959, under the direction of Chief Technician Robert I. Phillips, the training period for technicians was expanded from one to two years, and the formal educational portion was broadened considerably. The program formed an affiliation with Northeastern University for didactic lectures in the basic sciences. (For more recent developments, see Chapter 44 on the MGH Institute of Health Professions.)

Despite the chronic shortage of space for expansion, many innovations were possible largely because of the perseverance of department staff. In the late forties a room for clinical research was provided and enabled important work in angiocardiography. Selective arteriography began in the same room about 12 years later. Image intensification was first used in 1954, and its combination with television became a reality in 1961 when the use of television and cine-fluoroscopy started on White 2. Remote control fluoroscopy was added a few years later, and automatic film processing began in 1958.

The organizational structure of the department followed the approximate pattern started by Holmes when separate units were equipped in Phillips House in 1917 and in Baker Memorial in 1930. There was, however, a shift toward subspecialty groups within the department, an evolutionary development produced by the increased volume and complexity of certain types of examinations. The first such subspecialty was neuroradiology, headed by Paul F. J. New. An angiocardiography unit, headed by Robert E. Dinsmore, grew out of the increased use of radiology in the diagnosis of heart disease and the use of selective visualization of arteries in the diagnosis of a variety of diseases. (Angiography had been started in the early forties by Wyman and selective arteriography in the early sixties by Robert A. Nebesar and James J. Pollard.) Alfred L. Weber developed pediatric radiology into a separate section. Because of Frederick S. Tomchik's interest in the radiographic diagnosis of breast disease, requests for the procedure increased to the point that a separate area had to be planned for mammography. In 1968, when Murray L. Janower was put in charge of the general hospital division, it was thought desirable to divide all procedures performed in that unit into subspecialty groups consisting of chest, bone, gastrointestinal, and genitourinary. However, the Phillips House Division, headed by J. Malcolm McNeill, and the Baker Memorial Division, under Dr. Dreyfuss, continued to function as general radiology.

When Robbins announced in November 1969 his desire to be relieved of administrative duties, he also stated his wish to remain in the department, to become a clinical radiologist once more, and to devote more time to teaching.

He thereby continued a tradition that proved to be of great value to the department. After he died, in March 1980, several colleagues composed a touching Memorial Minute that ended with these words: "His legion of friends in the country and abroad and particularly those of us who worked with Larry Robbins at the Massachusetts General Hospital are indeed most fortunate to have experienced his special, charismatic combination of professional excellence, scrupulous integrity, personal modesty, and enduring loyalty. We shall miss him greatly."

> Adapted from *J. Malcolm McNeill's* history of MGH radiology and from a Memorial Minute, *Harvard University Gazette,* February 13, 1981

1971–1980

The MGH administration used the interval between Robbins' announcement of his wish to step down as chief and the appointment of a successor to review the department as a whole. After many committee deliberations the General Executive Committee recognized the wisdom of separating radiation therapy from the Department of Radiology and established a new department called Radiation Medicine in 1971 (see Chapter 35). The search for a new radiologist-in-chief ended in the selection of Juan M. Taveras, an eminent neuroradiologist, academician, and departmental chairman, who received his medical education at the University of Santo Domingo in his native Dominican Republic. During his first years in the United States he earned a second M.D. degree at the University of Pennsylvania Medical School while completing his radiology residency and was elected to Alpha Omega Alpha. He joined the faculty at Columbia University in 1950 and was director of radiology of the Neurological Institute until 1965 when he migrated to St. Louis to become professor and chairman of the Department of Radiology at Washington University School of Medicine and director of the Mallinckrodt Institute of Radiology. His curriculum vitae further includes an extensive list of publications—most notably, perhaps, his 1964 book, *Diagnostic Neuroradiology,* the standard reference in the field, which Taveras wrote with Ernest H. Wood—along with an impressive array of consulting and other professional activities. This, then, was the man who became the fifth radiologist-in-chief of the MGH and, concurrently, professor of radiology at the Harvard Medical School.

Taveras assumed his full-time duties in September 1971. He was most pleased to have Robbins continue as senior radiologist and teacher as well as chairman of the residency teaching program and selection committee. There was a certain ebb and flow of staff through the mid-seventies. Upon his arrival Taveras made several immediate additions. Stanley Baum came from the University of Pennsylvania Medical School to become head of cardiovascular radiology but returned to Pennsylvania four years later to become chairman of Radiology there; Christos A. Athanasoulis, who had joined the MGH staff in 1972, moved into Baum's position. Glen Roberson, who joined the neuroradiology section in 1972 and became its head in 1976, subsequently accepted a chairmanship at the University of Albany. Roger A. Bauman resigned from the U.S. Public Health Service to become assistant radiologist-in-chief for operations and computer activities in

1974. Majic S. Potsaid rejoined the staff in 1971 as director of Nuclear Medicine, working with Henry Pendergrass, the co-director. The latter decamped in 1976 to become assistant chairman of Radiology at Vanderbilt. Thereafter the staff stabilized, leading Taveras to note, in 1981, that "although a number of the senior staff has been offered chairmanships of departments of radiology . . . around the country, none has undertaken to leave the MGH."

When Taveras arrived in the department, much of the radiographic equipment was approaching the end of its useful life. He implemented an aggressive, carefully phased replacement program which was completed in six years. His extensive experience with radiographic equipment and construction contributed significantly to the success of the effort; by combining still valuable portions of radiographic rooms with new equipment, quality facilities were assembled—in several instances at far less cost than entirely new equipment.

In his tenth annual report in 1981, Taveras reviewed the developments of a decade:

The last ten years have seen the introduction of an entirely new and revolutionary imaging technology, namely Computed Tomography. This non-invasive imaging procedure grew tremendously in succeeding years following its introduction in 1973, when the first or second unit in the United States was installed here at the MGH. The growth of this type of procedure has been short of spectacular and after the first three months or so when it became apparent that this was an extremely useful clinical diagnostic method the unit was swamped with requests for examination. We have never been able to catch up with the demand even though another total body instrument was added (in 1976). Two instruments at a hospital like the MGH are far from fulfilling the needs even though both units are operated for 16 hours per day, plus an 8-hour shift on Saturdays. . . . Perhaps as important as the discovery and development of CT scanning technology is the fact that this opened up the field so that other imaging approaches utilizing the same computer algorithms could also be developed. These include emission computed tomography and digital ultrasound imaging and, more recently, nuclear magnetic resonance. At the same time other non-invasive methods continue to develop.

Continuing his summary, Taveras observed that "one of the interesting phenomena that is worth mentioning is that between 1946 and 1975 there was an average of 7% compound increase in the number of radiologic diagnostic procedures." Some of the figures were astonishing. For example, from 1971 when there were 164,671 examinations conducted in 29 procedure rooms, there was an increase to 204,843 examinations in 42 rooms by the end of 1973. "Then," Taveras wrote, "in 1975, the rate of growth began to decrease, and in the last three or four years the number of diagnostic procedures has been virtually stationary. However, at the same time that there was a decrease in the number of relatively simple procedures, there was an increase in the more complicated examinations which include angiographic procedures, computed tomography, nuclear medicine procedures, and ultrasound. The result of this is that if each examination is converted to what is ordinarily referred to as Relative Value Units, there has been a continuing increase in the number of RVUs so that, in fact, the trend in radiologic diagnostic procedures continues upward. I would predict that this trend will continue now that the greater emphasis on non-invasive diagnostic examinations is being demanded by everyone. The newest non-invasive, or only slightly invasive, procedure on the horizon is digital computerized subtraction angiography. This procedure will replace many arteriograms being carried out at present, but the net result will undoubtedly be an increase in the number of examinations because this can be carried out on an outpatient basis."

As the clinical load increased, so did the paperwork. Computers were pressed into service to handle the department's scheduling, film library management, and reports' transcription and distribution—all improving service to patients and referring physicians. The acquisition of new equipment, the renewal of old, the intense clinical demands—the department in 1980 saw some 700 patients per day—and research needs required modifications of old building facilities as well as new floor space, after 1974 accomplished under the watchful eye of Dr. Bauman. (See list, Chapter 7, for significant construction activities.) But Radiology, like virtually every other department at MGH, still felt cramped in its quarters. While noting considerable improvement in the flow of patients through radiologic facilities, Taveras conceded that "unfortunately, the expansion of the various imaging procedures taking place at the same time seems to gobble up any savings in space brought about by better rearrangement of the activities. For instance, we now need about 4 ultrasound diagnostic rooms of which there were none in 1971, and the equivalent of 4 rooms to accommodate CT scanners. Also, we now need 8 diagnostic rooms in the cardiac nuclear medicine area of which we had only one equivalent room in 1971."

Taveras responded to the escalating levels of complexity in radiology by continuing and refining the system of subspecialization begun during Robbins' tenure. Ultimately, 12 separate radiology subspecialty sections evolved, including gastrointestinal, genitourinary, bone, neuro, angiography, pediatrics, cardiac, ultrasound-computed body tomography, mammography, and nuclear medicine. Individual section leaders were entrusted with considerable administrative and professional autonomy under Taveras' guidance, and many rapidly developed national reputations in their specialties. Baum pioneered angiographic techniques for control of gastrointestinal hemorrhage, an instance of the sometimes inexact boundaries between diagnosis and treatment; Joseph T. Ferrucci, Jr., introduced techniques for examination of the pancreas, duodenum, and biliary tract and became the youngest president of the Society of Gastrointestinal Radiologists. Richard Pfister explored the mechanisms of reactions to iodinated contrast media; he pioneered antegrade pyelography via percutaneous catheterization and also accomplished needle puncture and aspiration of renal cysts under fluoroscopic control. William Strauss refined nuclear medicine methods for assessing cardiac functions. The dynamism and balance provided by these and other energetic staff members extended the reputations of the MGH Department of Radiology as one of the nation's best.

The Taveras administration also saw the creation, in 1972, of the Division of Radiological Sciences under the leadership of Edward W. Webster, the department's physicist and authority in radiologic physics and radiation protection; in addition to his research and teaching responsibilities, Webster served as the hospital's radiation safety officer and chairman of the MGH Isotope Committee. Meanwhile, the Radiology Department's research arm was strengthened by the transfer of the Physics Research Laboratory, under the direction of Gordon L. Brownell, from Medicine to Radiology. This group became known for its work in the elucidation of gamma dosimetry of radioisotopes as well as for developments in positron brain scanning; continuing work in positron imaging resulted in the construction of an advanced positron camera known as the MGH PCII.

Studies of the brain and of cerebral circulation under the stroke program center grant and studies of the heart have been done utilizing short-lived isotopes produced by the MGH cyclotron. The Physics Research Laboratory has also been active in applying computer techniques to nuclear medicine imaging.

There is little doubt that the past quarter century was a period of stunning growth and accomplishment for the MGH Department of Radiology. And there is little reason to suppose that this momentum will diminish in the foreseeable future. "We anticipate further development of imaging technology," Taveras predicted, "and I look forward to the clinical application of intravenous digital computerized subtraction angiography as well as, somewhat later, nuclear magnetic resonance. The latter promises to be nearly as revolutionary as computed tomography."

With the assistance of *Roger A. Bauman* and *Joseph T. Ferrucci, Jr.*

35. MGH and Cancer

Cox Building for Cancer Management

In 1968 the priority for construction at the MGH was an ambulatory division for cancer patients that would be the first facility at the hospital to adhere to the principle of one level of care for all. Howard Ulfelder, Joe V. Meigs Professor of Gynecology and then head of the department at the MGH, had been associated with this project from its inception, ten to fifteen years before. Appointed chairman of the building committee, Dr. Ulfelder's main role was raising funds for the construction of the Cox Building. He is especially proud of the new design philosophy that stresses the interior aesthetics and which, he has found, "reassures the majority of patients, who seem to equate the fact that we were interested enough to attend to their comfort, with the availability of expertise for their care."

Dr. Ulfelder was also instrumental in planning how the various clinics would be organized, considering, for example, that medical oncology at the MGH had consisted of a series of unrelated doctors' offices, some more organized than others. The purpose of the Cox Building, however, was not just to provide new quarters for previously existing facilities but rather to "see what cancer would require of a hospital ten years from now." In the process of supervising the move into the building, Dr. Ulfelder assumed the new title of deputy director for cancer affairs. He is involved with the clinical program, with some aspects of the research program and applications for its funding, and with the administration of the only building at the MGH that has a disease-oriented designation.

Not too strongly identified with any one of the disciplines related to cancer, Dr. Ulfelder feels that this was a plus in that within the Cox Building, radiation therapy, various facets of chemotherapy, surgical oncology, and research can all be equally emphasized in a beneficial environment for cancer patients. His recollections on the Cox Building follow.

During the course of planning new quarters for an overcrowded department of radiation therapy and the Tumor Clinic, the opportunity presented itself to review the entire panorama of cancer activities at the Massachusetts General Hospital. We found, as we expected, that every necessary or appropriate and desirable aspect of research, diagnosis, and treatment was represented already at the hospital, but that the logistics of utilization was sometimes awkward and communication between offices, clinics, and laboratories often meager. The planning committee proposed and the trustees agreed that any new construction or renovation should emphasize the following opinions:

—that in contacts with the medical world the cancer patient would most often be in ambulatory status as a visitor or transient and that this would in the future be even more the case.
—that the involvement of several kinds of special professional knowledge and experience—the multidisciplinary approach—was necessary for optimum care and that this would be used for all cases, starting with the stage of treatment planning.

—that the ambience that frames these activities, including the attitude and behavior of professionals as well as the physical environment, plays an enormous role in the support of patient and family confidence, in their ability and willingness to reestablish normal or nearly normal patterns of life, and in husbanding their energy and patience when these reserves were low.

With these objectives in mind, the Cox Building was designed to accommodate the entire department of radiation medicine and its awesome equipage, the Division of Medical Oncology, the Tumor Clinic and Registry, and some activities of Surgical Oncology as well. Laboratories for all three oncology units and for physics and pathology are located on the upper floors of the same building with the deliberate intention that this geography would not only facilitate rapid convocation of multiple experts when appropriate but also provide a constant mix of laboratory and clinical personnel that could not avoid provoking frequent informal communication and germinating ideas.

The pattern of patient movement throughout the building received special attention. Only on the lower level, ground floor, and second floor does the hospital staff deal directly with patients, and therefore the aesthetics of foyers, entrance halls, and waiting areas have been designed to be pleasing and minimize stark functionalism, particularly the "hospital look." Long walks and tedious waiting are avoided as much as possible. The truly sick or failing patients are not paraded before the generally well; they enter by chair or wheeled stretcher through another entrance or by an elevator accessible directly from the off-street driveway. Both social and psychologic support personnel are in residence; every practicable step has been taken to keep delays, confusion, misunderstanding, and tiring multiple appointments or repeat visits to a minimum.

The hospital now encounters more than 4,000 new patients with cancer each year. Over half will sooner or later be seen or treated by the medical oncologists, and almost half at some time receive treatment by radiation therapy; many, of course, become involved in both. Programs are constantly modified, and new features are incorporated as they demonstrate effectiveness. It is a complex and changing affair which for best results requires a spectrum of technical skills, apparatus, and drugs that can be justified only by the volume of the demand. In radiotherapy, for example, as wide a variety of specially trained physicians and individualized equipment is available as there is in surgery, where we have come to expect quite different facilities for thoracic, neurosurgical, urologic, orthopedic, and other types of procedures if best results are to be achieved in all situations.

As sections of the Cox Building were completed and equipped, beginning in the spring of 1975, they immediately began functioning. The first was a cobalt unit for radiation therapy chiefly for patients with cancer of the breast; it has since been followed by a second cobalt unit of somewhat different capabilities, and then a linear accelerator. Even with these operating, the installation continues of additional high energy units as well as the orthovoltage equipment used for the treatment of superficial lesions. All the necessary facilities for patient care such as simulators, the mold room, examining spaces, and so on are located on the same level in keeping with our original philosophy of concern for the convenience of the patient. On the third floor are the offices for the department and on the sixth and seventh, the laboratories where Herman Suit and his colleagues conduct the research programs in radiobiology and physics for which the unit is recognized. Worthy of special mention are the breeding and housing facilities for purebred strains of mice that are maintained continuously pathogen-free and in a defined flora status. By virtually eliminating sepsis, this stratagem makes it possible for scientists to study the effects of radiation exposure or any other debilitating maneuver with much less risk of confusing or complicating their ability to evaluate results in sound statistical terms.

On the second and sixth floors of the building, medical oncology, for the first time since the halcyon days of Ira Nathanson's leadership, has once again established a home for much of its clinical, training, and research activities. In the tradition of the late Rita Kelley, Davies Sohier, Robert Carey, and Sheldon Kaufman conduct what must surely be one of the busiest group practices in the hospital, particularly in the matter of corridor and telephone consultations. Their area on the second floor is designed to accommodate the entire range of medical oncologic practice whenever it is safe and feasible on an outpatient basis. By appropriate planning and scheduling, this has permitted the administration of extremely sophisticated chemotherapy, both adjuvant and palliative, to an increasing number of patients. In view of the multiplicity of programs in use today, this is a welcome advance toward greater efficiency and economy.

The laboratories on the sixth floor have become operative under Thomas Stossel, the new division chief. They are adjacent to and share some facilities with those of surgical oncology, where William Wood and Alfred Cohen study and apply their understanding of the immune mechanisms to animal and human tumors. The pathology of immune processes and the research questions it seeks to answer are under intensive study on the fifth floor where Ann and Harold Dvorak have installed their laboratories, and an animal farm is in construction on the eighth floor for the support of all these researches.

Multidisciplinism is most apparent on the first floor, where the old Tumor Clinic has emerged from its chrysalis as the Cox Ambulatory Services. Medical, surgical, and radiologic oncologic attentions are offered continuously, but in addition each clinical department has the use of the facilities during a scheduled time each week. This ensures that the different groupings of cancer patients will be seen and managed by interested and qualified staff members. This arrangement is also of great benefit to our varied training programs, but best of all it gives the specialty staffs an incomparable opportunity to consult with others whose time is spent exclusively in oncology and in the building. It means that the design and equipment must be multipurpose—that lights in the examining rooms, for example, must range from a system that is acceptable to a dermatologist to one that properly illuminates the larynx. Although administratively the units are not so ordered and restricted that the building can be designated a center or institute, in a very real sense the structure embodies the architectural expression of multidisciplinary cancer care.

For the MGH as a whole, inpatients—predominantly surgical cases—form the greater part of cancer care at any given moment. These and other large elements of our cancer program should never become incorporated into the ambulatory facility, but we can provide ready access to diagnostic radiology, clinical and tissue pathology, nuclear medicine, hematology, and many other necessary components of the total picture. Pediatric and hematologic malignant disease have their own places of management, and much cancer care is rendered in private offices of the MGH and by the Massachusetts Eye and Ear Infirmary staff.

Research in cancer is very much a part of the activities of this acute care general hospital. The Huntington Laboratories and many others have contributed to the solution of a number of basic problems, but the MGH is, of course, also able to initiate and foster clinical research of all kinds. In their simplest form such studies are engendered wherever a tumor registry is developed that at once easily provides data on all cases seen. Through the Tumor Clinic here, officially inaugurated in April 1925, reports have been generated that reviewed the case material in cancer of the breast, stomach, colon, uterus, cervix, ovary, vulva, vagina, larynx, pharynx, esophagus, and other sites too numerous to mention; papers dealing with disease entities like leukemia, lymphoma, melanoma, and bone and soft tissue sarcomas have also been published. Valuable conclusions have been reached with respect to staging and treating these diseases, and useful leads have been suggested for facilitating detection and diagnosis, identifying etiologic factors, and improving end results, both palliative and curative.

Over the years this type of case review study has undergone modification and refinement, much of it in efforts either to scrutinize selected questions or to control the composition of the group in order to characterize the effect of specific variables in statistically meaningful terms. Currently, and most particularly in the area of cancer therapy, there are in progress a number of protocol studies emphasizing prospective investigation, identical treatment patterns for all patients, proper controls, and the simultaneous involvement of many institutions in order to amass large numbers of patient profiles quickly.

Progression from straightforward case analysis and through controlled investigation to prospective protocol studies and the laboratory bench is illustrated by our experience with the stilbestrol disorders. (See Chapter 26 on Gynecology for details.)

Every conceivable kind of affiliation, formal or informal, has developed between the MGH and the surrounding medical community over the years. Much of this interaction has the goal of improved care for individual patients, but with increased frequency joint programs are coming into existence for student, staff, and technical education and for investigating methods of delivering care as well as the results of treatment. For the Harvard-affiliated institutions, the unifying effect of serving on one faculty responsible to one dean has encouraged collaborative efforts. Such a joining of skills and sharing of information has been and will continue to be productive. For example, in the stilbestrol studies, one case of the eight that were studied epidemiologically was from the Peter Bent Brigham, and the entire group of women investigated prospectively for benign anomalies resulting from fetal exposure was from the Boston Hospital for Women. Consultation has also been notable with the departments of biochemistry and preventive medicine at the Medical School.

Yet such occasions are determined almost by chance; they wait upon initiation by one or another of the involved investigators and require that he or she have some inkling of where to turn for assistance. More significant, perhaps, are a number of activities in which representatives of many departments and hospitals in their meetings and deliberations correlate resources and review program designs in order to avoid unnecessary and inefficient duplication of efforts or undetected contradictions and omissions.

With the opening of the Cox Building the MGH joins other institutions of the Harvard Medical School in recognizing two concepts: that the cancer patient requires a separate and specialized environment and that multiple specialties must be brought together in that patient's care. We believe that in institutionalizing these concepts we have built well for the future, until such time as cancer can be prevented or cured by simple means.

Adapted from an article by *Howard Ulfelder* in the *Harvard Medical Alumni Bulletin,* January-February, 1977. The three introductory paragraphs appeared in the same article and were written by the journal's editors.

Medical Oncology

Medical oncology established its roots in this hospital when the Huntington Hospital moved to the MGH as a separate laboratory headed by Joseph Aub. Under his direction the Huntington Laboratories became a nationally recognized research center in biology (see page 343). At the same time Aub gathered around him an active clinical oncology group. In those days Ira Nathanson, a surgeon, shared with Aub leadership of this group. Nathanson was one of the first people to treat inoperable breast cancer with hormones; the response to hormone therapy was occasionally dramatic and served to attract general internists to the use of hormones and thus to specialize in cancer therapy. Among the first of these was Rita Kelley who, having done some postgraduate work at the Huntington Laboratories, obtained her M.D. degree from Columbia and then returned to the MGH for her residency and the practice of a combination of internal medicine and hormone therapy, particularly in breast cancer. B. J. Kennedy was another early joiner in this effort, to be followed by William Baker, John Freymann, and Davies Sohier.

Later, when Paul Zamecnik was directing the Huntington Laboratories and fully committed to a research career and after Nathanson's death in 1954, Alan Aisenberg, who had been a resident at the MGH, was brought back from Wisconsin by Dr. Bauer to head up the Medical Oncology Unit. He has been a continuously productive scientist in his definition of the anergic state associated with Hodgkin's disease; his views on the biology and management of lymphomas brought him national recognition; and for years he almost single-handedly provided the consultative backup for the oncology fellows on the Medical Services and ran a busy Lymphoma Clinic.

It had been Bauer's and Churchill's view that the MGH should make its contribution to clinical oncology through the understanding of the biology of cancer and that the Huntington Laboratories were the vehicle for accomplishing this; Alexander Leaf shared this view. Nevertheless, the empirical approach with radiation and chemotherapy was showing evidence in some tumors of providing reasonably effective therapy. The MGH could not remain behind in clinical oncology as the volume of patients—approximately one-quarter of the new cancer cases in Massachusetts each year—applying for treatment increased.

The construction of the new Cox Building as a cancer management center irrevocably committed the MGH as a major clinical oncology center. Endowment for a tenured position to support the efforts in clinical oncology at the MGH as well as modest laboratory space (approximately 2,500 square feet) on

Cox 5 made it possible to search for a new chief of Medical Oncology. The small search committee agreed upon the need to find a person who would nourish academic and scholarly activities in the busy clinical oncology service. As a resident at the MGH Thomas P. Stossel had acquired a reputation for wit and originality; more to the point, he had joined the Hematology Unit at the Children's Medical Center under David Nathan and had done some internationally acclaimed research on phagocytosis. He tackled this important problem of host resistance with ingenuity and success. He carefully isolated the contractile proteins in lung macrophages and, discovering several new factors, reconstituted the purified component of the contractile mechanism responsible for phagocytosis and locomotion of macrophages. He was already an associate professor of pediatrics when he was induced to return to the MGH in 1976 as associate professor of medicine and chief of Medical Oncology. Stossel set about straight away to organize his laboratory research program and to attract fellows both for research and for clinical service. The excitement of his investigations attracted a spate of the very best MGH medical residents to join his group as research fellows.

In the meantime, Leaf had several discussions with Leonard Ellman, then chief of the Hematology Unit, about bringing someone in to strengthen research in hematology. When the choice of a productive investigator fell through at the last moment, Leaf decided to go along with the suggestion that several of the senior staff had made and to which Ellman had agreed, namely to combine hematology and oncology into one unit. Many of the leading programs in the country—at Barnes, Seattle, Columbia, UCLA—had combined "Heme-Onc" units. Most importantly, Stossel's training had been in hematology, and his personal research fitted both subspecialties equally well. He accepted the dual responsibility, and Ellman became director of the Clinical Laboratories. (See also Chapter 15 on Hematology and the Clinical Laboratories.)

Hematology-Oncology is thriving with the recruitment of excellent fellows, a strong research base, and the gradual development of a unit-based group practice; it shows signs of becoming one of the strongest of the medical units. Stossel has accepted editorship of the *Journal of Clinical Investigation,* which is both a great honor and major responsibility. It speaks well for academic medicine at the MGH to have the journal at this institution.

> With the assistance of *Alexander Leaf, Howard Ulfelder,* and *W. Davies Sohier*

Rita Kelley. Among the many people who devoted their energies and talents to the development of the Cox Center was Rita Kelley. She earned her medical degree at the HMS in 1947, completed her residency at the MGH in 1949, and joined the hospital staff in 1951. She participated very actively in the planning of the Cox cancer facility and, when it opened, belonged to the Medical Oncology Group Practice located on the second floor of the building.

Rita Kelley died in July 1981, after 30 years of service to the MGH and to thousands of devoted patients. The following remarks were made by Ned H. Cassem, chief of the Psychiatric Consultation-Liaison Service, at the memorial Mass celebrated in her honor on the 25th of July:

Rita Kelley—the model physician: supreme competence, keen insight, monumental industry, unerringly sound judgment, massive common sense. Teacher, scholar, Harvard Professor of Medicine, consummate clinical oncologist. A woman of great faith and towering integrity.

In Solzhenitsyn's novel *Cancer Ward* Dr. Dontsova complains to Dr. Oreschchenkov: "It seems unfair that I, an oncologist, should be stricken by an oncological ailment, when I know every one of them, when I imagine all the attendant effects, the consequences, the complications." The old man replied, "There's no injustice here. . . . This is the surest test of a doctor: to suffer an illness in his own specialty." (He reasoned thus because he had not been ill himself.) I couldn't help recalling this passage when Rita herself was stricken by cancer—though I never heard Rita complain about it. Cancer was a familiar enemy to her: While she was still a teenager it claimed the life of her father. Twenty years ago her sister Ann also died of cancer.

Like Dr. Dontsova, however, Rita certainly knew all of the complications, and knew, as she often reminded me, that she had three to four years to live. These comments she relayed to me as matter-of-factly as she might the data on an abstract case report. There was in her an almost ruthless honesty, a kind of straightforward, straight-from-the-shoulder bluntness which was at once a bit intimidating and yet reassuring. You always knew where she stood. Her judgments were always fair. Their very solidness was comforting. With Rita it was as though court was always in session; verdicts were sure to come promptly but the sentences were always meted out with gentleness and compassion. And she always gave us time off for good behavior. She had that unusual knack—whether it was telling a diagnosis or giving her opinion of our medical judgments—of telling, but telling "easy." She dispensed truth the way she prescribed medicine: If it was strong stuff or even hurt, it was administered only for our well-being. Though she was filled with compassion and kindness, she had no use whatsoever for sentimentality.

I don't know how to say this with exact accuracy but there could be a sternness about Rita—it was definitely part of her awesomeness; not that she would be unjustly critical, but her standards of quality were uncompromisingly high, so that I was always a bit worried about measuring up to them. For example, to my initial dismay but eventual amusement, I learned that she had almost no use for psychiatrists. After a while she trusted me to see an occasional patient and, as I became more relaxed, I must confess I couldn't in opportune moments resist teasing her by repeating to her extreme psychoanalytic interpretations of oral/anal/genital dimensions of human motivation. About two weeks before she died I spotted a copy of the *New England Journal of Medicine* at her bedside and located in it a verbatim quote of an especially rank analytic interpretation made to a child patient. With a twinkle in her eye (and to my delight) she took the bait and replied, "Now that is absolutely ridiculous" and followed with a short speech on the excesses of misguided psychiatric intervention—all quite accurate, of course.

Rita could not be teased as I'd tease my mother. She could be neither shocked nor scandalized. She was simply above either.

To me the most awesome aspect of Rita Kelley's life, and the most brilliant fusion of her intelligence, scholarship, tough durability, steadfast fidelity, emphatic gentleness, was her devotion to the care of her patients. She lives and will always live in my memory as an exemplar of the Physician. She gave her patients the best of medical wisdom, the confidence that she'd be there when needed, and, especially, safe passage in their difficult journeys with cancer.

Surgical Oncology

WILLIAM C. WOOD

In 1955 the Tumor Clinic was a metastasis from the former Huntington Memorial Hospital into the MGH but continued in many respects to be independent of the MGH. The chief, Grantley Taylor, was a colorful personality who was as well known for his quotably acerbic commentary as for the elegance of his radical dissections. He drew most of the Tumor Clinic staff from the clinical associates;

essentially, their only contact with the hospital was through that association. The house staff did not rotate through the Tumor Clinic.

When Claude Welch was appointed chief of the Tumor Clinic in 1957, E. D. Churchill suggested that John Raker be invited back from a rather unhappy assignment as chief of Surgery at the Philadelphia General Hospital to serve as associate chief of the Clinic. Welch and Raker had worked together before at the old Huntington Hospital and shared goals for the Tumor Clinic and for cancer surgery at the MGH.

Their first task was to amalgamate the Tumor Clinic into the mainstream of the hospital. Soon the house staff was rotating through the clinic, and gradually the staff visiting the clinic was changed so that the associates in surgery were replaced. William Rogers, who had joined Taylor after training at Memorial Hospital for Cancer and Allied Diseases in New York, shared with Welch and Raker a keen enjoyment for teaching resident surgeons. Students began to be included as well.

The next task was to inaugurate a cancer registry—no easy matter with nearly 3,000 new cases added annually and inadequate personnel to manage the clerical duties. The Massachusetts Department of Public Health provided some help, and Raker's heroic efforts kept the enterprise afloat. However, chronic under-staffing and minimal support ultimately led to the loss of approval by the American College of Surgeons. In recent years Alfred Cohen has headed the tumor registry; with his tremendous efforts plus additional resource allocations from the hospital, it is working very well and has been approved by the College.

Shortly after Welch became chief, a multidisciplinary postgraduate course in cancer was established and grew very popular. More recently, under Cohen's leadership, it has gradually evolved to an advanced course in surgical oncology, still held for three days just before Thanksgiving each year, with the faculty drawn from several disciplines but the perspective being surgical.

In 1966 Raker assumed the role of chief of the Tumor Clinic, since Welch was functioning as a Herculean clinical surgeon whose daily surgical list would often eclipse that of a medium-sized hospital. During this period there was no attempt to develop what today would be called surgical oncologists. Some in-dividuals, such as Raker, were extremely knowledgeable in the entire area of oncology. In general, however, clinical care of malignant disease in separate areas of the body was given by the surgeons interested in that particular part of the anatomy. Thus neurosurgeons, thyroid surgeons, breast surgeons, thoracic sur-geons, abdominal surgeons, and orthopedic surgeons functioned comfortably under the umbrella of the Tumor Clinic.

The papers published in the 1950s and 1960s were chiefly reports of individual efforts and were almost entirely clinical in nature and retrospective in view. Fundamental research in cancer was carried on by Paul Zamecnik and others, but these activities were divorced from the Tumor Clinic which remained almost entirely a clinical service.

In 1974 W. Gerald Austen established the Surgical Oncology Unit with Raker as the first chief. William Wood joined him in 1975, and in 1976 Cohen was added to the unit. Also in 1975 Howard Ulfelder, deputy director for cancer affairs of the MGH, oversaw the move of the Tumor Clinic, the Surgical On-cology Unit, the Medical Oncology Unit, and the Department of Radiation Therapy into the just completed Cox Building, which provided new facilities required by the growth and progress of the disciplines involved. More than that, by physical proximity, the integration of the various specialties in clinical care was greatly abetted.

Austen reflected on the maturation of the Surgical Oncology Unit by observing, "The development of surgical oncology as a specialized area in the department of surgery at the MGH has been an important accomplishment. The tradition had been that cancer surgery was an area that most members of the department were involved in. With the increasing sophistication required to care properly for these patients, as well as to be at the leading edge of investigation and education, some specialization seemed appropriate. There was certainly some apprehension in the department when we appointed individuals who were committed to spend essentially all of their time in cancer surgery. However, this concern was quickly dissipated by the exemplary behavior of Drs. Wood and Cohen as well as the realization by all that surgical oncology required this kind of emphasis. Surgical oncology is, in my view, doing well at the MGH. I believe that the future is bright and will require even more resources and staff."

Wood and Cohen have offices on the first floor, and their research laboratories on the sixth floor, of the Cox Building. With Austen's encouragement the emphasis of the unit was directed first toward teaching the surgical residents tumor biology and the role of radiation and chemotherapy in planning comprehensively for the care of the patient with cancer. The focus has not been on establishing another subspecialty but on better teaching at both the resident and postgraduate levels. The research interests of the unit have been strongly directed toward crossdisciplinary innovation as exemplified by the development of a program in intraoperative irradiation in conjunction with radiation therapists, limb-sparing surgery in conjunction with high dose irradiation for soft tissue sarcoma, and the use of allograft bone to spare the lower extremity in tumors of the pelvis in conjunction with the orthopedic service. Basic research work has involved studies of the surface antigens of breast cancer, colon cancer, and brain cancer cell lines.

The principal teaching session of the Tumor Clinic was a one-hour consultation clinic held Wednesday at noon. This served as a Tumor Board for the hospital. Over the years separate conferences arose among interested specialties: Lymphoma Rounds served as a consultation board, Thyroid Clinic served a similar purpose, and Pigmented Lesion Clinic was a focus for those interested in melanoma. This trend was encouraged in the Cox Building with the addition of rounds in bone and soft tissue sarcoma and weekly teaching rounds for surgical residents.

In 1979, following Raker's sudden death, Wood and Cohen were made co-chiefs of the Surgical Oncology Unit. The clinical and administrative responsibility of a unit with the oversight of resident teaching, 800 private surgical cases annually, and numerous clinical and basic research studies in progress has proved an exciting challenge.

Department of Radiation Medicine

Radiation therapy acquired departmental status at the MGH in 1971 as the Department of Radiation Medicine under the chairmanship of Herman D. Suit.

The early development and use of radiotherapy as part of the Department of Radiology have been covered partially in Washburn's and Faxon's histories, but reviewing some of the older data helps place the events of the past quarter century in perspective. In 1970, when the hospital undertook its review of the Department of Radiology, Milford D. Schulz produced a "Brief Resume of Radiation Therapy at the MGH since 1940," which provides excellent background to the current Department of Radiation Medicine. In that report Schulz wrote:

Radiotherapy at the MGH has over the years grown both in concept and practice. Conceptually, this growth has been the acceptance—albeit reluctant at times on the part of some—of the fact that needs and uses of this activity justify and in fact require, if it is to prosper and serve its purpose and the public as it should, recognition and developmental encouragement as a medical specialty. In 1940, radiation therapy was conducted as a somewhat anecdotal activity of the general radiologist and in part by the dermatologists (x-ray treatments), and in part by the surgeons (radium use). No staff member considered his activity to be devoted wholemindedly to the study of malignant disease and its control by ionizing radiation and the allied radiobiologic and physical bases of the processes involved, or to the basic investigation of the neoplastic process itself. . . .

In 1940, 3,781 treatments were reported as having been given. By 1945, this rose to 8,986, and in 1950 and 1955 the numbers were 10,108 and 17,226. In 1960 to 1965 the volume rose, with no improvement in the facility; there were 17,295 and 24,734 treatments in these years respectively. In 1969 . . . 32,180 treatments were given in a radiation therapy facility still unchanged since 1957.

During the years, staff in radiotherapy has changed much in character but little in size. From 1942 to 1959, there was but one full-time radiotherapist on the staff [Schulz himself, who had come over with the Huntington Memorial Hospital group when it moved to the MGH]. Since 1959, two, and since 1968 three [Schulz, C. C. Wang, and George Zinninger] full-time radiotherapists. On the level of technical help, the department has fared better. From two technicians and no secretaries, the non-professional staff has increased to four secretaries, one nurse, one nurse's aide, and seven technicians. Support in the form of radiologic physics has been available since the mid-1950s but is still limited, there being but one physicist and two associate physicists shared with Radiodiagnosis and Nuclear Medicine.

Training of young physicians in radiotherapy has developed slowly at the MGH. Until 1968, no resident was trained in therapeutic radiology only, but always in general radiology. There are now (1970) two such trainees. It must be noted, however, that in some measure because of the stimulation received at the MGH at least eight physicians have gone on—by dint of further training or concentration of effort and experience—to become radiotherapists and related scientists of some accomplishment. Dr. C. C. Wang is among them.

In recognition of the growing importance of radiotherapy in this hospital, there have been numerous attempts to break out of the limitations imposed by the physical facility. The first such real effort was the appointment of a committee . . . in 1959 . . . chaired by Dr. Earle Chapman. These and various other efforts have now at long last resulted in a definitive action by the Trustees to proceed with the development of a cancer management and radio-therapeutic facility which will truly serve the needs of the hospital and the community it serves.

As Schulz's narrative indicates, during the sixties the hospital gravitated slowly toward a policy of increasing support of a radiotherapy program. In its 1962 annual report the General Executive Committee acknowledged that "the increasing load of patient care that must be handled by the Department of Radiotherapy . . . strains our present facilities." In the 1965 annual report Knowles wrote, "For some years we have been concerned with our total effort in the field of cancer. We have felt the need to do better radiotherapy." Knowles raised the issue again in the 1968 report: "We look forward with increasing confidence to the future and have already started raising new capital for the next two pressing needs of the institution and its community, that is, for a modern radiotherapy facility and the development of a more balanced Department of Radiology with increasing facilities for radiobiology, radiotherapy, and research." In that same year a report of the Arthur D. Little Corporation emphatically presented the need for more space and better facilities for radiotherapy and radiobiologic research. Finally, in 1969 the trustees voted "to approve in principle the construction of a new building to house the now tremendously overcrowded radiotherapy facility." That vote, of course, resulted in the development and construction of the Cox Cancer Management Center, a facility made possible in large part by a gift from Mrs. William C. Cox. (See the section on the Cox Center in this chapter as well as Chapter 6 on the Committee on Research for related discussions.)

Meanwhile, administrative changes at the hospital were to some extent prompted by the 1969 decision of the Harvard Medical School to create separate departments of radiation therapy and radiodiagnosis. The immediate stimulus for the establishment of an operationally autonomous department at the MGH was Robbins' request to be relieved of his responsibilities as chief of Radiology. As explained in a previous chapter, Juan Taveras became chief of Radiology—*radiology* having effectively been redefined as *radiodiagnosis*—while Suit was appointed chief of Radiation Medicine and professor at the Medical School.

Suit began working immediately with Howard Ulfelder, chief of Gynecology, in developing plans and selecting equipment for the new center while recruiting additional staff and building units in radiation physics and radiation biology research. The Cox Center was completed in 1975; by 1976 equipment had been installed—including two Cobalt-60 therapy machines, two 18-MeV linear accelerators, and a 35-MeV linear accelerator—and the clinical activities of the Department of Radiation Medicine had been transferred to the new quarters. A new high intensity radiation biophysics laboratory was constructed, equipped, and staffed on the sixth floor of the Cox Center; in 1977 a radiation biology research group moved into the Edwin L. Steele Laboratory on Cox 7.

In his annual report for 1981 Suit wrote that since its establishment "the Department of Radiation Medicine has been in an exciting and rapidly moving period of upgrading and growth in clinical, research, and educational activities. The department is now widely accepted as a first-rate, world class center of radiation therapy. . . . A principal accomplishment has been the development and provision of manpower and facilities which make feasible the provision of quality medical care. Our medical staff will as of this summer be nine—a workload per physician almost at a reasonable level. The policy is one full-time clinical equivalent per 225 new patients seen per year. We have developed subspecialty practice modeled on surgical subspecialties, i.e., head and neck, GU, GI, thoracic disease, CNS, lymphoma, bone and soft tissue, breast. The resident training program is based on 11 positions for three- to four-year training. For the clinical physics program we have 7 Ph.D.s and 3 M.Sc. clinical physicists working full-time on clinical physics programs. . . . This excellent staff is strongly and effectively supported by an excellent group of nurses, technicians and secretaries. The physical facilities in which this group works are as handsome and effectively laid out as any center in the world. The facility was designed to provide a capability for handling 2,000 new cancer patients per year as a maximum. The equipment complement includes three high energy linear accelerators (35×1; 18×2),

Cobalt units (2), simulator, computer treatment planning unit, dedicated CBT unit. We are now seeing over 2,000 new cancer cases per year and the number of patients treated per day is averaging about 190 with peaks as high as 210. In addition there are 10–12 patients undergoing simulation per day."

Research quite naturally flourished in this climate of fine equipment and physical generosity. Among the department's major clinical research efforts was the Proton Beam Radiation Therapy program to evaluate the role of modulated energy proton beams in the curative treatment of selective cancer patients. The research was funded by the National Cancer Institute at the rate of about $700,000 per year—the grant was still active in 1981—with Suit and biophysicist Michael Goitein as principal investigators. "My judgment," Suit observed cautiously in his 1981 report, "is that at least for two categories of tumors the advantages for fractionated dose proton therapy have been shown sufficient to warrant this treatment as being designated the treatment of choice. This obtains for treatment of patients with malignant melanoma of the eye and tumors of the base of the skull or cervical spine which abut on CNS structures." In 1978 a program of intraoperative radiation therapy using electron beams began in collaboration with the departments of surgery, anesthesia, and nursing. The program was directed to patients judged to have soft tissue localized abdominal or pelvic tumors, for whom conventional therapy was unlikely to radiate the tumor or posed excessive risk of damage to normal tissues. After exposure of the affected site in the operating room the patient, under general anesthesia, is brought to the Department of Radiation Medicine. The exposed tumor tissue is directly irradiated by electron beam from the 35-MeV linear accelerator through the open incision under sterile conditions. By mid-1980 more than 50 patients had been so treated and some thoroughly impressive results achieved.

Meanwhile, four separate laboratory groups, each independently funded by the National Cancer Institute, were engaged in projects to study (1) Radiation Sensitization Applied to Radiation Biology (Edward R. Epp); (2) Extracellular Modification of Hyperthermic Lethality (Leo E. Gerweck); (3) Tumor Response of Hyperthermia and Irradiation (Muneyasu Urano); and (4) Tumor Response to Local Irradiation (Dr. Suit).

Thus the science and practice of radiotherapy has traveled fast and far at the MGH, and the man whose obstinate labors had sown the early seeds of inspiration had the satisfaction of watching them sprout. Schulz reached retirement age—if not state of mind—in 1976. The Department of Radiation Medicine marked the occasion by establishing an annual event in his honor, the Milford D. Schulz Lectureship in Radiation Therapy. He continued to serve as consulting visiting radiation therapist.

With the assistance of *Milford D. Schulz, C. C. Wang,* and *Herman D. Suit*

Cancer Research: Joseph Charles Aub

PAUL C. ZAMECNIK

Where the Ohio River runs past the hills of Cincinnati, there was born in 1890 a boy named Joseph Charles Aub. At an early age he took for granted that he would follow the example of his well-known and popular uncle, after whom he had been named, and would choose medicine as his life's work. He went off to Harvard at the age of 17, weighing 87 pounds and having just graduated into long trousers. He felt small and insignificant in the presence of more articulate undergraduates, among them Walter Lippmann and Alan Gregg. His yearnings for football were sublimated into service as coxswain for a freshman crew. In the humanities, he was conscious of the presence of Ralph Barton Perry and Charles T. Copeland, but particularly of George Santayana, who awakened in him a love of art and even for a time influenced his way of speaking.

It was, however, George Howard Parker, one of the pioneers of American biology, who provided the greatest influence at this time. It was Parker's habit to give a promising student a research problem to pursue, and he put Aub to work studying the mechanism by which a flounder shifts its eye after birth. (Although initially the eyes are on both sides of the fish's thin body, one eye soon migrates over to the other side. Parker wanted to know how the flounder's eyes on the same side managed to synchronize instead of being divergent in their movements.) Aub found from dissecting flounder after flounder that not only did one eye move over to the other side but in so doing also twisted, so that the eyes were able to move symmetrically rather than in opposite directions. This was a new finding, and a heady stimulus toward a career in original work.

He finished college in three years, choosing to press on toward his immediate goal of becoming a doctor. In 1911 he entered the Harvard Medical School, at that time still a local school largely dominated by local people, but with certain notable exceptions. Such a person was Walter Cannon, a pure American product who had, while still a medical student, begun to use the newly discovered roentgen tube for studies of intestinal motility. By the time Aub studied physiology in 1911, Cannon had become interested in the effect of epinephrine on the gastrointestinal tract, and he invited students of his class to come into the laboratory to try their hands at research. Aub, along with Stanley Cobb and Carl Binger, took up this offer. Cannon suggested that Aub and Binger study the influence of smoking on the flow of epinephrine, and the experiment took the form of working with nicotine and cats. A catheter was passed up the femoral vein of the cat until it was opposite the adrenal; then samples of blood were sucked out and tested for the presence of epinephrine, by means of its effect on smooth muscle contraction. In this way it was clearly shown that nicotine stimulated the flow of epinephrine. Aub's first publication, with Cannon and Binger, reported this finding in the *Journal of Pharmacology and Experimental Therapy* in 1912. Thus at the age of 22, Joseph Aub had chosen the direction he was to follow all his life and had already become a partner in a contribution to existing medical knowledge.

At the end of his first year in medical school he joined a small group of Harvard College students and spent the summer in Labrador with Sir Wilfred Grenfell. There he saw beriberi and pellagra in severe forms, and hospital beds filled with unfortunates with edema and paralysis. He also came into contact with an Eskimo population ravaged by measles and tuberculosis introduced by the white man. This experience had a deep impact on a fresh medical student pressed into service in the interests of a seriously ill population.

Before quite completing his medical school requirements, Aub was appointed an intern at the MGH, and an association with David Linn Edsall (then professor

of medicine and later dean of the HMS) began which both men prized and enjoyed for many years. (During the 1960s Aub collaborated with R. K. Hapgood in a biography of Edsall, published in 1970.) At the time of the internship examination, this young medical student's fame had preceded him, because a month previously he had recognized the unusual leontine features of a case of leprosy in the outpatient department and had identified it under a microscope. The internship was an arduous 18 months. At that time the slush bath for typhoid fever patients and cupping for inflammations were standard therapy, and heroic nursing care often tipped the scales when dealing with serious infectious diseases.

Then followed a happy scientific experience working at the Russell Sage Physiological Laboratories at Bellevue with Eugene DuBois and Graham Lusk. These were the years from 1915 to 1916, and the concepts of basal metabolism and calorimetry were just beginning to be understood and applied to human problems. Aub quickly appreciated the clinical potentialities of these tools. The papers of Aub and DuBois on "The Basal Metabolism of Dwarfs and Legless Men with Observations on the Specific Dynamic Action of Protein" and of Means and Aub on "A Study of Exophthalmic Goiter from the Point of View of the Basal Metabolism" illustrate this important development and forecast a growing interest of Aub's, embracing the metabolism of all the organs of internal secretion. As part of his experience in New York, Aub collected circus people—pituitary dwarfs, chondrodystrophics, and giants for his studies with DuBois. Some of these people later became devoted patients and lifelong friends; one of Aub's delights years later was to invite students to shake hands with "the Angel," a gentle acromegalic wrestler of frightening dimensions and countenance, endowed with huge hands plus unusual strength in spite of this affliction.

On his return to the MGH in 1916 to take up a new arrangement known as a residency in Medicine, Aub joined Paul White in studying the effect of thyroid disease on the heart and quickly showed that the electrocardiogram in hypothyroidism was quite characteristic, with a low voltage in keeping with the cardiac difficulties of that disease.

When World War I involved the United States, he joined the MGH Unit and spent 20 months in France. He attempted to study traumatic shock in the freshly wounded at the front under the aegis of Walter Cannon; and when the war was over, Aub joined Cannon in the Department of Physiology at Harvard and took up, in a less harried way, study of the nature of the critical metabolic event in traumatic shock. He made the important observation that low venous oxygen tension was an early sign, which indicated that when oxygen had been used up in the peripheral blood, shock was imminent. He pointed to the lowered metabolism, the reduced blood flow, and the rising blood creatine level as further criteria of the metabolic state of shock.

In the early twenties lead poisoning was a serious human industrial disease, and Edsall, a man of wide-ranging interests in medicine, was looking for a young man with imagination willing to tackle this problem. Aub was such a young man—with a restless mind, eager for a new challenge—and he took up this quest. He quickly recognized that the metabolism of lead ran parallel to that of calcium, and that anything that influenced calcium excretion would favor lead excretion. He also learned to administer calcium to stop lead colic, in a classic therapeutic experiment. With talented colleagues, he showed that the origin of lead palsies occurred in the muscles, and that the nerve lesion came only secondarily. He found that lead combined with phosphate on the surface of the red cells, and that the red cells became like hard rubber balls instead of the normal soft-surfaced ones; these hardened red cells broke up more readily, and an increased peripheral blood destruction occurred. This was probably the earliest specific explanation for a hemolytic anemia. He found in cats that lead that was inhaled was much more toxic than lead that was swallowed. All these findings were of great importance to the lead industry, and the control of lead dust alone provided a great step toward the elimination of one of the most common of industrial diseases. The monograph on "Lead Poisoning" by Aub, Minot, Fairhall, and Resnikoff summarized this work and remains a model for research in industrial toxicology.

One of his colleagues points to Aub's singlemindedness toward science in those early days. This was not necessarily the case, however. There was a time when he and Paul White were equally known for gallantry in escorting young ladies across the ocean, as recorded in the best-selling book by Cornelia Otis Skinner and Emily Kimbrough entitled *Our Hearts Were Young and Gay,* written in retrospection some years later and then converted into a popular movie. When one of the girls developed measles on board ship, she was saved from detection by the immigration officers with the help of the young doctors.

In 1924 Aub returned from physiology to medicine—he liked both fields, and his entire career was an effort to bring them together. This was the time when Means was bringing into being the new metabolic disease ward, known as Ward 4. The age of physiologic medicine was just beginning, and with Aub's classic studies of calcium and phosphorous metabolism this period of medicine came into full flower.

The use of parathyroid hormone to eliminate lead gave Aub the idea of the existence in the body of a small, easily mobilizable storehouse of inorganic salts and resulted in his discovery that bone trabeculae function as this readily available storage depot. In a pioneer study DuBois and Aub accurately described and diagnosed a patient suffering from hyperparathyroidism. Aub encouraged his surgical colleagues, Edward D. Churchill and Oliver Cope, to search with persistence and patience for a parathyroid adenoma, which they cleverly located in a substernal position, after earlier disappointing searches had been made in the cervical area. In a short time Ward 4 and Aub became a world center for the study of hyperparathyroidism. In these studies the careers of Fuller Albright and Walter Bauer shot skyward on a high note of success.

In 1928 the Harvard Cancer Commission invited Aub to become director of the Huntington Memorial Hospital for Cancer Research, to succeed George Minot. Aub proposed to attack the problem in a fundamental way and to regard cancer as an aberration in growth control. This was a bold course on which to set an entire laboratory effort, since it involved a search for normal control mechanisms as well, and the short-range relevancy of such studies to the cancer problem was not immediately apparent. There followed a period marked by lean years, good largely for gathering gray hairs and crows' feet about the eyes. A generation passed before this forward-looking but difficult point of view met general acceptance among the cancer research laboratories of the world. In the interests of understanding growth regulation, Aub made laborious studies of the sex hormones and of the pituitary secretions in normal children, children with growth abnormalities, and those with frank endocrine tumors. His investigations with Ira Nathanson of the estrogen excretion of young girls, including some close to home, opened a new page in our understanding of the endocrine events heralding the onset of the menarche.

One day in 1936 he and Alfred Calhoun had injected radioactive lead (Pb^{210}) into a dog and following the dog's demise had laid a section of its femur against an unexposed x-ray film for a period of a month. The radioautograph was never published but was certainly a pioneer of its kind. Also in 1936 Aub and a young MIT physicist, Robley Evans, initiated an interesting investigation of radium excretion, which involved patients who had ingested radium salts in the course of pointing their brushes in painting luminous watch dials and others who had taken radium salts for arthritis. Because of radium's close metabolic resemblance to lead and calcium, an effort was made to promote radium excretion. These studies were not remarkable for reducing the radium content of the patients' bones to a significant extent because radium ingested so long before had become fixed in the metabolically inert bone cortex. However, for a physicist who had inhaled a radium salt in a recent laboratory explosion, the excretion-promoting program proved much more successful. These investigations lighted the first therapeutic candle for the atomic era, and at a meeting at the Argonne Laboratories 20 years later Aub was hailed as the "daddy" of all the subsequent work on the elimination of radioactive substances.

In the thirties George Wislocki was professor of anatomy at Harvard and a man of charmingly unusual biologic research tastes. One day he interested his friend Aub in joining a study of the seasonal changes in the internal secretions of the deer. Aub saw in the deer a marvelous opportunity to investigate the effect of the pituitary and male sex hormones on the synthesis of a mass of bone which, in the antler, reaches as much as 20 pounds in a single season. There followed several years of delightful collaboration. Initially, a deer a month was shot on Naushon Island off Woods Hole, through the generosity of Harry Forbes, who served as host for the expeditions. Wislocki took the endocrine glands, Aub the antlers, bones, and urine, if any. Venison steaks were enjoyed by all. Any fleet-footed younger members of the party were instructed to run for the deer as soon as the shot was fired, but they were never swift enough to find a full bladder. One of the by-products of this investigation was the development of an air gun for shooting testosterone (and subsequently flaxedil) pellets into the deer's hide to paralyze the animal temporarily and facilitate taking samples. An unanticipated demand for reprints of this paper came from wildlife veterinarians the world over.

The closing of the old Huntington Hospital in 1941 brought a turmoil of readjustment but a happy solution in the return of Aub and his laboratory to the MGH. In the MGH environment, as World War II began, Aub gathered a team of investigators and began to reevaluate the old criteria for shock, using newer techniques. As an unexpected finding, it was observed that clostridial toxins were a constant accompaniment of traumatic shock associated with muscle ischemia in dogs. Immunization in advance proved to be a useful procedure. A similar situation was soon reported from certain war fronts, and in civilian life an important parallelism in some surgical conditions was later observed.

An interesting and little appreciated contribution to the technique of blood storage during World War II came about in the following way. A number of volunteer medical students had been given radioactive iron in order to tag their erythrocytes, and they had agreed to serve as blood donors for patients coming into the MGH in traumatic shock. Unfortunately, no such clear-cut cases appeared, and in time the iron-tagged students were about to graduate and depart for distant places. As Robley Evans and John Gibson sat with him in sad contemplation of this inglorious fade-out of a promising experiment, it came to Aub in a serendipitous flash that this labeled blood might be used for the study of red cell survival under varied conditions. An extensive program on red cell storage grew out of these initial experiments. It was immediately observed that bloods kept at room temperature for a day or two and then subjected to refrigeration had a shorter survival time on reinfusion than those kept refrigerated from the time of withdrawal. The Navy accepted this finding promptly and flew drawn blood to the war fronts stored in refrigerators, while the Army continued for some time to ignore the lesson.

Aub always had a feeling for a good problem. When he retired for the first time in 1956, at the age of 66, he undertook a comparison of the surfaces of cancer and normal cells. This led to the original de novo observation that an obscure class of plant compounds known as phytohemagglutinins caused preferential clumping of cancer cells. At this point Aub retired for the second time, and this observation, carried out with his colleagues Drs. Sanford and Ryser, slumbered for several years in the pages of *Cancer Research* before being taken up and expanded into what is presently one of the most actively moving and exciting fields of oncology. This late-blooming scientific flower may be Aub's single most important contribution to science, one that justified his faith in the study of growth as an avenue toward an understanding of cancer.

The above remarks have touched on Joseph Aub's additions to medical knowledge. He was also in full measure a physician, friend, father, and "uncle" to a generation of admirers. What characteristics do these varied activities have in common? There was to begin with love of family, then enormous scientific curiosity coupled with a high order of mental acuity—this was a key to his scientific success. There was also an unusual degree of empathy toward his fellow man, confidence in the abilities of young people, and awareness of the gift of medical knowledge received from his mentors, to be added to, refined, and passed on to his students. Finally, there was an impish sense of humor: An internship examination committee, of which Aub was a member, was having a hard time with a bright applicant who appeared to know the answers to all questions. Aub raised his index finger and asked the candidate to explain what was wrong with it. Suddenly the latter became inarticulate. How was he to know that a monkey had bitten this finger a quarter of a century earlier, leaving it withered, stiffened, and slightly crooked?

Joseph Aub died on December 30, 1973. Of his generation in medicine he could say with Virgil, "These things I saw and part of them I was." He sat with grace at all tables; nourished ugly ducklings while their feathers were changing; served as family doctor and confidant to many colleagues; fought a gallant, losing battle against the laboratory coffee break; gave up smoking many times; and was often late but on entry never failed to brighten a dull room.

From a speech given on the occasion of the presentation of the Kober Medal for 1966 to Dr. Aub, published as a notice in the *Transactions of the Association of American Physicians*

John Collins Warren Laboratories of the Huntington Memorial Hospital

The Faxon volume of MGH history told of the dissolution of the Huntington Memorial Hospital of Harvard University and the dispersal of its parts to various Harvard-affiliated facilities. In 1942 the Huntington Medical Laboratories, the major component of the John Collins Warren Laboratory complex, moved to the MGH, with Joseph Aub as their director. In the foregoing chapter Paul C. Zamecnik writes of Aub's leadership of the Huntington Laboratories, of the imprint he made on the direction of research, and, finally, of his retirement from administration—if not from scientific investigation—in 1956. At that time Zamecnik was appointed the new director, a position he held until 1979. He offers the following chronicle of more recent events:

By this time [the mid-fifties] in the evolution of cancer research, the gap between clinical investigator and full-time laboratory scientist had grown too large for all but the rare individual to bridge. The direction of the laboratories was thereafter concentrated on the development of new knowledge related to the biochemistry of the growth process; and the clinical arm of the Huntington began to suffer from lack of internal support of full-time clinical investigators. A central feature of the growth process was recognized to be the synthesis of protein. The Huntington Laboratories became known as the birthplace of understanding of the mechanism of protein synthesis.

A large share of the dissection of the complex steps between free amino acid and completed protein came from the efforts of the Huntington group in the decade of the 1950s. Included among the investigators at that time were Ivan Frantz, Jr., Robert Loftfield, Philip Siekevitz, Elizabeth Keller, Mahlon Hoagland, Jesse Scott, Mary Stephenson, John Littlefield, Marvin Lamborg, Lisa Hecht, and David Allen. The first cell-free synthesis of cholesterol originated from the work of Nancy Bucher. The immunologic deficiency associated with Hodgkin's disease was pinpointed by Alan Aisenberg. Lewis Engel, an organic biochemist, came in 1946 to give depth to the studies on the relationship of steroid hormones to cancer. He found that there was no simple steroid aberration which could account for the development of cancer of the breast and serve as a urinary diagnostic test. For the next 20 years, however, Dr. Engel enriched our knowledge of the pathways of steroid synthesis, conversion, and degradation.

The Huntington group at the MGH was the first large full-time nucleus of basic science investigators. Following their clinical residencies, a parade of medical investigators of later distinction spent time immersed in these laboratories. They included Lloyd H. Smith, Paul Russell, Hermes Grillo, John Burke, Charles McKhann, and Charles Huggins, Jr.

Among the clinical investigators of the latter years was also Rita Kelley, who had developed her lifelong devotion to the cancer problem as a technician at the Huntington, fresh from college in 1940. . . . William Baker's and Davies Sohier's backgrounds were rooted in the Aub years. Claude Welch had been a student house officer in the old Huntington Hospital, and John Raker had followed him in that position a decade later. Milford Schulz had been a Fellow in Radiotherapy at the Huntington Hospital when the million volt machine had first been built. Many other members of the MGH had drunk at the old Huntington Hospital fountain, rich in knowledge of the natural history of cancer, with the largest outpatient clinics in the malignant disease field of any hospital in New England. Thus we all owe a debt to the Huntington for enriching the New England area in sophistication in the cancer treatment and investigation field. If it has, at the present time, lost the roots which John Collins Warren planted, it has served a purpose. Its place in the Harvard framework has now largely been taken by the Farber Center, a re-creation in the quadrangle area of the Medical School of the concept of a hospital uniquely devoted to malignant disease in its human expression, surrounded by laboratories populated by investigators focusing multiple disciplines on this still unsolved problem.

The self-effacing Zamecnik neglected to mention in this summary the tremendous significance of his guidance on the direction of research first in the Huntington Laboratories and then, by that example, on the MGH community at large. His work on the mechanism of protein synthesis opened doors and suggested avenues for others. He was first to establish that ribosomes are the site of protein synthesis and to develop a cell-free system for the study of the mechanism of protein synthesis in the test tube; it was an elegant and early application of the modern scientific approach to understanding the process of growth through the combined disciplines of cellular anatomy and biochemistry. This research became the cornerstone upon which Zamecnik and his colleagues in the Huntington Laboratories built during the sixties and seventies. Their achievements provided stimulus and focus for the development of a strong basic research presence within the MGH. Zamecnik sat on the Committee on Research for more than three decades, arguing the cause of basic research with unusual power and eloquence.

Zamecnik's many original findings in basic biomedical research were directed to an understanding of controlled and uncontrolled growth in man and animals. His peers in the area of cancer research signalled their appreciation of these accomplishments by electing him president of the American Association for Cancer Research in 1964–1965 and awarding him the American Cancer Society National Award in 1968. He was also the recipient of numerous other honors.

A friend of Zamecnik, who wishes to remain anonymous, sent the following paragraph: "Zamecnik and his associates were the first to devise a cell-free system in the test tube in which protein synthesis could be demonstrated. This enabled them to study the individual components of the system and thereby elucidate the mechanism of protein synthesis. What finally emerged was an understanding how the genetic code is translated into enzymes, hemoglobin, and structural proteins. The unprecedented expansion of fundamental biological knowledge which we are now witnessing and which in time will be of immense benefit in the prevention and cure of disease, stems from the work of pioneers who have the vision and ability to open up new territories. Zamecnik is one of these pioneers."

The first paragraph of Zamecnik's last published annual report of the Huntington Laboratories (1977) expresses as well as any piece of prose the aura of excitement and promise that surrounded the Huntington researchers as they patiently pushed back the boundaries of ignorance: "The increasing complexity of the machinery of growth and reproduction now being revealed in work from many laboratories never ceases to leave this writer in awe—and yet this infinite subtlety of construction cannot be otherwise, if one is to explain the development of a fertilized ovum into an adult human being. The sector of scientific inquiry related to study of the tumor-inducing viruses of animals has recently become a glowing crucible in which new concepts relevant to the excessive growth potential of the tumor cell are being refined. It is impossible to search for molecular characteristics of tumor viruses without simultaneously examining their counterparts in the normal cells they invade and subvert. Thus, scrutiny of the molecular biology of tumor viruses enriches our knowledge of the genetic operations of normal cells, the details of which are still largely unknown."

36. Blood Transfusion Service

CHARLES E. HUGGINS

The MGH was particularly fortunate to have Morten Grove-Rasmussen as director of its Blood Bank and Transfusion Service from 1952 until his death in 1973. Grove-Rasmussen had come to the MGH from Denmark shortly after World War II as a surgical fellow. Because he was married and had a child, he needed more financial support than his fellowship provided. Lamar Soutter, who was then director of the Blood Bank, took him on as an assistant because the expanding activities in the service required more medical supervision. Grove-Rasmussen learned very quickly and came to like the transfusion service so much that after a year he gave up all thoughts of a surgical career and became a full-time assistant director of the bank. He carefully accumulated expertise in the field of red cell serology and eventually gained a worldwide reputation. He spent a good deal of time studying rare blood types and developed a list of blood donors' sera that could be used for the positive identification of these types. He sold them to drug companies at a considerable profit for the hospital.

When Soutter left in 1952, Grove-Rasmussen was appointed head of the bank. Although he was never a licensed physician or a member of the Massachusetts Medical Society, he participated effectively in blood banking affairs on both state and national levels. Meanwhile he gradually became a New Englander and acquired property on the shore of Martha's Vineyard where he built a house.

Like so many other MGH entities, the Transfusion Service had several homes. In 1955 it resided on the ground floor of the old Domestic Building; in 1964 it moved to Temporary Building II. Finally, in 1969 the service came to rest in new quarters in the Gray Building. The first floor area is used primarily for reception of blood donors, blood collection, and component preparation; the second floor houses processing and cross-matching laboratories.

All of this moving about, though disruptive, was not permitted to arrest scientific development. During the 25-year period of this history, blood transfusion changed from a laboratory-administrative activity to a medical specialty. A quarter of a century ago all attention focused on the question of whether there was any apparent incompatibility between donor blood and that of the recipient. If not, whole blood in a glass bottle was administered to the patient. With the development in the early sixties of multicompartmented plastic bags of good quality, it became possible to separate whole blood into its constituent elements. Component therapy makes it possible and practical to give the patient only those elements of blood that are actually needed. Red cells may go to a patient with anemia, plasma to a burn victim, platelet concentrate to a leukemic, and so on. Separation of blood into components also increases greatly the number of patients that can receive a particular component; for example, group A red cells may be given safely to recipients in the A or AB groups, and so forth. By increasing the pool of potential recipients for blood of any particular group, it is possible to operate with lower inventories, and waste of blood from outdating is thereby minimized.

Whole blood cannot be preserved in the refrigerator for longer than 21—at best 35—days following collection. It had been known for many years that if plasma were separated from the formed elements of blood it could be frozen and kept for long periods without further deterioration of its content of protein or labile coagulation factors. By contrast, red cells frozen without cryophylactic agents are totally destroyed after thawing. In 1950 Audrey U. Smith, in London, made a major breakthrough in showing that if glycerol were added to red cells before freezing, it was possible to store and thaw them without damage; she also reported that it was necessary to remove the glycerol after thawing to permit the red cells to be resuspended in a physiologic environment. These discoveries enabled preservation of small volumes of red cells; however, the preservation of "full" units was quite impractical.

During the course of basic investigations into the causes of, and methods for protection against, injury during freezing and thawing of large volumes of tissue, the MGH Transfusion Service found that it was possible to add in a single step a solution of the cryophylactic agent dimethylsulfoxide (DMSO), or glycerol, to permit freezing, storage, and thawing of "full" units with minimum damage. At that point it became clear that if a simple method could be devised for removing the DMSO after thawing, red cells could be preserved at very low temperatures. We discovered that if red cells are diluted with sugar solutions they form very large clumps. Subsequently, if saline solution is added, the clumps resuspend completely. This phenomenon, called reversible agglomeration, made it practical to preserve large quantities of red blood cells for clinical use.

Frozen red cells have areas of advantage over conventional forms of blood in that they can be stored for indefinite periods. This is very useful for inventory maintenance, storage of cells for one's own use at a later date, and storage of very rare forms of blood. During the course of deglycerolization the white cells are very largely removed from the red cell residue. This has proved to be beneficial for kidney transplant recipients and leukemic patients who may need large quantities of platelet concentrate at some later date. Removal of the plasma has been very helpful to patients who have antibodies against substances that may be contained in plasma, and there have been indications that the incidence of post-transfusion hepatitis can be greatly reduced by the use of frozen red cells.

Dr. Grove-Rasmussen established the Reference Laboratory Committee of the American Association of Blood Banks in 1956 with the objective of centralizing information from the entire country about the location of donors with very rare forms of blood. With the advent of freezing technology for red cells, the system was expanded to include storage locations. Grove-Rasmussen helped found the first frozen storage depot at the U.S. Naval Hospital in Chelsea. The MGH became the second such repository, and rare types of blood have been shipped as far as New Zealand. In 1965 the Navy set up frozen blood banks in Da Nang as well as on board two hospital ships; the Air Force maintained a similar capability in the Philippines. The MGH supplied the first 150 units of O-negative blood to these stations. Several MGH surgeons—Gerald S. Moss, Frederick Ackroyd, and William Abbott—spent time in Vietnam and oversaw the operations of the banks. A study was undertaken to determine if it was possible to supply frozen red cells from the U.S. to Vietnam, and deglycerolize them, faster than walking donors could be bled; the answer to both questions was yes.

In July 1972 tissue typing—or, more properly, the Histocompatibility Testing Laboratory—under the direction of Thomas C. Fuller, moved from the Department of Surgery to quarters in the Blood Transfusion Service. This laboratory functions in very close liaison with the Transplantation Unit. All cells of the body except red blood cells have on their surfaces human leukocyte antigens (HLA). Patients awaiting kidney transplantation who may have formed an anti-HLA antibody via either pregnancy or blood transfusions will destroy the transplanted kidney in a very short time if the kidney comes from a person with a corresponding HLA antigen. Thus it is critically important to determine the HLA types of both potential donor and recipient. In addition, an actual cross-match between white blood cells of the donor and serum of the recipient is performed with the hope of avoiding acute graft rejection. Since the principles by which one types white blood cells, screens for the presence of unexpected antibodies, and does cross-matching procedures are similar to those for handling red blood cells, it seemed logical to move the Histocompatibility Testing Laboratory to the Blood Transfusion Service.

In the early 1950s the majority of blood for transfusion was obtained by replacement donations from families of patients or by paid donors when families could not fulfill the need. As American society became more mobile, the percentage of replacement donations gradually declined. A decision was therefore made in 1967 to establish a volunteer blood program outside the traditional replacement concept. George A. Parkhurst was hired as a community liaison officer to recruit groups and individuals to donate blood at the hospital. As the program proved increasingly successful, the number of paid donations dropped substantially. Then, in 1976 we obtained through a number of contributions a beautiful blue and yellow, custom-fitted Blue Bird school bus. This Blood Donor Mobile Unit goes out virtually every day to factories, schools, and other organizations. The collection program has been extremely successful and now accounts for between 15 and 20 percent of all blood used at the hospital. Since 1978 the MGH has coordinated its blood donor program with the American Red Cross so that the two do not compete for the same precious resource.

Grove-Rasmussen died unexpectedly in 1973. Charles E. Huggins, who had been clinical director of the Blood Transfusion Service, became the new director. Since administrative items were proliferating, he asked Thomas C. Fuller and Harold E. Warford to be assistant directors for scientific and administrative matters respectively. This team oversaw several improvements including the opening, in 1973, of an Out-Patient Transfusion Service in the blood donor clinic, which permits patients to come, receive blood quickly, and leave. In 1976 the transfusion service obtained specialized equipment for collection of granulocyte white cells from normal donors for transfusion to patients lacking white blood cells because of infection; and two years later the service acquired an IBM Blood Cell Separator, a device that makes it possible to remove blood from a donor, stabilize it against clotting, and mechanically separate by differential centrifugation virtually any blood element.

In 1979 isolated reports indicated that many different types of patients with plasma protein abnormalities or autoimmune antibodies might benefit greatly from exchange of the clear, yellow liquid plasma of their blood. By using different settings on the IBM separator, one can remove four liters of an individual's plasma and replace it with four liters of a 4.5% albumin solution in 90 to 180 minutes. Initial experiences with plasma exchange procedures on patients with myasthenia gravis, acute Guillain-Barré ascending paralysis, and Waldenström's macroglobulinemia with hyperviscosity have been most gratifying. The service now has four IBM separators and generally does two to four plasma exchange procedures a day.

Overall, then, there has been both growth and refinement of activity in the Blood Transfusion Service. In 1955 it issued 13,212 units of whole blood; in 1979 34,520 units of whole blood, packed red cells, and frozen, thawed, deglycerolized red cells were issued. In the same period 26,912 units of fresh frozen plasma, platelet concentrate, and cryoprecipitated antihemophilic factor were used clinically. Albumin, gamma globulin, and other plasma protein derivatives accounted for an additional 45,460 units. A total of 106,901 different blood components and derivatives per year made the Blood Transfusion Service of the MGH the most active of any hospital in the world. Meeting the tremendous increase in demand for blood required a very considerable increase in personnel staffing at all levels, a feat that was accomplished over the years.

With the assistance of *Lamar Soutter*

37. Bacteriology Laboratory

LAWRENCE J. KUNZ

The past 25 years have witnessed extensive changes in the practice of medical bacteriology, not only at the MGH but also in hospitals all over the world. The spectacular advances that have been made in both medicine and surgery during this quarter century have resulted in increasing emphasis and demands on the practice of clinical diagnostic microbiology. The ever-expanding number and types of antibiotics and the need for testing the susceptibility of microorganisms to them represent only one of the several major impacts on hospital bacteriology. More challenging, however, has been the need to devise methods for recognizing microorganisms that were formerly ignored in diagnostic culture but have now become increasingly serious threats to patients whose natural defenses have been compromised by new modes of therapy such as steroids, antitumor drugs, and immunosuppressive agents.

Not only has the Bacteriology Laboratory under the direction of Lawrence J. Kunz provided leadership and direction to facilitate the design of new techniques and the guidelines for their application but, because of the increasingly large numbers of cultures processed during this period, the laboratory also has been able to provide substantial information needed for the identification and inter-pretation of previously nonexistent or unrecognized problems of infection. Much of this innovation has been made possible through collaboration with one or another medical colleague, usually a member of the Infectious Disease Unit, and in later years with the assistance of a computer system. The expansion of the role of the laboratory in the care of patients would not have been possible without the provision of increased laboratory space made possible by the occupancy of the Francis Blake Bacteriology Laboratories in September 1968 in the then new Gray Building.

Among the groups of microorganisms specifically studied during the early part of this quarter century, certain enteric bacteria were considered especially inter-esting because new importance was being suggested both by taxonomic studies by academic microbiologists and by new emphasis by clinical colleagues on pro-duction of disease. With the assistance of William H. Ewing of the National Center for Disease Control, methods were devised for easily recognizing and identifying these bacteria. The benefits of this technology were quickly realized in the detection of *Salmonella* infections acquired by certain hospitalized patients who had undergone special treatments. Thus, with Orjan T. Ouchterlony, a visiting professor, it was discovered that brewers' yeast contained three different types of *Salmonella* as contaminants. David J. Lang helped uncover the fact that carmine dye contained small numbers of *Salmonella cubana* which was, never-theless, able to infect some patients with preexisting gastrointestinal problems. William R. Waddell had reported earlier that certain patients seemed to be espe-cially susceptible to *Salmonella* infections after stomach surgery, probably because of a decrease in stomach acidity. Reviews of the effects of two different groups of enteric bacteria provided the medical community with—for many physicians and bacteriologists—new insight into the importance of these bacteria. These reviews were prepared through major efforts of Bernard N. Fields, Pierce Gardner, Arnold N. Weinberg, and Morton N. Swartz of the Infectious Disease Unit.

Similar studies resulted in the rediscovery of various streptococci as important agents of infection, previously appreciated but somehow forgotten during World War II and thereafter because of the great success in the treatment of serious streptococcal infection by the earliest widely used antibiotic, penicillin. David S. Feingold initiated studies of streptococcal infections and encouraged greater emphasis by the laboratory on precise identification of various species and groups of streptococci. This study was continued by Richard J. Duma, again with other members of the laboratory of the Infectious Disease Unit and of the Bacteriology Laboratory.

Similarly, yeasts, anaerobic bacteria (which require an oxygen-free environment), and an unknown agent that causes infection associated with cat scratches have been studied and their effects reviewed. Strangely, yeasts which were first studied in the Bacteriology Laboratory in 1961 were not evaluated in clinical disease until almost 20 years later when members of the Department of Pathology and the Infectious Disease Unit reviewed infections caused by the yeast *Torulopsis glabrata*. The role of *Mycobacteria* in certain infections was reviewed by Harvey B. Simon and other colleagues.

Between 1955 and 1980 the workload of the Bacteriology Laboratory increased 500 percent for several reasons relating to the increased susceptibility of certain patients undergoing new treatments and to the resistance of many microorganisms to antibiotics and other antimicrobial agents. Fortunately, the Laboratory of Computer Science under the direction of G. Octo Barnett was able to provide computer systems, first for the chemistry and subsequently for the bacteriology laboratories. The latter system went into operation in 1970; it was one of the earliest, most comprehensive, useful, adaptable computer systems designed for use in a microbiology laboratory. Both the computer (hardware) and the programming (software) of the system are becoming outmoded, and design of a new system is underway.

The original objective of instituting a computer program in bacteriology was to collect, store, analyze, and interpret the bacteriologic data that are automatically generated in the results of tests performed in the laboratory on specimens from patients; such information was the source of our earlier analyses and reviews of the effects of microorganisms on patients' illnesses. By the time the system was completed, however, the workload of the laboratory had increased so greatly that the primary use of the computer was shifted to facilitating the generation, storage, and transmission of the results of laboratory tests to the patient care area of the hospital for insertion into the respective patients' charts.

Manipulation of laboratory data for research purposes, which became a secondary objective, remained an important function of the computer and continues to be so. One of the primary uses of the laboratory for research purposes has been to study the interrelationships of various antibiotics on the large population of many species of bacteria found in the MGH. Robert C. Moellering, Jr., of the Infectious Disease Unit has used the laboratory computer and the data derived from it for research purposes and has made many important contributions on a worldwide basis from the design of his inquiries and the observation and interpretation of the analyzed data. (Another secondary and important function of the computer has been to designate and record charges for various tests performed for all patients from whom specimens have been submitted and to provide, without intrusion of human error or neglect, for the appropriate collection of these hospital charges.)

Despite what was considered to have been a progressive attitude toward innovation and experimentation in laboratory technology, the laboratory has participated only cautiously in the acquisition of automated instrumentation for the performance of bacteriologic tests. Kunz believes that he has been scientifically discriminative and that this perspective and reserve will be justified by decisions forthcoming in the 1980s.

38. Chemistry Laboratory

SIDNEY V. RIEDER

At the beginning of this most recent instalment of MGH history, 1955, the Chemistry Laboratory was situated on the fourth floor of the old Domestic Building. Charles DuToit occupied the position of director, G. Margaret Rourke that of head technician. The laboratory personnel comprised about a dozen persons. Although modest by later standards, the laboratory had already started expanding, stimulated by the introduction of new techniques and equipment. For instance, the Chemistry Laboratory was among the first of the clinical laboratories to introduce electrophoresis of serum proteins; it also began to employ a newly introduced technique, flame photometry, for the measurement of the serum cations, sodium and potassium. It began to perform the thyroid function test referred to as PBI (protein bound iodine) with the aid of automation, the Auto Analyzer, which had been developed by the Technicon Corporation.

In general the Chemistry Laboratory engaged in cooperative research projects with the clinical staff. But as research laboratories proliferated in the hospital, Chemistry began to assume a service function as well, performing many tests for these enterprises.

After DuToit's death in 1958, Lot Page became the acting director until 1961 when Sidney Rieder assumed the role of director. Since Miss Rourke resigned her post that same year and the workload had increased tremendously, some reorganization of the laboratory seemed in order. The role of head technician was divided initially between two people, Olive Holmes and Mary Zervas, and they were soon joined by Robert Champlain. By this time the laboratory was expanding in exponential fashion with an increase in testing of approximately 20 percent per year. More automation was introduced—notably in the area of electrolyte determinations, permitting four to be made from the same specimen—and many changes were made in methodology.

In 1965 the Chemistry Laboratory moved to quarters in the temporary steel-walled structure on the Bulfinch lawn, a move necessitated by the construction on the site of the Domestic Building of what would be the new Gray Building. The total personnel in the laboratory had by that time increased to about 35 or 40 people who operated the laboratory on an around-the-clock, every-day-of-the-year basis. During the next few years the need for computerization made itself apparent, and a time-sharing program was developed with the Cambridge-based firm, Bolt, Beranek and Newman. This program, started in 1966, was expanded by the MGH Laboratory of Computer Science in 1967. It was also in 1967 that a fellowship program was instituted within the laboratory to train postdoctoral biochemists in the field of clinical chemistry which had, by then, expanded energetically.

In the fall of 1968, as though in reward for the years spent in the temporary facility, the laboratory moved into the Gray Building. There, on the fourth floor, Chemistry acquired spacious new quarters to accommodate a staff that had grown to somewhere between 50 and 60 people and operations that were still increasing at a phenomenal pace. Computer capabilities were further extended so that by the fall of 1969 complete reporting of laboratory results was begun, and the operations within the laboratory was beginning to be computerized. Meanwhile, new techniques such as atomic absorption, automated enzyme analyses, and gas-liquid chromatography were introduced to accommodate the need for drug and metal analyses and to respond to the ever-increasing demand for new, and expanding use of existing, tests.

39. Pharmacy

The growth and intensification of medical care that characterized the years 1955 through 1980 left their mark on the MGH Pharmacy as on other areas of the hospital. Pharmacy employees increased in number from 42 to 90. The budget for medical supplies, $500,000 in 1955, stood at $7 million in 1980. The average number of outpatient prescriptions per day jumped from 400 to almost 1,000 in the mid-seventies, and then dropped back to approximately 500 when the Massachusetts Eye and Ear Infirmary established its own outpatient dispensing pharmacy in October 1976. Responding to the increased demand for services, the Pharmacy expanded its hours of coverage: in 1961 it began staying open until 10 P.M., and in 1974 it went on a 24-hours-a-day, seven-days-a-week schedule.

For most of this active and challenging quarter century, the Pharmacy was under the guidance of John Webb. His predecessor, John T. Murphy, directed the Pharmacy from 1943 to 1959—in the earlier phase of his administration, under the title of Apothecary—when he became chief pharmacist to the director of pharmaceutical research and development; at the same time Murphy assumed responsibility for the Central Sterile Supply Room and for the requisitioning of surgical instruments, activities for which he had both a natural flair and love. Webb, who had been assistant director since 1956, was promoted to the directorship of the Pharmacy, a position he holds as this volume goes to press. Webb is a man held in esteem by the people in his domain. "He is a leader in his profession," wrote his colleague Ruta Straumanis (emphasizing that her statement represented a composite of reflections from a number of people in the department), "an original and creative thinker whose ideas precede the popular trends by years, if not decades. Examples are his interest and promotion of unit dose packaging in the early 1960s and infusion pumps in the 1970s and his current interest in a miniaturized intravenous drug administration system, a concept that is slowly gaining acceptance.

"Mr. Webb's administrative style appeals most to those who enjoy freedom and responsibility. He sets high standards, but treats his staff as equals. He expects excellence but gives much freedom in developing individual talents. However, he never lets his staff forget why they are here: the patient. His style is responsible for the department's reputation for stability and tranquility. He is people-conscious, and his employees find him approachable. He is an attentive, compassionate, and thoughtful listener, willing to give support. His staff admire his even temper, diplomacy, and tact, and the fact that he never takes out his frustrations and pressures on them; they also appreciate his wit and good humor."

While overseeing the operation of the large and diversified Pharmacy, Webb has also been a contributing member of professional organizations and served as vice-president of the American Society of Hospital Pharmacists. He is clinical professor of pharmacy and director of the Masters program in hospital pharmacy administration at Northeastern University. He is, in addition, the author of numerous articles.

Under Webb's supervision, and often with the cooperation of other departments, the Pharmacy operations have sustained several modifications in the interest of efficiency, effectiveness, and economy in delivery and administration of medication. Plastic made its appearance in the mid-fifties, ending decades of labor-intensive procedures involved in the sterilization of glass syringes and rubber intravenous tubing. Gummed labels came into use in the sixties and relieved pharmacists from the chore of making glue. The old system of identifying prescriptions for outpatients in the ambulatory clinics by numbers and letters was discontinued in the mid-fifties because it was easy for the prescriber and the dispenser to transpose numbers. In 1962 John Stoeckle suggested putting the generic name on the label to let patients know what drugs they were taking; the proposal was finally implemented in 1976.

Stimulated by industrial engineering concepts, Webb devised the MOSAIC drug distribution system which went into operation in 1963. The program required pharmacists to visit patient floors daily; in addition to improving relations between the Pharmacy and the nursing and medical staff, MOSAIC reduced the workload for nursing, clinical administration, accounting, and other areas of the hospital. The development of "satellite" pharmacies further augmented the Pharmacy's contacts with clinicians. A Radiopharmacy was established in the Nuclear Medicine Department in 1970; another satellite opened in the OR in 1972; the Burnham 5 satellite, serving the needs of the Children's and Gynecology services, began service in 1975; a Medical Services unit opened in 1977, and another on White 11 in 1980. Consequently, the MGH Pharmacy staff reads with amusement papers published by other hospitals in 1980 about the "new" concept of a pharmacy satellite in the OR.

Led by Webb, the Pharmacy was an early proponent of unit dose packaging, since it seemed reasonable that the manufacturer could package and label more economically than could the pharmacist on a manual or, at best, semiautomatic basis. Webb published several papers to encourage the industry to change its packaging procedures.

The Pharmacy became interested in preparing intravenous admixtures in the mid-sixties. Though a logical extension of drug compounding, the preparation of these admixtures had for years been the responsibility of a specialized intravenous nurse team. It had also been felt that residents gained valuable experience by doing this work on the Medical Service. It was not until late 1980 that man-hours were formally transferred to Pharmacy to prepare intravenous admixtures for approximately 400 patients. However, in the intervening years the department prepared specialized intravenous admixtures such as hyperalimentation, cardioplegic solutions for the operating rooms, and preparations for the Children's Service which had no intravenous nurse coverage. In connection with the last item, William A. Gouveia, a graduate student in hospital pharmacy who belonged to the staff of the Laboratory of Computer Science, developed Project CURE (Care Unit Research and Evaluation), a computer-based program for intravenous admixtures for pediatric patients. The computer signalled potential incompatibilities or excessive doses, greatly simplifying the pharmacist's tasks. In 1979 David Bailey, assistant director of Pharmacy, worked closely with the Laboratory of Computer Science to modify and update the system; CURE became Project AIM (Automated Intravenous Medications).

Meanwhile the Pharmacy Committee devoted many hours to drafting guidelines for the administration of drugs by intravenous infusion, and Pharmacy staff were constantly called upon to advise medical and nursing personnel on questions pertaining to drugs given intravenously. Many of the problems involved pharmaceutical chemistry. In 1969 Webb published a paper on incompatibilities anticipated by changes in the pH of solutions; other contributions of this order were to follow.

It appeared to Webb that infusion pumps would answer some of the problems associated with intravenous infusion. Accordingly, he proposed their use to the Pharmacy Committee in 1967. According to his own account, the recommendation received "less than enthusiastic response, but did gain the support of one member." The only member of the medical staff to evidence an active interest was John D. Crawford of the Children's Service. From modest, controlled beginnings with pediatric patients, the use of infusion pumps gradually spread to other areas of the hospital.

The hospital receives numerous calls from people worried about poisonings, usually anxious parents referred by pediatricians. In 1966 a telephone tie line was established to direct these calls, at assigned times, to either the MGH or one of three other local hospitals. The MGH calls come to a special number in the Pharmacy. Vincent Cervizzi devoted countless hours to directing this program; he and his team demonstrated that pharmacists could play an important clinical role in the community.

The proliferation of "street" drugs, the increase in drug abuse, and the frequency of theft and forged prescriptions during this period forced procedural changes. The Pharmacy began in the early seventies to record issues of sequentially numbered prescription blanks; each floor or clinic was required to keep the forms locked in a drawer. The Pharmacy prints an identification number on each narcotic label to aid the Boston police in determining the source of seized drugs. Physicians are now required by law to print their names beneath their signatures on prescriptions and to include a special number assigned to them by the Bureau of Narcotics and Dangerous Drugs.

This truncated account has been selected from a much longer list to give some sense of the scope and diversity of the Pharmacy's services during the quarter century under review. The department has, as well, been involved in educational programs. In 1955 the hospital had a residency program in cooperation with the Peter Bent Brigham Hospital and the Massachusetts College of Pharmacy. This was the forerunner of the MGH's own program which was accredited by the American Society of Hospital Pharmacists in 1966. Webb maintains academic affiliations with both Northeastern University and the Massachusetts College of Pharmacy.

Webb credits an excellent staff with the successful accommodations to expanding and changing responsibilities during his administration. "It is people who make the hospital, and this is particularly true of the Pharmacy," he wrote. "It would be difficult to overstate the value of Ruta Straumanis to the Pharmacy. Starting out as my secretary, responsible for the office, her even temperament, remarkable memory, and overall zest for living made it only natural for her to assume ever greater responsibility.

"It was not unusual for Pharmacy employees to stay for relatively long periods of time. The presence of such people as Kenneth Rosenthal, Alfred Fiore, Karl Wood, and George O'Sullivan gave continuity to the department. There was also a balance created by a staff made up of all age groups. Over the years many females were attracted to the department in part because there was no sexual discrimination. It took no effort to adjust to the feminist movement of the sixties and seventies. Because there was no racial discrimination, it was also easy to adjust to federal legislation prompted by the civil rights movement. The annual Christmas party smorgasbord, representing the cultures, races, and nationalities of the people who work in the Pharmacy is always popular."

With the assistance of *John Webb* and *Ruta Straumanis*

Part VI. Other Departments and Services

40. Nursing Service

Historians have attended more carefully to MGH nurses, their education and service, than they have to most other elements of the hospital. Previous authors in this series have kept the chronicle up to date. More inquisitive readers can refer to Sylvia Perkins' comprehensive account of the School of Nursing—which, by extension, accounts for the Nursing Service as well—prepared for the School's 100th anniversary in 1973. The volume, entitled *A Centennial Review,* constitutes the most ambitious historical effort in recent years concerning any aspect of the MGH. Its useful presence prompts the observation that despite a high level of historic consciousness among hospital staff little history actually gets into print. Evidently the demanding work of medicine precludes time for sifting through and ordering the past. Thus the current editors are especially grateful for an exception that relieves them of the necessity for backtracking and permits them to pick up the narrative thread where the last volume left it dangling.

Dr. Faxon's chapter on nursing may have left some readers in suspense because he reported that "from 1943 to the present time (1955) the hospital has been handicapped by shortage of nurses, so that during no year has the hospital been able to operate at full capacity. Wards and rooms were closed for periods and nurses moved from one part of the hospital to another to meet the need." The scarcity, he explained, was a national phenomenon: Employment opportunities in public health, industry, doctors' offices, and as private practice nurses offered better pay, shorter hours, more holidays, and no night duty, thereby enticing nurses away from strenuous hospital work. "The reduction in beds which was often necessary produced financial difficulties, deprived the community of needed facilities, and produced long waiting lists."

After Faxon completed this chapter, there ensued the usual delay between preparation of a manuscript and setting it into type—a lapse of time that enabled him to insert an asterisk directing the eye to a terse footnote: "In May 1957 all hospital beds were available." The footnote requires amplification. The supply of nurses had not, in fact, increased between 1955 and 1957. The MGH had, however, improved its position in the competitive market. In 1957 the trustees voted a sharp increase in wages along with bonuses for evening and night duty. Commenting on the opening of all beds, General Director Dean Clark observed, "This success reflects to a very large extent the philosophy adopted this year by the Nursing Service in dealing with the so-called nursing shortage. According to this philosophy, the supply of graduate nurses in the United States is going to be limited for a long time to come and may well get still worse before it gets better, and so instead of merely worrying about the shortage, we had better get busy learning how to do the best we can with what we have."

The tone of Clark's prose—particularly that cranky remark about the "so-called" shortage—stemmed from his conviction that poor deployment of human resources and inadequate nursing education had more to do with the conditions than a scarcity of bodies. "A lot of nonsense has been written and spoken," he complained, "about giving nurses too much education and 'pulling them away from the bedside.' It is my firm conviction, and the events here this past year bear me out, that with the right kind of leadership in nursing service administration—directors, supervisors, and head nurses—cooperating fully with staff physicians and hospital administration, the utilization of available professional nurses and other nursing service personnel can be so much improved that much of the shortage in mere numbers can be overcome. That kind of leadership, however, requires more and better education, not less, because the skills which are involved in making the best use of personnel in a complex institution like a hospital can be taught successfully, and indeed, probably *have* to be taught." Thus, as the story of MGH nursing resumes, the trustees and administration had faced the shortage squarely, and it is probably fair to say that for the first time MGH nurses received compensation on a scale approximating the value of their service to the institution and its patients. Having adopted and sustained this financial stance, the MGH has not had to close down wards or beds again.

But, as Clark's comment suggests, wages only begin to tell the story of nursing at the hospital since 1955, for these were years of transformation in practice and education. Essentially, of course, nursing responsibilities have not changed in the past century: Now as ever it is the nurse's role to care intelligently and compassionately for the sick and to assist the physician. But as medicine has evolved since the mid-fifties, so have the functions that go with caring for the sick and assisting the physician. During the past 25 years the MGH was active in the development and testing of educational and administrative devices that allow nurses to discharge effectively those traditional responsibilities in the complicated medical and social setting that is the modern hospital. The nursing profession was called upon to respond to many forces: In the hospital specialty units, technology, new medical practices, and third-party payment systems altered patterns of patient care and demanded new medical and administrative skills; social phenomena such as the rise of professionalism, the women's movement, and the instability of urban populations also influenced nursing, especially in large metropolitan hospitals.

The character of individual leadership at the MGH proved to be a tremendous asset in coping with the multiple aches of adaptation. Clark's plea for the right kind of leadership in nursing service administration was in no way a criticism of his own staff where, he assured readers, the leadership was topflight. For 20 years, from 1946 to 1966, the remarkable Ruth Sleeper, director of the Nursing Department (which then embraced both the service and the school), presided over a staff numbering more than 1,000 and an educational program serving several hundred graduate and undergraduate nurses in any given year. She was blessed by a competent associate director, Edna S. Lepper, who effectively ran the service, thereby liberating Sleeper to devote most of her energies to the school. The immensely capable Sleeper improved communications between the administration and the Nursing Department by articulating the problems of her department boldly, carefully setting them in the larger context of the hospital, and never striking an adversary pose. She possessed the political gift for balancing potentially conflicting loyalties.

As her report for 1956 demonstrated, Sleeper shared Clark's suspicions about the nature of the nursing shortage; no doubt she had helped shape his views. "Although the demand for nurses is most often expressed in terms of a number shortage," she wrote, "the demand for stability of service and ability to function in the changing situation are of equal importance. In fact, a significant part of

the national and local shortage is without doubt created by the constant movement of nurses, and the inability of some nurses to meet the changing patterns
of staffing and patient care." Sleeper further enumerated some of the alterations
and their cumulative impact upon the role of the nurse: "More admissions tend
to result in a more acute service; more doctors tend to plan more care for nurses
to give; a higher ratio of auxiliary workers to nurses inevitably modifies the
function of the graduate nurse.

"Traditionally the average graduate nurse sees herself as the one who gives
direct patient care. This activity with its patient and medical relationships is a
major source of satisfaction to a nurse. Through the direct patient care many
nurses expect to achieve their professional goals. In the Phillips House alone
does the staff nurse at MGH have consistent opportunity today for this type of
care. In all other units the staff nurse and the student nurse intern find themselves
for the most part a director of auxiliaries, or occupied with medication and special
techniques. Although both recognize the importance of these functions each
tends nonetheless to resist her separation from the patient and the relationships
which to her are *Nursing.* . . .

"If our present system with its diversely prepared workers is to succeed, the
nurse must be helped to see and accept her new role. She must learn how to
find opportunities for patient contacts in this new role. She must have support
and counseling which will help her to work successfully with auxiliary groups.
With the other nursing personnel she must find new ways of working which will
enable the nursing team to give safe and adequate care to increasingly large
numbers of patients. There must be equipment as needed, automation as it can
be found practical, and reassignment of functions as rapidly as personnel can be
trained." Sleeper's few paragraphs spelled out the major issues confronting the
Nursing Service and, by implication, the school and its curriculum. Characteristically, she located her description perfectly between advocacy of the department and responsibility to the hospital. (Since the school had additional concerns, it will be considered separately with the reminder, however, that until
1966, it shared the service's administrative shelter.)

Accommodations to the new realities of the hospital demanded imagination
and energy. The trustees' 1957 decision to grant pay increases boosted the morale
of the Nursing Department. As though to prove its worth, two years later the
service demonstrated its ability to stretch personnel and handle more patients—
a feat that was possible because of greater stability among staff nurses. But
measurements of stability were relative: The 1948 turnover rate had been a
staggering 102 percent; by 1959 it had dropped to 65 percent thanks, largely,
to better pay.

The nursing staff responded warmly to the appointment of John Knowles as
general director in 1962. According to Mary Macdonald, Knowles had already
captured many affections among the nurses. "He made no bones about the fact
that he liked nurses and, until he met [his wife], I am told that the feeling was
remarkably reciprocal!" Knowles successfully fended off the first attempt at the
hospital of unionization of its employees in 1967 when the State Association of
Licensed Practical Nurses won the right to hold an election at the MGH. Macdonald provided this account. "I have read that St. Francis of Assisi had the
capacity to charm the birds. He had nothing on John's ability to charm the
drones in his beehive! On a cold December morning, he stormed into my office

at 6:00 A.M. A unionizing campaign of one segment of the nursing department was in process and he had come in to meet with the night crew in an attempt to stay their course. He greeted me with a series of expletives and pulled up a trouser leg to expose an obvious tooth bite. He went on to relate that his dog—who had never encountered him in the kitchen at that hour of the morning—mistook him for a prowler and took immediate corrective action. I am told that he went to the meeting, leveled with the staff on the true posture of the MGH toward its employees and, in closing, pulled up the same trouser leg and, with the same expletives, exposed his wound as proof of his personal concern. At the close of the day, the final tally of votes was 96 for John and 4 for the union." The vote delighted Knowles who interpreted it as "a tremendous event in the history of this hospital in terms of the vote of confidence in the institution as such and recognition of the leadership that this hospital has never failed to exert in the improvement of the lot of its employees. Our salaries, fringe benefits and working conditions are second to none in this city and indeed in this country."

Knowles did not get by on charm alone. His administration produced significant changes in administrative design. When he started his expansion of the General Executive Committee in 1964, Ruth Sleeper was the second "outsider" to be invited in recognition that she, too, represented one of the largest professional groups in the hospital. The gesture, official acknowledgment of the extent to which the hospital depended upon its nurses, was not lost upon the nursing staff. When Knowles resigned, Macdonald—by then head of the service—observed, "It is a well-recognized fact that nursing grew in stature as a health care discipline during his term in office."

Sleeper retired in September 1966. Sylvia Perkins, her associate for many years, summarized her tenure in these words: "The winds of change accelerated and blew unrelentingly during the thirty-three consecutive years of her association with the MGH. No one realized better than she that the fortunes of the hospital and the competent delivery of superior nursing were essential to the development of the School.

"The MGH Trustees recognized in her one of the best and most helpful pilots in the institution. The hospital's administrative officers respected her as a sound and sensible co-worker, who kept in mind the central functions of the Hospital and appreciated the obligations of the Nursing Department. Miss Sleeper's prestige in Nursing was a major factor in their acceptance of some unpalatable changes."

Upon Sleeper's retirement, the trustees chose to assign the Nursing Service and School to separate individuals. Lepper became chief of the service; Macdonald succeeded her in 1968. Natalie Petzold was designated head of the school. In an effort to bring more stability to the service and more satisfaction to the nurses, Macdonald and her associates implemented a gradual transition from organization based on buildings to one linked to service functions. "In our planning," Macdonald explained in her 1971 report, "we aimed at the development of a more horizontal structure which would permit increased responsibility, authority, and accountability at the operational level and which would serve to amalgamate the interests and needs of patients and staff, regardless of their geographic location in the hospital."

Many readers have by now probably remarked upon the proliferation of the word *problem* and its synonyms in this brief chapter. Be advised that compared with official reports, we have been miserly in our usage. The sober fact is that nursing—at the MGH and at other urban medical centers—is a problem-plagued service and has been since 1946. In 1969 Knowles gazed gloomily into the future: "The problems of nursing service and nursing training, as well as nursing education, particularly at the graduate level, are expanding in complexity as the shortage of manpower and nursing expertise becomes more acute." The difficulties have persisted to the present time. Though the MGH Nursing Service has supplied sufficient personnel to keep all hospital beds available, instability remains a chronic problem. Competitive wages, in-service education, specialty-trained nurses, the development of the medical team with its nursing component, and administrative ingenuity have not been able to offset entirely the special pressures that the MGH and similar institutions place upon nurses—pressures ranging from the emotional stresses of an acute care facility to such primitive hazards as plunging into violent city streets at the end of night duty.

Though the turnover rate dropped a dramatic 12 to 27 percent in 1977, staffing remained problematic. In 1978 the Nursing Service reported "some unsettling trends in nursing circles—i.e., a diminishing number of nurses who are attracted to full-time positions in an acute care setting; a singular reverse in the number interested in intensive care nursing; a marked predeliction on the part of many to seek employment on a per diem basis, with the innate advantage of flexibility in scheduling through arrangements with the outside employing agencies; and the exit of large numbers from the work scene to complete the requirements for professional degrees in nursing and other fields."

Obviously, then, the problems of shortage have not been solved and, given the structure of the labor market in nursing, there is little reason to anticipate solutions in the near future. But the longevity of the situation produced an expedient shift in attitude at the MGH. What might be described as the wringing of hands that characterized the late 1940s and early fifties has yielded to the realistic philosophy outlined by Clark. This approach has enabled the Nursing Service, by virtue of excellence of leadership, to manage in adversity.

It is something of a miracle that through all the turmoil the Nursing Service has continued to provide first-rate care. That most important person in the hospital, the patient—probably unaware of the shortage and unconcerned with distinctions between RNs, LPNs, aides, and student nurses—receives a general impression of competence and personal attention. And countless doctors secretly recall incidents from the fledgling months of internship when the calm and quick-wittedness of some seasoned MGH nurse rescued them from embarrassment. The Nursing Service has not mistaken the ability to cope with conditions for solutions, nor are its leaders inclined to accept institutionalization of the problems. The search for solutions continues.

41. School of Nursing

Given the necessary and indissoluble link between the nursing profession and the institutions of nursing education, it is no wonder that the fortunes of the School of Nursing have fluctuated during the past quarter century. Two categories of challenge have confronted the school: First, it has had to prepare young women and men to act effectively in a vast and varied contemporary medical world, equipping them with an array of clinical, administrative, technical, and personal skills. That, of course, is the proper business of education: a continuous, dynamic dialogue with practice and periodic tinkering with the curriculum. It had been going on at the MGH for about a century. As the preparation of a 1908 nursing student differed from that of a 1934 student, so a 1945 graduate would discover unfamiliar fare in the 1970 program.

The turbulent sixties gave rise to curriculum redesign guided at first by Ruth Sleeper and continued by Natalie Petzold. "Advances in all clinical fields have of course produced changes in the content of the curriculum, as well as in the emphasis given some subjects and in the order of their presentation," wrote Sylvia Perkins in her history of the School. "In 1973, for example, the first-year student spent nearly half her time in gaining a basic knowledge of the physical and biological sciences, of mathematics as it relates to chemistry and pharmacology, and in the study of group dynamics and the role of the nurse in society. The rest of her time—somewhat more than half—was devoted to the principles and clinical practice of nursing, against this background. The second-year student concentrated on clinical experience in mental health nursing and on the study of social and emotional factors relevant to the health of the family unit, and on the nursing care of ambulatory patients and of those undergoing surgery. In her third year, the student continued her study of human relations and group dynamics, but gave the major part of her time to clinical experience, particularly in the areas of medical, surgical, orthopedic, and neurological nursing, and gained some experience in team leadership and group dynamics."

Along with the constant need for fine tuning of the curriculum, the school during this period found itself afflicted with the difficulties that beset all educational institutions: skyrocketing costs, fluctuating enrollment, a student population representing diverse backgrounds, and new societal expectations of higher education. When the two sets of problems—in the nursing profession and in the educational world—are superimposed, it is easy to see why the subject of closing the school became a matter of discussion by the hospital and the school. Perkins described the dilemma as follows: "Both recognize that continuing the education of nurses is a national necessity, but they recognize also that the diploma school is not designed to offer instruction in all the fields whose study is desirable for members of the profession today. To function at her highest level and to make the maximum contribution to the needs of the community, the nurse must have the broad education provided by a college or university. A college or university, on the other hand, does not have the close association with a hospital that is essential to the nurse's preparation."

The Coordination Program between the MGHSN and Radcliffe College, set up in 1946, had been developed to combine excellence in classroom and clinical experience. But its progress was troubled. The program proved unworkable by the early sixties and was discontinued after the last class graduated in 1966. A collaborative effort with Northeastern University enjoyed an even shorter life—from 1962 to 1966—in part a victim of its own success. (Northeastern withdrew from the partnership to start its own college of nursing.) Meanwhile society, and consequently the nursing profession, grew increasingly credential conscious; the bachelor's degree replaced the high school diploma as the sine qua non of career advancement. Aspiring nurses selected university-based degree programs over hospital-based certificate programs. Applications to MGHSN tapered off. Intensive recruitment efforts and the tight job market of the early seventies eased the enrollment situation only to be undercut later in the decade by uncertainties and rumors concerning the school's future.

For all the talk about closing the school, the trustees hesitated to do so. Though nursing diploma schools were going out of business all over the country, the continued crisis in nursing personnel suggested to MGH administrators a redesign of the educational machinery rather than a precipitous shut-down. They appreciated the school's role in ensuring a steady supply of students and nurses to the hospital. There was also an item of sentiment: the school had a long and honorable tradition. And so, even as questions about closing were being raised, the MGH provided the school with its first adequate facilities in 92 years. The quarters, a renovated school building, are in Ruth Sleeper Hall, the first MGH building ever named in honor of a nurse.

The discussions about the school intensified in the early seventies. As time passed they became part of a larger order of considerations involving a number of educational programs in the hospital. Finally, in 1978, the hospital acquired degree-granting capability. With respect to nursing education, the pernicious problem of credentials found a cure at the MGH. A three-year program will be offered to liberal arts college graduates with sound science backgrounds; graduates will receive a master of science in nursing degree. This development, coupled with the explicit goals of the American Nursing Association to have all entering professional nurses possess at least a bachelor's degree in 1985, brought about the phasing out of the MGHSN diploma program. The last class graduated in May 1981.

Boston may be a city that cares about tradition, but when a tradition outlives its proper function, reason prevails over sentiment. The masters program in nursing at the MGH is now conducted within the framework of a new Institute of Health Professions of which nursing is but one course of study—although the most heavily subscribed course if the institute's prophecies prove accurate. The MGHSN has therefore surrendered its identity to a larger organization. The school's last few years were often painful, and Director Petzold did not disguise "feelings of insecurity and impending sense of loss and separation" in her bailiwick. But since Petzold and her faculty fully supported the principle of transition from a diploma to a degree program, they devoted long hours in committee work to make the new course a success while maintaining the standards and the quality of the school's resources for enrolled students until the last diploma class graduated. The transition from school to institute was nearing completion, as activities were underway to admit in September 1982 the first class of students to the graduate program in nursing. Roslyn Elms, Ph.D., R.N., alumna of the school (Class of 1959), was appointed professor and program director of the new program, and faculty were being recruited.

One tradition has passed, but another more important tradition remains in force: The philosophical ground against which decisions about nursing education are set has not shifted from Petzold's elegant description of 1971: "Though it has often been said that educational programs in nursing exist because of social need, we have accepted a mandate to do more than 'exist.' A school of nursing must strive for excellence in implementing its primary goal of helping students to develop their personal and professional capabilities to become well qualified and able practitioners of nursing; and in doing so must be responsive to the voices of change, the sounds of need, and some visions of what 'might be' and 'what ought to be.' "

With the assistance of *Natalie Petzold*

42. Social Service Department

Josephine Barbour, the former chief of the Social Service Department, introduced her annual report for 1963 with refreshing candor:

Annual reports of the Social Service Department for the past few years seem to have a repetitiveness. "The same facts and problems have constantly appeared, such as the increase each year in referrals to the department; large amounts of money arranged to meet ancillary costs of medical care; more patients with more severe psychosocial and medical problems; and continued lack of community resources to meet these problems particularly at times of crisis. On the administrative side there are staff turnover, crowded working quarters, new studies and projects, heavy teaching responsibilities, and the understanding support of administrative, nursing and medical colleagues and the Social Service Advisory Committee.

On further analysis of the thirty reports from staff, one finds that in such a changing, dynamic and individualized service as helping in the social aspects of living, people who are ill, deprived and depressed and often facing major surgery, there is infinite variety and in spite of discouragement, a striving for new ways of helping and adapting to stress situations.

If one were lacking in historic curiosity, this statement would suffice as a summary of a few years; it could even be pressed into service as a synopsis of the department's entire life which began in 1905. That should not be taken to mean that Social Service has functioned without changes. Along with the rest of the MGH it has expanded in size and in scope of activities; it has also sustained various structural alterations. But the fundamental problem of medical social work is the same as ever: to help patients derive maximum benefits of health care.

Though the physical afflictions that draw people to the hospital have to some extent changed since the turn of the century—tuberculosis, for instance, is rare today—the disruptions that disease often precipitates in the lives of patients and their families differ only in surface detail. As Eleanor Clark, current chief of Social Service, observes, "Our goals today are exactly the same as those outlined by Dr. Cabot [Richard C. Cabot, the MGH physician who originated the first hospital-based social service at the MGH in 1905]. Our responsibility is to assist the patient in making the best use of medical care, whether it be preventive, curative or rehabilitative."

Given the persistence of human problems and the stability of the department's approach to them, specific dates do not ordinarily assume the significance of milestones in Social Service history. Unlike medicine which marks years by events such as the discovery of the association between DES and cancers, or surgery which recalls the first successful replantation of a severed human limb, the collective memory of Social Service is populated with individuals—their anguish, their families, their humor, their failures, their courage—the "infinite variety" of Miss Barbour's description.

However, 1955 was an exceptional year, a date that commands instant recognition among old guard MGH staffers. No one who was at the hospital then can erase the images of the polio epidemic, what Barbour called "the unforget-

375

table, haunting picture of over four hundred polio patients." The Social Service Department set up a special polio office to extend support to victims and their families. Since recovery from polio was a slow process often requiring several returns to the hospital for complications or surgery, social work in many cases extended well beyond hospitalization into convalescence, rehabilitation, or adjustment to permanent disability.

The same year also was the occasion of a happier event particular to the Social Service Department: celebration of half a century of hospital-based social work at the MGH. The ceremonies occurred October 20–22, 1955. Over 600 guests, including former department members and students, other social workers, clinicals, hospital administrators, and health professionals, attended. The program centered around discussions devoted to examinations of issues facing medical social work as a profession. (There was also an appropriate quantity of reminiscing about the department's early days.) Selected papers and reports, including the historic contributions, were published in a commemorative volume entitled *Fiftieth Anniversary Celebration, Social Service Department, Massachusetts General Hospital.* [Former students and workers from Hawaii sent masses of orchids and other exotic flora for decoration, and the serious proceedings were occasionally punctuated by levity. The festivities ended, Social Service workers returned to their patients—among them the polio victims.]

At the time of the celebration the department consisted of 35 professional staff, four case aides, and 12 secretaries. The Social Service Department handled an average monthly caseload of 1,418, figures that yield an average of approximately 36 cases per worker each month if case aides are counted as full-time and fully responsible workers. While these numbers record the magnitude of work, they say nothing about the density or diversity of human situations. Josephine Barbour was chief of the department, a job she had inherited from Ida Cannon in 1945. In March 1981, Eleanor Clark, Barbour's successor (and only the third department chief during its long lifespan), reflected upon Barbour's administration: "Jo Barbour was a student of Ida Cannon and modeled her administration of the department on Miss Cannon's methods and ideals, adapting to the changes of volume, increased number of beds and patients and, therefore, patient needs and staff. She was justified in maintaining the administrative structure, the most important aspects of which are being emulated today by departments across the country. For example, from the beginning social work in the hospital was organized as one unified department with staff assigned to specific units and responsibility delegated to the working unit. The most current management theory endorses this organizational system." Clark, therefore, viewed continuity of method as testimony to the soundness and imagination of the department's originators.

A further tribute to Barbour's foresight was her wish to find as her replacement a person with sophisticated understanding of human behavior who would encourage the integration of new psychosocial concepts in the assessment and treatment of all patients, medical and psychiatric. That was a very rare point of view in hospitals at that time. This viewpoint was shared and supported by John Knowles and resulted in the appointment of Eleanor Clark who had been the supervisor of the Psychiatric Unit.

Social work, like the health professions, was tending toward smaller units of specialization. Barbour's conviction that hospital social work must resist those centrifugal forces rested on her understanding of the social worker as an integrating person on the medical team. The gravitation of social work into separate fields should not continue within the hospital because it implied the risk of *dis*integration rather than enhancement of patient care. Clark shared Barbour's concern and worked consciously to protect the integrity of social work as practiced and taught at the MGH. She stated the policy clearly in her first report as chief: "Unlike many institutions where medical, psychiatric and research social workers function quite independently of each other, this Department has long been one administrative unit. This has many assets, the most important being the improved continuity of care for patients. It is our belief that the needs of patients are best served through a generic casework point of view and we will further this concept in several ways over the next few years."

During the past 25 years the staff of the Social Service Department has more than doubled. In 1980 the department employed 114 people, including 55 social workers with masters degrees, 30 casework assistants, and seven registered nurses. The greatest proportion of that growth occurred during the sixties in response to needs presented by Medicare and Medicaid patients and to the hospital's development of community-based health centers. Clark became head of the department in December 1964. On July 30, 1965, President Johnson signed the long awaited Medicare bill which would become effective in July 1966. The new chief, therefore, had many additional responsibilities. The Social Security amendments of 1965 creating Medicare and Medicaid provided payment for health care for many who had been forced to neglect their health needs. As these people came to the in- and outpatient units of the hospital, their extensive social problems became apparent and innovative programs were needed.

For example, several weeks before Congress approved the Medicare bill, but when its passage seemed virtually certain, the MGH authorized and funded a Transfer Office with the objective of maximizing community-based care for all patients who could possibly go home and to ensure transfer to appropriate continuing care facilities when necessary. The office came under the direction of the Social Service Department and was staffed by social workers and nurses supervised by Joanne O'Brien. An interdisciplinary team surveyed nursing homes to evaluate their capacity to care for patients discharged from the MGH and consulted in tailoring individualized plans for each patient. The Transfer Office is believed to have been the first hospital service of its kind; it operates today under the name of Continuing Care Planning Unit, but its functions remain essentially unchanged and have been replicated in hospitals throughout the country.

The department's increased involvement with the community was further expanded with the hospital's establishment of satellite clinics in Charlestown (1968) and Chelsea (1972). The social workers' knowledge of the problems and social organization of these communities and their avenues of communication with the neighborhoods facilitated program planning and the acceptance of the new system of primary health care offered by the hospital.

The 1970 annual report suggests the dimensions of the problems that confront MGH social workers:

Of the more than 12,000 patients served by social workers this year, an increasing number present themselves to the hospital with social difficulties so complicated that these issues present more hazardous conditions than the medical problem which admits them to our system of care. Poverty, isolation, and depression are predominate problems in our case load. Alcoholism, drug usage, requests for assistance with unwanted pregnancies, and problems of family breakdown leading to neglect or abuse of children are increasingly frequent reasons for referral. Several authors have reported that traditional social agencies fail to encounter or assist many of this population. Perhaps it is our medical setting which encourages the most needful to our door and endows our institution with trustworthiness which makes it possible for them to enter into a relationship with us aimed at the solution of these life problems. The work toward a solution is a difficult and costly process of therapeutic intervention with the patient, his family and the community. Obstacles in the community are great. The social systems of the community are so hampered by bureaucratic burdens that delays in obtaining services are common and often involve weeks.

Overall, the MGH patient population is older than it was 25 years ago, and there are fewer children, a statistical profile consonant with the demography of the country and with better preventive measures for children. Alcoholism has made recent inroads among adolescents and women, there are more problems with drug abuse—both street and prescription drugs—and MGH patients are sicker than they used to be. The high occupancy rate in the hospital over several years has activated an informal priority system for the allotment of beds: Patients with less severe ailments may be referred elsewhere. These trends, along with social legislation, have resulted in more numerous referrals to the Social Service Department.

The introduction of Medicare and Medicaid required the hospital to allocate additional resources to the Social Service Department. Greatly increased numbers of patients necessitated major increases in staff. Innovative methods of intervention proved useful: Group treatment and family intervention techniques were adapted to meet the needs of hospitalized patients. Federal reimbursement for health care generated major increases in the complexity of the regulatory process, causing the department to be constantly involved in negotiations with external agencies in order to maximize benefits for patients. During this period of expansion and reshaping of clinical methods, Grace K. Nicholls, associate director of the department, led the way in setting high standards of clinical practice. She brought to this new responsibility a rich clinical background coupled with teaching experience at Smith and Simmons Schools of Social Work. She put her knowledge to good use in selection of staff and in tailoring for them learning opportunities that enhanced their full educational potential. Under her chairmanship, formal quality control in the form of peer review was introduced in 1967.

Poor patients are not alone in requiring the assistance of social workers, a fact recognized by the Social Service Department long ago. The stigma that middle- and upper-class patients often attached to the notion of social work gradually faded. In 1967 a full-time social worker was assigned to Phillips House.

During the seventies the high volume of need, shrinking external resources, and the mission of the department to provide patients with high quality care in as efficient a manner as possible led to several system changes within the department. Under Clark's leadership MGH social service led the way among hospitals in the nation in introducing measurements of productivity based on units of service provided. A non-social worker joined the management team of the department for the first time when Nathaniel Butler became the business manager.

An automatic screening and referral system has recently been introduced—a necessity predicted by Ida Cannon in 1920. A department secretary sorts all admissions cards according to criteria based on diagnosis, age, demographic characteristics, and living arrangements. (Location within the hospital and method of payment are not among the criteria.) All patients identified through this process are contacted on the day after admission unless the physician formally indicates that intervention would be inappropriate. The Social Service Department believes the program to have been about 95 percent effective since it went into full operation in May 1980. Analysis of the admissions cards catches about 20 percent of the hospital population. The first screening, in which a social worker talks with the family or patient and reviews the record, reduces the number by 7 or 8 percent, leaving a balance for whom the Social Service Department provides assistance with discharge.

The growing numbers of vulnerable, elderly people seeking MGH services, in the ambulatory clinics as well as within the hospital, have prompted the Social Service Department to develop a novel Family Care Program. This "foster home" service offers an alternative to institutional living for adults who do not need continuous skilled nursing care or 24-hour-a-day care provided in most nursing homes and who would rather live with a family but for various reasons have no nearby family or friends to care for them. Social workers and nurses interview prospective patients and host families to weed out those who fail to meet qualifications and to match patients with families. The screening is a delicate process once it has moved beyond objective criteria into the realm of human sensibilities, but the results of two years and approximately fifty placements are encouraging. Aside from the more obvious human benefits, the Social Service Department has been pleased with the financial efficiency of the Family Care Program. Host families receive a monthly payment under Medicaid sufficient to furnish a modest supplementary income, yet the costs are lower than a nursing home.

One may reasonably wonder why the MGH became involved in such a program. After all, it is a funny thing for a private hospital to be doing. The question must be asked of the hospital as a whole because, although the Social Service Department may propose programs, they become operative only with the support and blessing of the administration. In large part the answer lies in the MGH tradition of responsibility. The boundaries of institutional responsibility have been moving outward ever since Dr. Cabot began impressing upon the hospital the idea that its obligation did not terminate when the patient passed through the door from the ward into the world. Cabot made a medical rather than a moral judgment; he argued that if patients were not helped to use medical care properly, then physicians worked in vain. When the perception of responsibility extends beyond the hospital walls, intervention becomes appropriate at the junctions between the hospital medical care and the patient's social context. It has surely been essential to the success of social service that the original impetus came from within, from a doctor, and that the department has since enjoyed the support of the hospital's medical and nursing establishment. With all her intelligence and energy, Ida Cannon, an outsider and a lay person, could not have implemented such a plan without Cabot.

Viewed in terms of an institutional definition of responsibility, the Family Care Program is a logical development, a device created to fill identified needs. That the program has proven to be cost effective (and if undertaken on a national scale could conceivably result in substantial health care savings) is not accidental.

The Social Service Department as patient advocate keeps a stern eye on health care costs. The multiplicity of services it provides is designed to reduce the patients' and society's health care bills by making medicine work for them, keeping them out of hospitals and other expensive institutions insofar as possible.

Social Service, of all MGH departments, is the one most immediately identified with patient care. One can easily overlook its active programs of teaching and research. Medical social work, like nursing, was once an untrained, intuitive field. Today a professional requires a master's degree which usually involves two years of academic and field training. The contemporary knowledge base is broader, and the student acquires a wider range of skills with which to assess and intervene. The MGH Social Service Department maintains long-standing affiliations with departments of social work at Simmons College, Smith College, Boston College, and Middlesex Community College. The department also participates in the new MGH Institute of Health Professions which offers a 12-month certificate program in social work. (The department judged that there were already sufficient masters' programs in the vicinity. The Institute course fills the health care gaps in those programs and gives students the option of transferring credits and pursuing a master's degree elsewhere or accepting a non-master's position in a social work department.) Eleanor Clark and Grace Nicholls serve on the faculties of the Institute, Smith College, and Simmons College.

Research in the Social Service Department takes two forms. The first is primarily examination of its own functions, routine monitoring of quality and quantity of departmental work. Regular audits of casework control quality, while recording of services monitors quantity. Over time the results of the studies permit fine tuning adjustments which improve the service at MGH and—since the MGH unit is often a model—elsewhere. Moreover, every new program is piloted and evaluated before it goes into full-scale operation. Department staff also engage in more conventional research, usually as members of an interdisciplinary team. Social workers are currently involved in Avery Weisman's Project Omega (a study of terminal illness and death), the Center Without Walls (a multi-institutional study of Huntington's disease), and Edward Campion's geriatrics research project.

With 75 years of experience to guide them, social service workers are better equipped to help patients. The uninterrupted rise in numbers of referrals to the department speaks more eloquently than any testimonial of its value to the hospital. The Social Service Department has become indispensable to the proper discharge of responsibility as the MGH defines it. It is difficult work because there is never an end in sight. Social workers do not possess the magic of doctors to heal; the problems they deal with are not susceptible to pills or the scalpel. Yet for those who stick with it, the work is gratifying. As Clark observes after 27 years of work with MGH patients: "To see what can be accomplished by carefully engineering the resources of society and familial attitudes, along with fine medical intervention—there's very real satisfaction in that."

With the assistance of *Eleanor Clark*

43. Dietary Department

The year is 1980. Computers whir and click, gleaming CAT scanners disclose long-held secrets of the brain, sound waves pass painlessly through skin, muscle, and bone, sending back images of a beating heart to a video screen. Meanwhile, down in the MGH kitchens, a scene faintly redolent of the Middle Ages unfolds. Whole carrots, celery stalks, parsley bunches, and beef shins simmer gently in a vast kettle. Joints of meat sputter away in a cavernous oven. A vegetable specialist patiently rinses and sorts his way through a mountain of fresh spinach. Ovens discharge their cargos of bread and rolls, while the baker mixes up a batch of 1,100 raisin bran cookies.

The hospital's fare won't put any local gourmet restaurants out of business, but MGH meals embarrass the efforts of most airlines and college cafeterias. American eating habits have sustained a minor revolution during the past quarter century, venturing beyond the meat-and-potatoes diet into more exotic ethnic terrains. MGH planners have updated the menus accordingly, bringing dishes like shish kebab and lasagna into the hospital. "Lots of 'home cooking' goes on in the kitchens at the MGH and it is reflected in the menu," commented a *Boston Globe* reporter dispatched to sample the products of local hospital kitchens in 1977. It should be emphasized, however, that the homely aspects of MGH cookery do not include the casual sanitary practices of ordinary household kitchens, to say nothing of the average restaurant galley. Since hospital patients are highly susceptible to infection, extraordinary care is devoted to the storage and handling of food and to the cleanliness of the kitchens.

As any payer of grocery bills knows, food costs have soared since 1955, gathering great upward energy during the 1970s. In Dietary Department terms, in 1965 a $17,000 inventory supported the distribution of $965,000 worth of food; comparable figures for 1979 were $95,138 and $2,076,137. The department could not indulge in the money-saving tactics available to individuals: It could not join the meat boycott or turn temporarily vegetarian. And a patient who orders chicken does not pay any less than one who eats roast beef. Through it all, the Dietary Department managed to hold to its budget, often below the national inflation rate and substantially below that for the hospital as a whole.

With regard to space, the natural urges of the department to expand and modernize were partially gratified. Dietary acquired new receiving and storage areas in the Gray Building (after having been marooned in Temporary Building I for seven years) along with a kitchen on Bigelow 7 to serve White and Bigelow inpatient floors. The new kitchen is a satellite, an efficient distribution point for hot foods brought up from the main kitchens by elevator; cooking on the new premises is limited to "fast food" items—broiled or grilled meats and fresh or steamed vegetables—cooked to coincide with the service line.

The service and "gourmet" functions of the Dietary Department tend to upstage its responsibility for nutritional care, a mission that the American Dietetic Association defines as "the application of the science and art of human nutrition in helping people select and obtain food for the primary purpose of nourishing their bodies in health or in disease throughout the life cycle." As Louise Hatch and Annie Galbraith—former and current directors of the Dietary Department and Dietary Internship, respectively—observed in a 1973 article, "In this hospital, it is still the responsibility of the physician to prescribe the diet. . . . When a modified diet is in order, the dietitian who interviews the patient evaluates the appropriateness of the prescription for continuing use in terms of the patient's clinical status, life style, and ability to cope. If indicated, recommendations for revisions of the plans and more realistic goals are discussed with the attending physician, social worker, or other staff." The department's expertise in diet modifications was widely recognized. Demands for the MGH diet manual, a handbook for health professionals in clinical practice, were so voluminous and persistent that Hatch and Galbraith were persuaded to prepare it for publication. The manual appeared in 1976; by 1978 it had gone into a third printing.

Almost every annual report during the past 25 years includes some reference to an increased demand for modified diets running the gamut from tube feedings through infant formulas to sodium-restricted diets. A 1975 tabulation of five years of daily records on MGH clinical units revealed "continued increase in the number of diet instructions and referrals (i.e., Baker Memorial = 600 in 1970, 2,000 in 1975)." As might be expected, the department's Nutrition Clinic serving outpatients in Boston experienced a comparable increase in traffic. Nutrition units in the Bunker Hill and Chelsea health centers have been very popular and innovative in their programs; in 1977, for instance, the Chelsea unit ran a series of classes for Spanish-speaking diabetics. In 1979 the two centers reported over 10,000 visits to nutritionists.

Nowhere in the MGH is there a more cohesive family spirit than in the Dietary Department. Credit for this warm feeling belongs almost wholly to Louise Hatch, the department's director from 1949 to 1979. Along with the skills required for managing large budgets and getting thousands of meals from market to tray, successful functioning of the department depended to an extraordinary degree on sound human instincts—which Hatch utilized in abundance. She also fostered a sense of togetherness through annual department newsletters, a tradition she started early in her career as director as a means of keeping personnel and alumnae in touch with one another.

Nothing speaks for the quality of Louise Hatch's administration more eloquently than the number of long service records that accumulated during her 30 years of tenure. Given the nature of many kitchen chores, one might expect a higher rate of turnover than actually occurred in the Dietary Department. Service records of five and ten years were not exceptional at all. Larry Stevens, the baker, has been on the job for more than 20 years. Frank Campanella (who believed religiously that "nothing tastes any good without garlic") was a cook in the White kitchen for more than 30 years. Baker kitchen chef Anthony Martinez picked up his 40-year service pin in 1979, but his record was topped by Tom Connolly, chef of the White kitchen, who celebrated his fiftieth year with the Dietary Department at the same time. (Connolly arrived from Ireland and started working at the MGH in 1926, a few years before electric refrigeration displaced iceboxes, a decade before the dishwashing machine, and 15 years before the dedication of the White Building.) Associate Director Mae Dozier, another departmental linchpin, came to the department the same year as Hatch.

Louise Hatch herself was 34 years in the department. Describing her qualities is as complicated as defining what makes a good mother. All the cliches of good management (intelligence, perseverence, efficiency) apply, but as much can be said of many computer systems. The qualities that characterized Hatch's leadership were distinctly human: personal warmth; an uncanny intuition about people coupled with a strong sense of justice—a combination that disposed her to recognize good people when she saw them and to reward fine performance; a precious ability to distinguish between the important and the trivial; and a sense of humor. Most important of all, perhaps, was that she never lost sight of the fundamental human need for dignity. She approached every individual in her charge with respect.

Hatch retired in 1979. She relinquished her gentle hold on the Dietary Department with grace, confident in the abilities of Annie Galbraith to carry on. When the moment came to announce her retirement to the staff, spontaneous speech failed her. She had anticipated that difficulty and had come prepared with a letter which she read aloud. In it she wrote: "All the words I have ever spoken to anyone about the excitement of life's adventures come back to me now. And I realize that the difference between my seniors and me is that they have not been blessed with the same associations that I have cherished during my 34 years at the MGH. I cannot tell you—you just have to know—how much I appreciate your part in weaving the pattern of my life."

With the assistance of *Louise Hatch*

44. Institute of Health Professions

Mention the word *education* in connection with MGH and the reflexes of the mind respond with Harvard Medical School, for that is the oldest and most famous of the hospital's teaching affiliations. Given the mutations of medicine during the past quarter century, the clinical training of physicians and surgeons is not the same as it used to be. References to changes in the clinical instruction of medical students are sprinkled throughout this volume in the histories of units and services.

It is also common knowledge that the MGH has been training nurses for more than a century (see Chapter 41). But the public seldom realizes that the hospital actually serves a veritable smorgasbord of educational programs. (The public is probably not alone in its ignorance; few MGH staff would be able to recite the complete educational menu.) Some idea of the range of teaching activities can be gleaned from the following list extracted from the February 1971 issue of the *MGH News:*

—*internships* in dietetics, social service, pastoral care, clinical psychology;
—*residencies* in pharmacy, hospital administration;
—*formal on-the-job training programs* for electrocardiograph technicians, house-keeping aides, respiratory therapy technicians, medical transcriptionists, surgical technicians;
—*affiliated programs* in cytotechnology with the Boston School of Cytotechnology, language clinic courses in language therapy with practice teaching in the Medford Public Schools, physical therapy with Boston University, Simmons College, and Northeastern University, radiologic technology with Northeastern;
—*informal on-the-job training* for laboratory technicians, unit secretaries, recreation workers, industrial engineers, autopsy attendants.

Though these several programs bear little resemblance to one another with respect to content, they rest upon the same fundamental principle that guides the education of doctors and nurses, namely that theoretical or classroom learning requires the complement of supervised clinical experience. The courses also share an important similarity of history: They came into being as the performance of various duties enjoined sufficient knowledge and skills to compel special training.

The MGH Institute of Health Professions started as a gleam in John Knowles' eye. Despite the institution's fame as a teaching hospital and its obvious commitment to education, it did not qualify as an educational institution as defined by the Commonwealth of Massachusetts, a distinction of financial import that became a topic of conversation during Knowles' administration. Certain educational costs, such as those involved in training medical students, were not borne by the hospital, but others, such as those of the nursing school, largely were.

Inevitably, some portion of those costs was reflected in patients' bills, aggravating complaints about high charges for medical care in teaching hospitals. A few sentences in Knowles' 1969 report on "Progress and Planning at the MGH" contain the germ of the idea that grew into the MGH Institute of Health Professions in 1978: "One particularly important long-range problem is the identification by State licensure of the MGH as an *educational institution*. This will not interfere with our traditionally strong ties with Harvard but will qualify us for vastly increased financial support which we do not enjoy at the moment (e.g. Federal funds for capital construction, lowered rates for medical and scientific journals that our library purchases, and private foundation support not presently available)." The issue was still on his mind two years later when he was quoted as saying—prematurely, as things worked out—that "we would seek licensure as part of Harvard."

Developments in what came to be known as the allied health professions favored the argument for licensure. In many areas academic degrees became requisites for employment and career advancement. Lacking degree-granting authority of its own, the MGH had circumvented that situation by entering into cooperative programs with local colleges and universities. In addition to those listed above, the School of Nursing had been involved at one time or another in affiliations with Simmons, Radcliffe, and Northeastern. All the joint programs proved problematic for one or more reasons: Administrative mechanisms were clumsy and time-consuming, difficulties arose over transfers of academic credits, and so on. Most importantly, it became apparent that the separation between academic learning (acquired in the college classroom) and clinical experience (in the hospital)—a disjuncture magnified by separate faculties—created a less than satisfactory education program. The contrast with the situation for the teaching of medical students, where the hospital teaching staff held appointments with the Harvard Medical School, made the shortcomings of other affiliations more apparent.

When Knowles left the MGH for the Rockefeller Foundation, discussions about state licensure were still tentative. His successor, Sanders, actively pursued the possibility in the belief that the hospital owed an obligation to its students and to the medical profession to standardize its educational processes and to offer degrees valid in other institutions; given the changes in the economic climate, however, he was somewhat less optimistic than Knowles about the financial benefits of academic accreditation. Nonetheless he pressed ahead with the help of Henry J. Mankin, chairman of the Committee on Teaching and Education during the period critical to negotiations, and of Richard J. Olsen, the hospital's educational planner. By 1973 the myriad questions inherent to licensure had been transferred from the full committee to 12 program development subcommittees "to determine the desirability and feasibility of developing formal curricula in respiratory therapy, physiotherapy, language therapy, social services, technological assistance, and a number of other areas covering a wide range of activities." An office of educational planning was set up to oversee the process.

The MGH thus assumed the task of designing a new species of educational animal—new because, while some other hospitals had attempted mergers between academic and clinical instruction, there was no precise precedent for the range of programs that the MGH contemplated. Moreover, development was not a simple matter of collecting existing educational pieces and inventing an administrative apparatus for them. Save in the instance of nursing, the MGH had provided only the clinical contents of programs, not the academic matter. It is interesting to note that the design process involved the simultaneous refinement of practical details (i.e., strategies for seeking licensure, decisions about which programs to include, curriculum development, administrative architecture) and a conceptual substratum.

It was determined almost at the outset of serious planning initiatives that Knowles' idea of seeking licensure through Harvard was not viable. Harvard, however, fully endorsed the principle of the MGH as a degree-granting institution. Robert H. Ebert, dean of the HMS, observed in 1975, "It would be a great help to have an allied health science school at the MGH since you have a far more appropriate environment for such a school than does Harvard." In short, the hospital had to develop credible academic programs on its own. Then decisions had to be made about which of the programs ought to become part of what was being called the education division. The School of Nursing posed a special and sensitive problem: While there was no doubt about the desirability of a masters program in nursing, the hospital hesitated to violate the school's traditional integrity by drawing nursing into the proposed education division. There was some initial sentiment in favor of the school's developing its own masters program and seeking separate licensure, but this notion yielded to persuasive arguments, especially the probability that nursing would be the most heavily subscribed course.

By the end of 1974, four of the program development committees had determined that degree programs were not appropriate to their specialties, leaving eight fields: nursing, dietetics, speech pathology, language therapy, social work, respiratory therapy, physical therapy, and radiologic technology. Speech pathology and language therapy later combined into a single two-year program.

Meanwhile, philosophic objectives assumed increasing clarity. This statement was issued in May 1976:

All the students' educational experience toward their degrees in the health care fields will be centered on patient care. This focus, the location of the programs in a hospital setting, and the emphasis on interdisciplinary cooperation should all contribute to sound education, to practical and worthwhile research, and to critical examination of professional theory. . . .
The academic and organizational plans for the Education Division are designed to integrate theoretical instruction with practical experience. It is hoped that the program plans reflect the strengths of both academic and hospital programs and that constant testing of theory through clinical practice will develop, and strengthen both theory and practice. The proposed programs are intended to promote interdisciplinary cooperation among students and faculty in classrooms and clinics, to educate together future clinical teachers, managers and practitioners from various disciplines so that they will be well equipped to plan and work together after graduation.

Acquisition of degree-granting authority is no simple matter in Massachusetts. The MGH submitted its petition to the state Board of Higher Education in July 1975. There followed a review procedure including a public hearing in May 1976, another review of financial plans for the enterprise by the Rate Setting Commission, and deliberations by the Public Health Council concerning the question of Certificates of Need. In March 1977 the Board of Higher Education granted the hospital the authority to award the following degrees: Masters of

Science in dietetics, nursing, physical therapy, and speech pathology; Bachelors of Science in radiologic technology and respiratory therapy. (Social work is the only certificate program.) Finally, on the last day of the 1977 legislative session, the General Court passed a bill to exempt hospital research and educational activities from the Determination of Need process. The path for realization of the education division had been cleared, and the nuts and bolts work started in earnest.

During 1978 the trustees appointed an Interim Steering Committee and an acting provost, Nancy T. Watts, and authorized a fund-raising campaign. Julian F. Haynes, who had been dean at the University of Maine, was named provost in 1979. Faculty were appointed and began drawing up specifications for course content. By February 1981 the faculty numbered 35, all individuals holding clinical appointments at the hospital in tandem with academic appointments in the division—or, rather, as it was now called, the MGH Institute of Health Professions. In 1980 the Rockefeller Foundation provided $500,000 for a student fellowship fund in honor of the late John Knowles.

Operational plans called for a phasing-in of programs beginning with the courses in physical therapy and social work. The first students were admitted in September 1980; six enrolled in the masters program in physical therapy and about 20 in the social work course. Nursing was the next item on the agenda. When all programs have been activated, the institute anticipates a total enrollment of about 300.

The MGH thereby entered the 1980s as a "health multiversity," for the first time in its educational history a legitimate academic institution.

45. Treadwell Library

JACQUELINE BASTILLE

The Treadwell Library has been responsible for providing published information to professional MGH staff since 1847 when the trustees appropriated $250 for the purchase of books by Henry I. Bowditch who was chosen librarian. In 1858, under the will of John G. Treadwell of Salem, the MGH library received his medical books and the sum of $5,000 as an endowment; soon thereafter the name of the Medical Library was changed to Treadwell Library. The 100th anniversary of that event was the occasion for a celebration in 1958. An attractive booklet was produced to mark the observance and to serve as a guide to the library and its history. In October, during the Ether Day program, 60 medical librarians and hospital staff were guests for sherry in the library and for luncheon on the Bulfinch lawn. Edward D. Churchill recounted the history of the library at the program for the award of service pins to hospital employees, and cases in the library displayed its collections of bookplates and historic volumes.

Since its 100th birthday party the Treadwell Library has sustained a series of changes that give the lie to the conventional image of the library as a stodgy, intractable institution. Like the clinical and research enterprises at the MGH, the Treadwell entered the era of high technology, pressing into its service computers and photoduplicating devices. More significantly, exigencies of space coupled with publishing trends prompted drastic revisions of fundamental policies regarding the acquisition and storage of library materials.

After World War II the medical library grew in size, acquiring at least ten new titles for each one they discarded; the Treadwell's collection increased by 50 percent during the 1960s. Providing space for such growth was impractical if not impossible. Retrieving information grew very complex. If MGH staff were to have quick, easy access to the information vital for patient care, teaching, and research, the role of the library had to change to provide a flexible collection, carefully selected to meet the greatest and most current needs.

Genevieve Cole, who succeeded Eleanore A. Lewis as librarian in 1957, started to make improvements toward these ends. New journal titles were added, missing or mutilated issues replaced, book purchases increased, and reference tools brought up to date. In essence, the Treadwell staff made heroic efforts to keep abreast of the multiplication of medical materials by employing the traditional library methods at its disposal. But as the literary tide kept rising, neither the old procedures nor the premises upon which they were based were adequate to the task.

The Treadwell tentatively entered the space age in 1962 when it acquired a photocopy machine, a contraption that significantly facilitated the dissemination of published materials. Another machine came to the library in 1970 as copying activity increased. The service continued to grow until it was second only to providing books and journals. Previous visitors to the library had spent hours taking notes from journals; now they simply copied the information to read later and file for future reference. A per page charge created some income for the library. A quarter of a million pages were photocopied in 1973; by 1980 the figure was nearly one million.

In 1965 Congress passed the Medical Library Assistance Act authorizing the National Library of Medicine to conduct a program of grants to public and private nonprofit institutions for the improvement of basic medical library re-sources—and, incidentally, acknowledging the crisis that most such libraries faced. Two years later the Countway Library of the Harvard Medical School was named the regional library for New England, while the Treadwell was designated a "level two" or resource library in the pyramidical network that had been devised by the National Library. The development of this network provided easier access to biomedical literature. A teletypewriter was installed in the Treadwell to speed requests for loans from the Countway or from other libraries throughout the nation.

As the collection expanded, the need for additional space became critical and forced a decision to transfer the volumes of Dr. Treadwell's bequest to the Rare Book Department of the Countway Library on a temporary but indefinite loan. In 1972 the books were readied for removal to Countway where they were housed in a humidity-controlled environment. This constituted the first step in changing the traditional storage-house role of the Treadwell.

The second step also occurred in 1972 when the National Library of Medicine named the Treadwell a MEDLINE Search Center. The MEDLINE data base consisted of several current years of the printed *Index Medicus* which indexes the world biomedical literature. The capability of searching this data base on-line, using strategies impossible in a manual search of the printed volumes, marked the beginning of the computer age for the library. At last it possessed a tool enabling quick, effective access to individual items in the expanding store of medical literature. Ms. Cole retired on this triumphant note in 1973.

The new director, Jacqueline Bastille, undertook formal planning for a system-atic transition from the storage-house library to a more active, flexible, and extroverted institution. Developing a long-range strategy coincided with a re-quest to prepare a provisional plan for one library to serve the MGH community as well as the degree-granting programs then under discussion and inaugurated in 1980 as the MGH Institute of Health Professions. Given those objectives, the first step was to pare down the size of the collection so that volumes could be efficiently shelved and easily retrieved. Pre-1960 books were examined; those with historic value were sent to Countway, others were sold. Nineteenth century journals with brittle paper and broken spines were discarded. Pre-1955 journals were stored in an outside facility whence they could be summoned via messenger service within 24 hours.

The Treadwell began to exercise careful selectivity in the purchase of new books. Very few new journal titles were added until a year-long study of the use of each publication had been made. The Library Committee approved a selection policy based on demand—measured by both quantity and quality—rather than on anticipation of need. Little or unused books and journals became candidates for disposal. This policy helped to control the size of the collection while de-veloping a resource responsive to changing needs.

Access to a library is usually provided by an ordered scheme so that materials may be described, searched, and retrieved according to prescribed rules and conventions. Having defected from the Dewey Decimal system during the 1920s, the Treadwell subscribed to the Boston Medical Library Classification scheme until that, too, became clumsy. By 1975 it had become very difficult to group books for easy access and productive browsing because of the enormous changes in the specialties of medicine and in the basic sciences. The library, therefore, adopted the widely used, authoritative National Library of Medicine classification scheme combined with the Library of Congress Classification. The slow process of reclassifying books was started using catalog data from CATLINE, the automated data base of catalog records produced and maintained by the National Library of Medicine.

In 1980 the Treadwell joined NELINET, a network of New England libraries that serves as a broker for the on-line interactive services of OCLC. This cut the time required to prepare a book for the shelf to an average of nine minutes— less than one-third of the time required by the previous procedures—while permitting excellent control of the inventory. Even more significant was a decision in 1980 to sign a contract with a data base vendor to develop an on-line catalog of the Treadwell collection. This facilitated the merging of the catalog of the Nursing School Palmer-Davis Library with the Treadwell's in 1982, eliminating the need for a cumbersome and expensive union card catalog. Control of the journal records was also automated in 1980 by an on-line interactive system called LINX, an innovation that promises to be of enormous value to both users and staff who have spent so much time in the past tracking elusive and ever-changing information on specific journal titles.

Throughout this period the Treadwell suffered a severe shortage of space. The 1976 renovation of existing facilities in the Moseley Building improved efficiency and, consequently, user confidence but involved no territorial gains. However, in 1979 the Treadwell was relocated from Moseley (which was demolished), where it had resided for 63 years, to Bartlett Hall. A modest area increase, from 5,600 to 7,800 square feet, and an adaptable space allowed the architects to design a highly functional, comfortable, and attractive facility. But the new location on the perimeter of the campus discouraged frequent visits, and a user survey revealed a decrease of 35 percent during the first year in Bartlett Hall. The statistics demonstrated a need for developing special services to staff on patient care floors. Such a program was scheduled to begin in 1981.

A series of studies accumulated data on user satisfaction, on the frequency with which periodicals were consulted, on the resources held in departmental and unit libraries, and other relevant matters so that the planning processes might be soundly based. Meanwhile, as the character of the Treadwell evolved and the equipment required for its successful operation in the new mode became quite sophisticated, the staff acquired proficiency in computerized search techniques and passed these skills on to various groups of MGH staff in orientation sessions.

By 1980 the Treadwell was a streamlined library facility. Its staff were flexible, imaginative problem solvers committed to developing the exciting capabilities of the computer systems in the service of the hospital's programs of health care, research, and education. All goals stated at the beginning of Bastille's directorship had been addressed but one: developing a practicum for the special training of health science librarians. It was not, however, a forgotten item. The accomplishments of the past 25 years maintained the level of excellence set by Grace Myers at the turn of the century and required by the MGH. The Treadwell will experience even greater changes in the future as it becomes a "library without walls," providing information to MGH staff however, wherever, and whenever they need it.

46. Volunteer Department

As might have been expected, the decade after the Second World War produced a precipitous decline in volunteer activity at the MGH. Whereas volunteers had logged over 135,000 hours in 1945, nine years later that number had fallen off to 48,000. As doctors, nurses, house staff, and other MGH personnel returned from their wartime assignments, many volunteers assumed that their efforts were no longer needed and dropped off the rolls. They were wrong, of course, but it was hard to fault their logic. And although the MGH had a history of voluntarism, it had not been accustomed to a large volunteer force; in fact, by prewar standards the 1954 record was impressive. It did, however, appear to be on a steady, possibly descending course.

Then came the summer of 1955 and the terrible polio epidemic. The demands that managing large numbers of critically ill patients, particularly those on iron lungs, made on the entire hospital had the effect of remobilizing the volunteer force. Registered nurses returned as volunteers to assist the hard-pressed staff on the polio units with feeding, bathing, and other tasks that patients could not accomplish for themselves. Volunteers sat at information desks, answered telephones, and extended hospitality and friendship to families in a lounge area that had been set aside to meet their needs in this trying situation. Volunteers entertained patients, organized birthday parties, ran errands, folded gowns, and did countless other chores that otherwise would have fallen to professional staff, whose skills were more appropriately applied in medical work, or would not have been done at all. Though volunteer activity customarily slackened during the summer months, people gave up vacations and worked double or triple shifts during the polio siege and reversed the normal curve. The epidemic demonstrated dramatically the potential of voluntary services in peacetime.

When the first polio victims were admitted to the MGH, Mary Ruth Wolf had been on the job as director of the Volunteer Department for less than a year. The epidemic arrived "as though to welcome me with a vengeance," she wrote in her book *The Valiant Volunteers* (MGH, 1980). Luckily, her previous experience with the American Red Cross during the war and directing recreation programs in military hospitals after the war had prepared her to meet the needs of the MGH. Having worked with gravely damaged young men and their families, she understood the stress endured by polio victims and the heartaches of their relatives. She also knew how to direct volunteers to be supportive without becoming overly involved and "burning out." While presenting her with the greatest challenge of her career, the epidemic indicated the presence of greater reserves of volunteer energy than she had anticipated, and she determined to draw upon them.

Wolf's approach to volunteer services, while good-humored, was decidedly no-nonsense. She acknowledged the importance of describing duties in such a way as to maximize the effectiveness of volunteers within the hospital. In her first report she reviewed the purposes of the department:

1. To supplement the activities of the regular hospital staff by releasing profes-

sional personnel from duties that do not require professional training, thus increasing service to patients;

2. To augment services to staff and patients which would otherwise be impossible in the routine program and budget of the hospital;

3. To further the public relations of the hospital through the message that an active, informed, and satisfied volunteer will carry to others.

However simple these objectives may have appeared, Wolf insisted that accomplishing them required particular qualities of character, above all maturity. "Commitment is not a one hundred percent feeling," she observed in her book. "We all suffer occasional doubts, anxieties, ambivalences. It is natural at times to feel angry, depressed, afraid. But a volunteer, while at work, should be in enough control of his feelings so that they become secondary when he faces a patient suffering deep depression, anger and fear—the inevitable concomitants of a hospital stay, along with physical pain.

"The volunteer who functions only out of a sense of duty is ineffective. The volunteer who seeks satisfaction in helping others as a substitute for some personal inadequacy is ineffective. A volunteer has to search in his own heart and soul to develop a sense of conviction and commitment to the basic idea of voluntarism."

Armed with this balanced, straightforward attitude as well as a warm, humorous, and energetic personality, Mary Ruth Wolf ran the MGH Volunteer Department for 22 years. In the year of her death—which occurred unexpectedly shortly before her pending retirement—825 volunteers had contributed 71,738 hours, an increase of more than 22,000 since 1954. Almost as extraordinary as the growth of the volunteer force was the gradual transformation of its composition, particularly with respect to men. Men had donated services during the war; for many who did not qualify for military duty, hospital work provided a means for contributing to the war effort. Once the crisis had passed, however, the traditional notion of volunteer work as "women's work" reasserted itself, and most of the men withdrew. By 1954 only five remained in the program. Happily, this particular article of conventional wisdom began to fall by the wayside toward the end of the fifties, and in her annual report for 1959 Wolf remarked upon the 61 men who had volunteered that year. By 1980 225 men were on the department rolls.

Maeve Blackman, who succeeded Wolf as director, was equally gratified by the gradual, steady increase in male participation. Reviewing those who had served in 1980, she noted slightly more than half were students who wanted either to gain experience in the hospital setting or to test their vocation to the medical profession. Most other men were retirees who wished to maintain a work-day pattern in their lives. But she also noted those who did not fit into either category: "One, who is still volunteering after 10 years is an insurance salesman who began volunteering when he was experiencing 'burn out.' He took off one half day a week and volunteered in our Emergency Ward. To his surprise, his sales on the other days more than made up for those lost by the time he spent in the hospital. His mental attitude and health improved, and eventually he moved his hours of service from daytime to the evening program. Another volunteer owned a construction company. His child's life was saved by the MGH Children's Service. From that time, for the next five years, he drove down from

New Hampshire to volunteer one night a week in pediatrics. Nothing was beyond Joe Fabbri—changing a diaper, feeding a baby, rapping with young men who were feeling like scared little boys inside, or slipping down to Cambridge Street for pizza. Joe left when he moved his business to California, but the spirit he typified is carried on by others."

Nevertheless, women have consistently outnumbered men during the past 25 years. Among them is a new breed of volunteer: the woman who wishes to enter, or re-enter, the job market after several years as a homemaker but is uncertain how to accomplish her goals. Volunteer service has often helped with the transition, providing a place to discover and develop skills and to build self-confidence. Meanwhile, fears that the rush of women into paid employment might deplete the volunteer ranks have not materialized.

Another phenomenon of this era was the substantial number of MGH employees who stayed after work as volunteers. Laboratory technicians eager for personal contact with patients sometimes elected evening assignments in patient care or pediatrics units; secretaries, administrators, nurses, building service employees, and others did duty in the General Store or the Flower Shop. From time to time the flow moved in the opposite direction, and a volunteer found a job in the hospital.

This abundance of voluntary enthusiasm might have been wasted without the guidance of Wolf, Blackman, their respective staffs, and the Volunteer Department's Advisory Committee. No matter how earnest their intentions, volunteers cannot roam the hospital and visit patients at random; the consequences could be disastrous. The department therefore developed orientation programs, prepared guidelines, and structured voluntary efforts to dovetail with the hospital's needs. As more and more students appeared during the summer months in search of field experiences, the department circulated questionnaires to the staff to discover what might be available for them. Blackman, who ran the student program before she became director, took special delight in youngsters who "graduated" from the volunteers into the health professions. Her experience with them shaped her view of the director as a "developer of people." A new interpreter and translation service drew on the pool of linguistic talents represented by volunteers: In 1976 they could offer help in eight languages. The volunteers' most ambitious undertaking was the opening, in 1976, of the first in-hospital flower shop in New England. It has been an unqualified success.

Miss Wolf was among the vanguard of volunteer directors who believed that the administration of such programs engaged special expertise. She became a charter member of the American Society of Directors of Hospital Volunteers as well as its equivalent in New England. From 1961 to 1971 she ran a four-week program to teach technical knowledge and skills within the hospital and, though the course finally lapsed, MGH volunteer administrators continued to provide consultation on individual bases.

The value of volunteers to the MGH can never be calculated by formulas involving hours and dollars. Volunteers supply services that the hospital cannot afford to buy. It has no budget for tour guides or for people to read stories to children or to comfort patients waiting for cancer treatments. That the trustees and administration appreciate the extra human dimension that is the gift of volunteers is symbolized by the Jessie Harding Award which the MGH has presented to an outstanding volunteer annually since 1962. The award honors a woman who had been a volunteer for over 20 years without missing a single day of her schedule. "Rare indeed was it to see her without either her basket—filled for deliveries—or pushing a wheel chair in order to gather lovingly—and interestedly—a patient who needed to be returned to his quarters. . . . Perhaps she was on her way to get a patient who needed an x-ray, or was scheduled at Physical Medicine; but, if the patient was young, uncertain, or scared, Jessie Harding had the ability to spread calm assurance." The Jessie Harding Awards have gone to: Doris Taylor Black, Henry Cotton, Ruth E. Clark, Adelaide M. Coleman, Edith M. Palmer, Charles W. Heard, Mr. and Mrs. Thatcher P. Luquer, Dorothy J. Kranes, Ann S. Higgins, Helen A. Sullivan, Louis Yoffee, Olivia Constable, Ann Marie Duffy, Charles M. Meyers, Olivia Finlay, Louise Riemer, John Paul Barry, and Angela Ricker.

Voluntarism is not a one-way street. The hospital gives something in return in what can be regarded as a fair exchange of intangibles. Over the years volunteers have found many forms for expressing satisfaction drawn from their work, but none put it better than a student who wrote: "I volunteered to see if I wanted to work in a hospital. I found my volunteer work with the traveling store on the units very rewarding. I met and made friends with many people. I had the satisfaction of feeling good when patients and staff thanked me with a smile for doing something for them. I smiled back because I realized how important a smile can be. Also, I learned something about tolerance, endurance, and acceptance of pain from the patients, and was grateful to be healthy."

With the assistance of *Maeve Blackman*

Ladies Visiting Committee

The Ladies Visiting Committee, appointed by the trustees in 1869, is believed to be the oldest of the MGH volunteer groups. For the past 25 years it has continued quietly to pursue its many projects throughout the hospital: visiting patients with books from the Warren Library, with a selection of art reproductions from the Art Wagon, with toys and Christmas gifts for young patients, with items from the Travelling Store, and with needlework kits and instructions. The Ladies Visiting Committee embellishes hospital corridors and waiting areas with artwork and supplies and arranges plants and flowers in the lobbies and the chapel. Special decorating is done for the holidays, and assistance is given with interior decorating projects such as the renovation of the White lobby. The Ladies Visiting Committee has also provided a place for refreshments to waiting patients in the admitting areas as well as to outpatients awaiting therapy in the Cox Cancer Center.

The opening of the Coffee Shop in 1964, the newly located General Store in 1969, the Flower Shop in 1977, and the Beauty Services in 1981 have all been major milestones; in response to the need and desire of the hospital community for expanded shop services, the Ladies Visiting Committee has found itself most definitely "in business." The income from the shops, in addition to funds left in trust, has provided the wherewithal over the past ten years alone to give over $350,000 to various projects throughout the hospital. From carriage rides for convalescent patients in the 1870s to bus rides to see the Tall Ships in the 1970s, Ladies Visiting Committee funds have provided an extraordinary variety of services. In addition to regularly budgeted expenses for such projects, the committee has also contributed in times of emergency such as during the polio epidemic of 1955 and during the more recent exodus of families from Southeast Asia. For example, the funds provided a stipend for a Hmung interpreter to work with some of the newly arrived Asian families unfamiliar with English as well as with hospitals such as the MGH.

Increased revenue from the shops has also enabled the Ladies Visiting Committee to fund the foster grandparents project; provide equipment and toys for playrooms and waiting areas for pediatric patients; enable cancer patients in need to obtain free parking; write and print foreign language guides in Spanish and Italian; provide complimentary TV service for needy child patients; fund pagemasters and a modern typewriter for the Volunteer Department; and assist with the special needs of patients seen by the Social Service Department. While the list is far from complete, it does suggest the broad horizons of the Ladies Visiting Committee's involvement.

Writes one long-time volunteer: "Our members continue to find themselves actively engaged in the corridors and rooms of the hospital—visiting patients, handling the bookkeeping of our assorted enterprises, hanging pictures, arranging General Store window displays, wheeling patients, books, or the Travelling Store, arranging flowers, working with the architects of the Ambulatory Care Center on the planning of the new shops, serving coffee, stripping thorns from hundreds of roses on Valentine's Day, tying dozens of bows at Christmas—in general providing a watchful eye and a listening ear to the extraordinary number and variety of people who travel within the MGH each day."

Service League

In 1951 the Ladies Visiting Committee approached physicians' wives with a special problem: Foreign visitors were arriving at the hospital well versed in their specialties but ill prepared to find suitable housing or make their way around Boston; their families, isolated by language and cultural differences, were often very unhappy. The wives responded by forming the Staff Wives Association and began planning a series of get-acquainted events to ease the visitors' adjustment. Association members "walked the streets from Quincy to Wakefield," as one recalls, seeking sympathetic real estate brokers and developing a housing service. By 1955 the staff wives had established a Reception Center for International Visitors—the first, and possibly only, facility of its kind in any hospital. By the mid-seventies more than a hundred professionals—physicians, technicians, nurses, social service workers—from 35 countries registered with the center each year.

Before they arrive at the MGH, visitors receive a personal letter with tips on getting along in Boston. If the family's requirements are known, an apartment may have been scouted in advance. A "Welcome to Boston" kit of information about the city is given each new arrival at the Reception Center. Families are invited to take a trip to the "furniture barn," where donated items can be borrowed for the duration of the visitors' stay. The Service League (as the Association has been called since 1961) may provide legal consultation for problems with leases, loans, or status within the United States. The League also organizes events such as an annual picnic, beach and pool parties, and teas, and invitations to family Thanksgiving and Christmas celebrations. Blocks of tickets to the Boston Symphony and to sporting events are made available to visitors.

The real beneficiaries of these efforts are the families of the visiting professionals. There was, for example, a Muslim woman, wife of a physician, who was prohibited by strong cultural mores from stepping out of her house unescorted. Because she had no acquaintances in Boston, league members were her only contact with the world beyond her front door.

Though founded with the particular purpose of assisting foreign visitors, the league diversified to provide many thoughtful services to patients and staff alike. It assisted in a massive screening in the 1960s of children from Chelsea and Charlestown as part of the Headstart program. Members also assisted in the Bicentennial tours of the hospital, Ether Day celebrations for employees, and in the Coffee Shop which the league cofounded in 1964 with the Ladies Visiting Committee. One of the league's greatest contributions has been the staffing of information desks at strategic locations throughout the MGH. The need for such a service is revealed by records kept at one desk: An inquiry is logged every two minutes.

Trustees of the Massachusetts General Hospital, 1955–1980

F. SARGENT CHEEVER, M.D. *Chairman*	1975–1982 1978–1982
*MARC J. ROBERTS, PH.D.	1976–1979
*MRS. RUTH M. BATSON	1976–1979
*PROFESSOR CHARLES M. HAAR	1979–
*LAWRENCE E. FOURAKER	1979–1983
JOHN L. COOPER	1978–

*Appointed by the Governor of the Commonwealth

Index